Role of Obesity in Human Health and Disease

Edited by Venketeshwer Rao and Leticia Rao

Published in London, United Kingdom

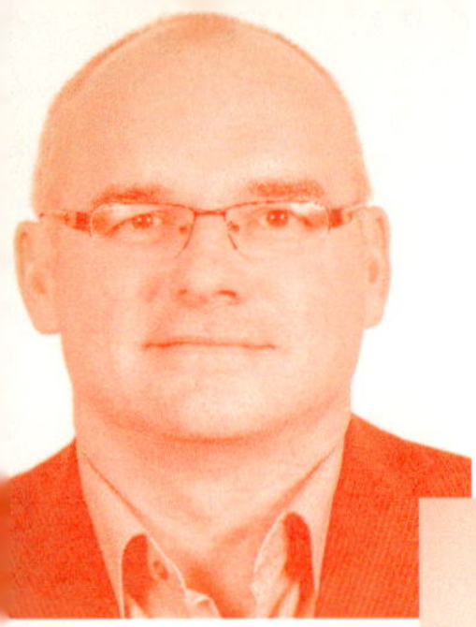
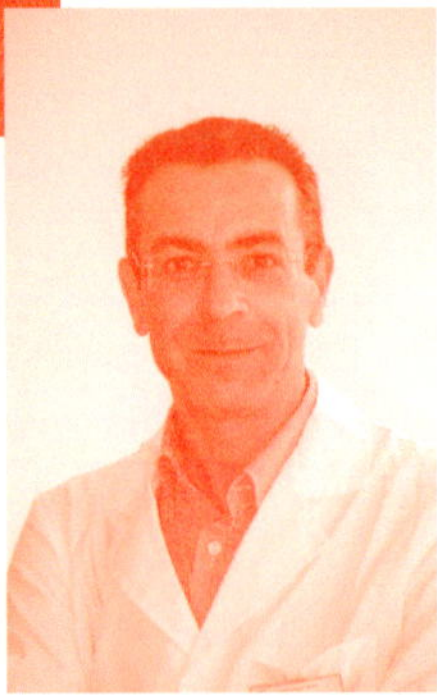
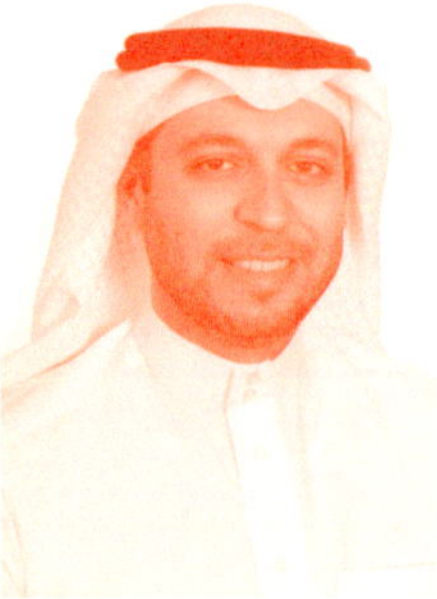
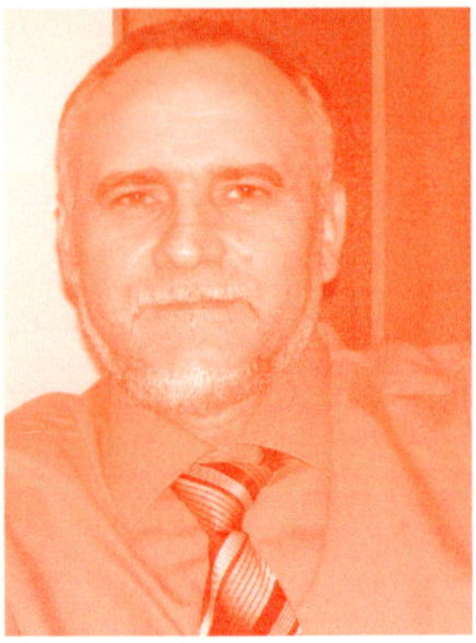
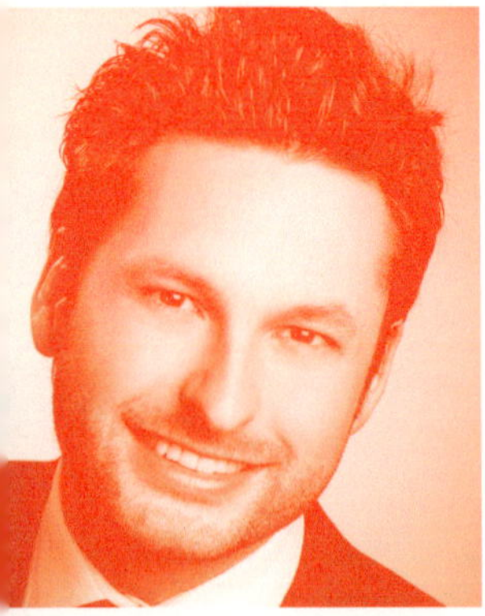
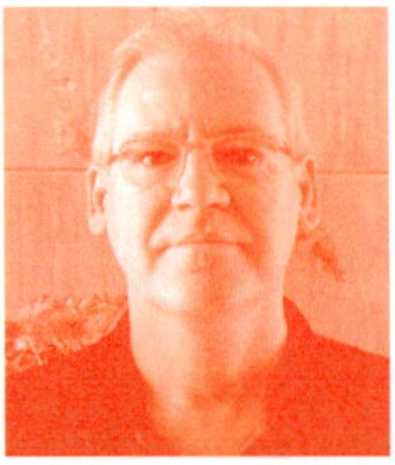
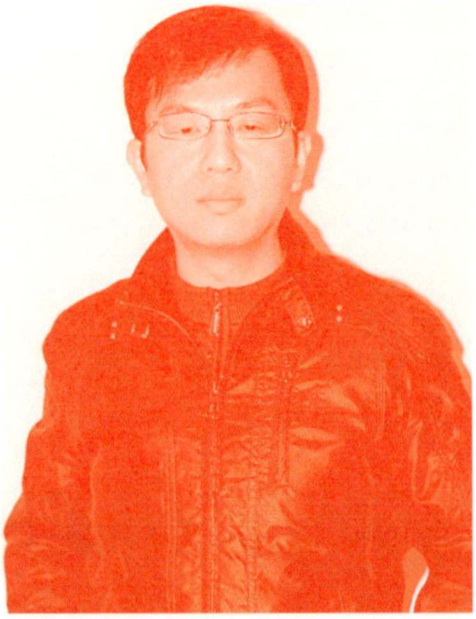

IntechOpen

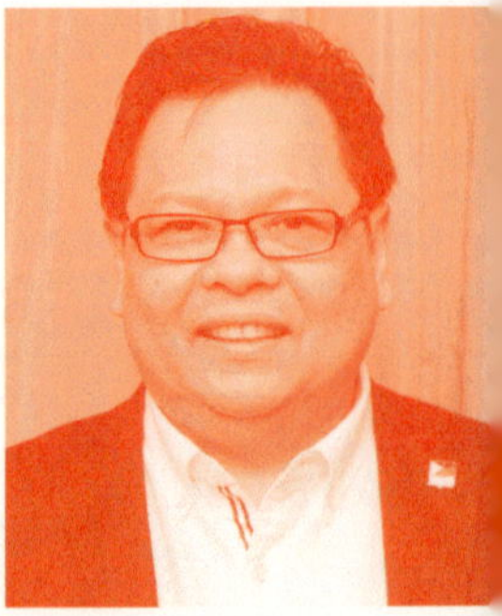
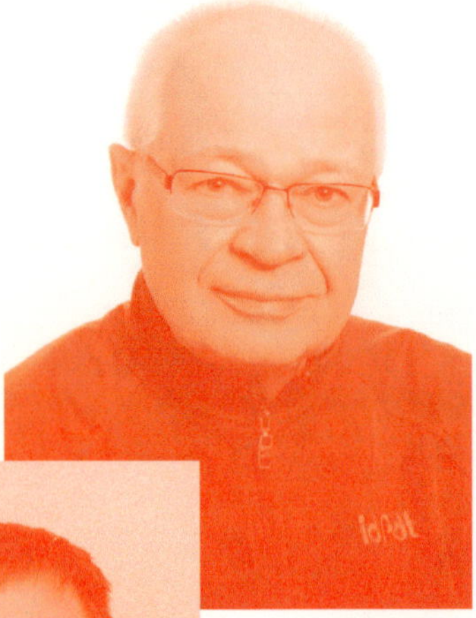
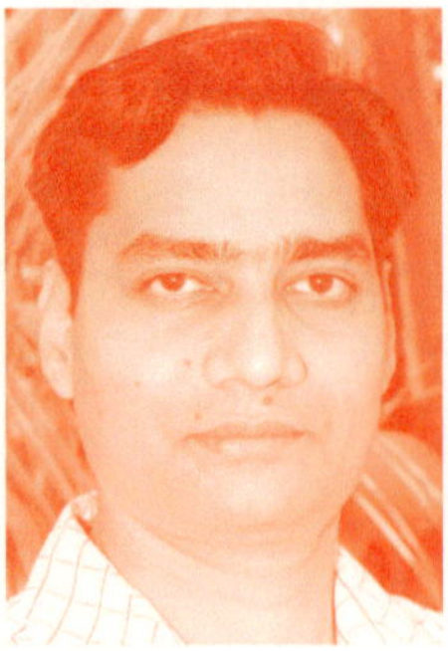
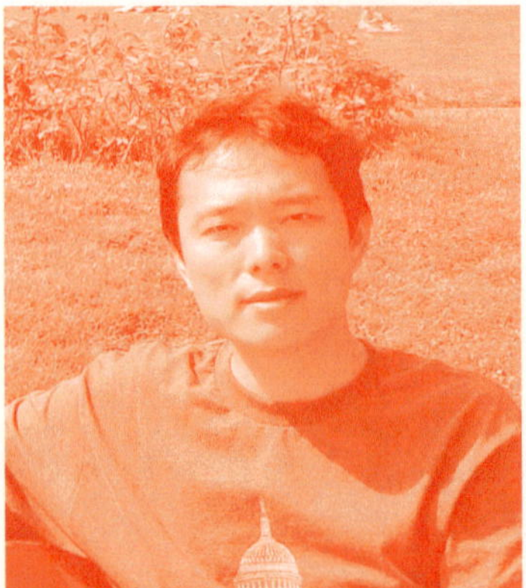
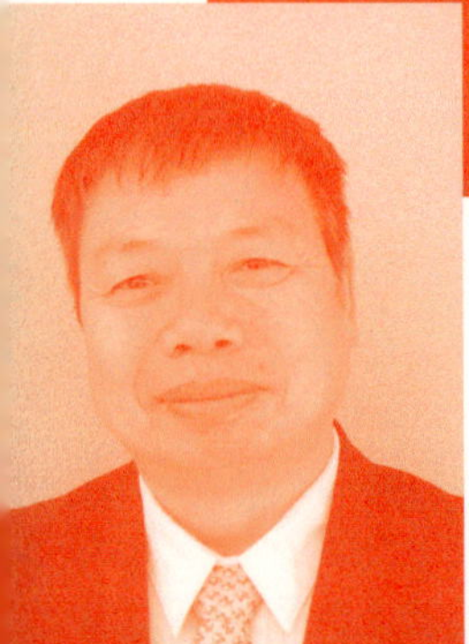
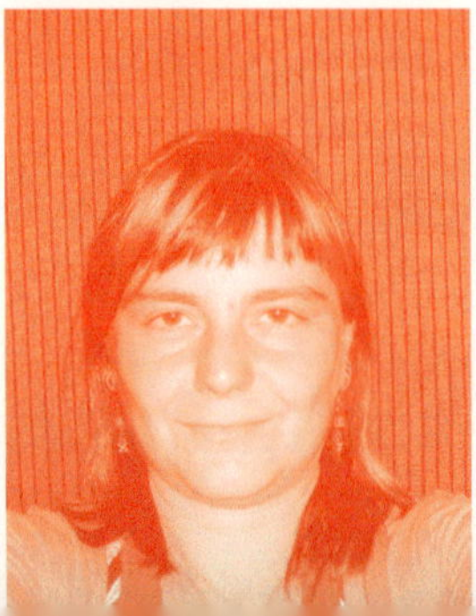

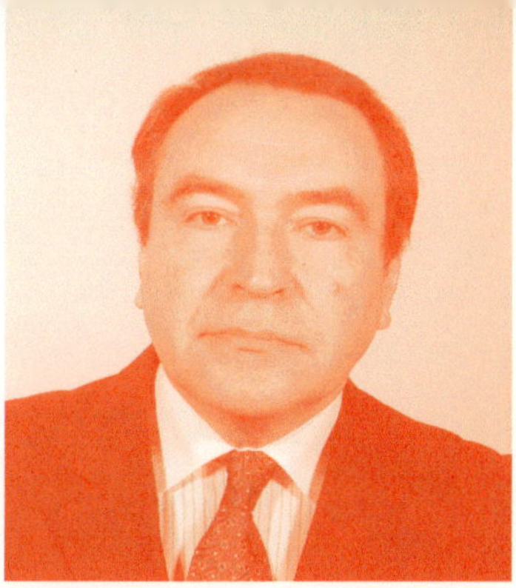

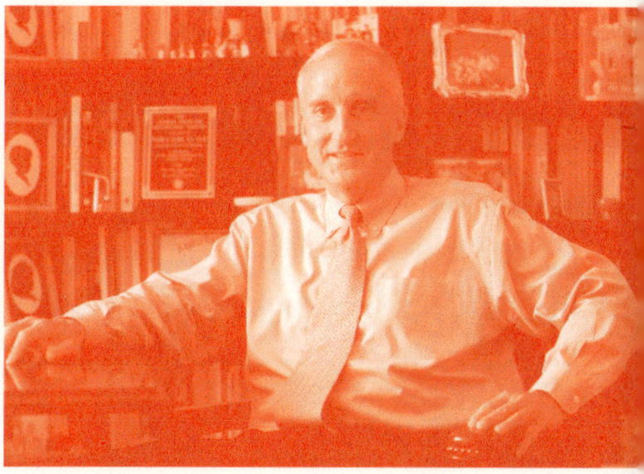

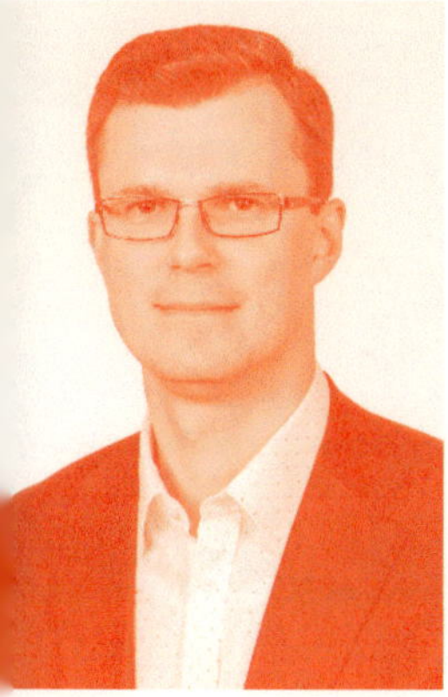

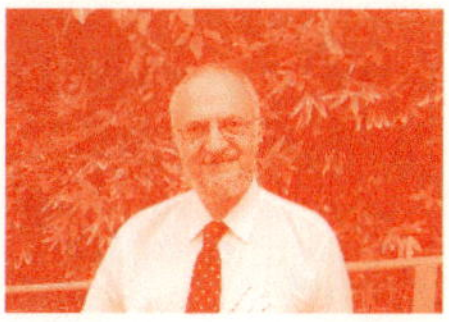

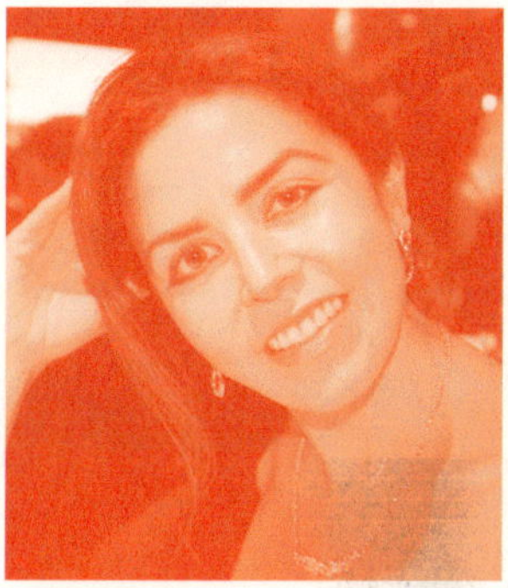

Supporting open minds since 2005

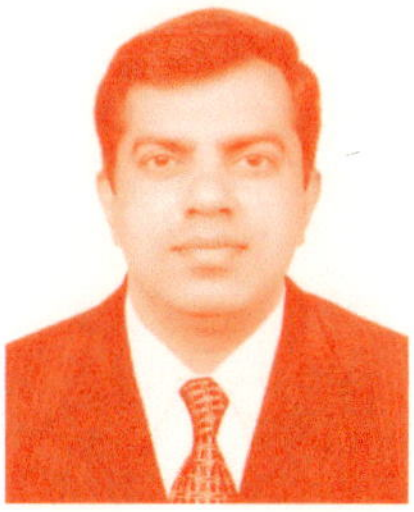

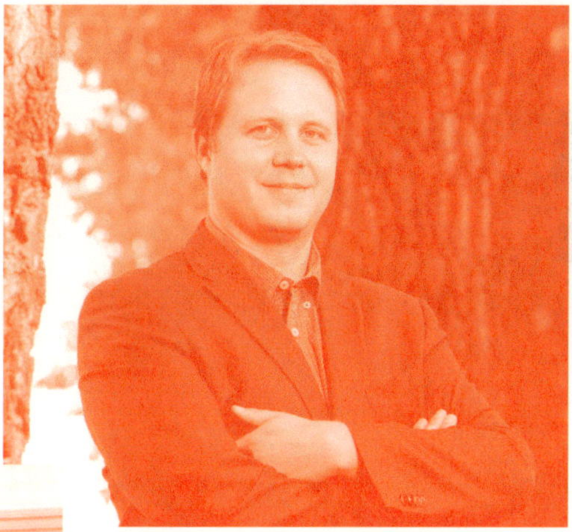

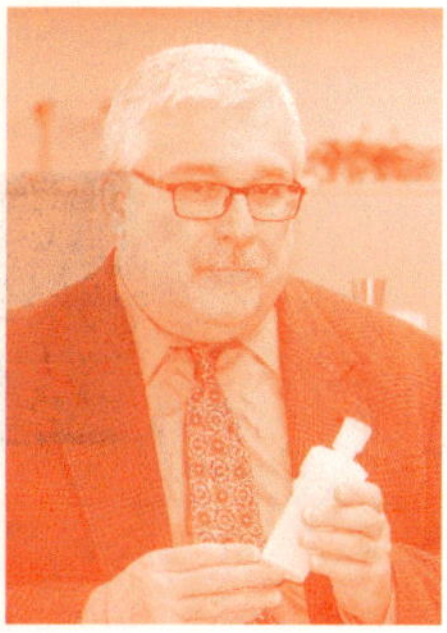

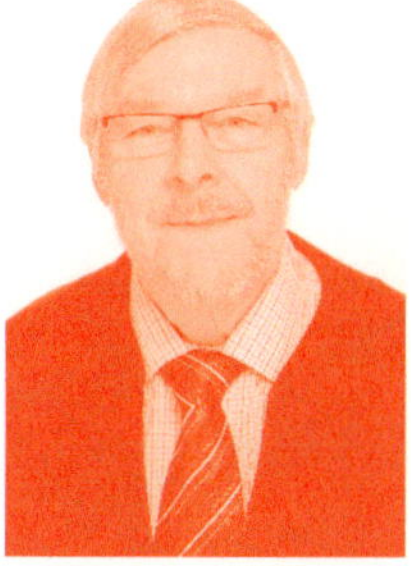

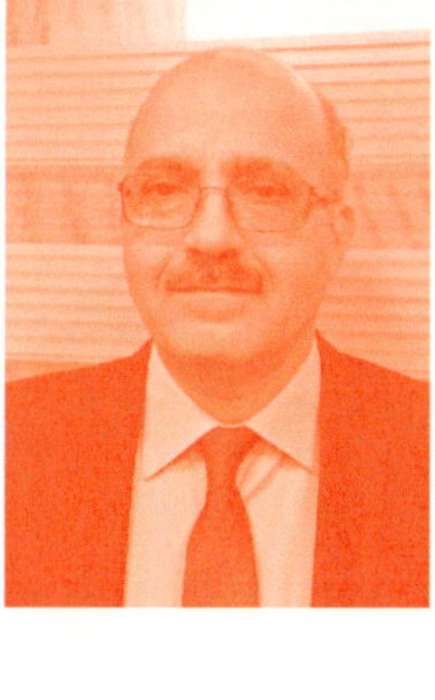

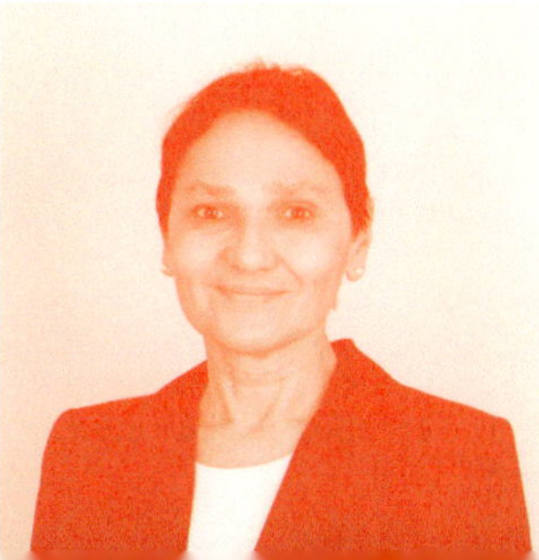

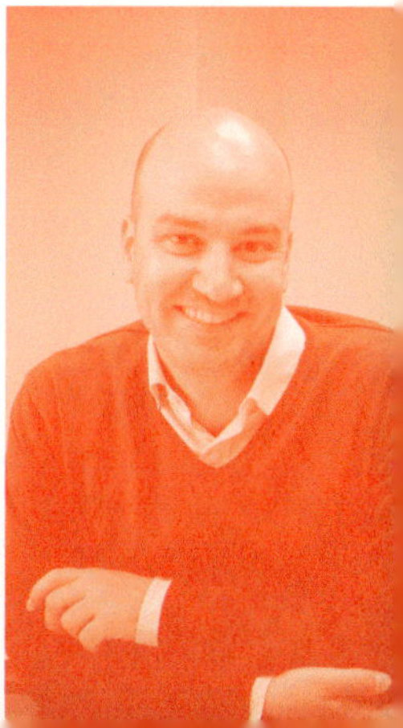

Role of Obesity in Human Health and Disease
http://dx.doi.org/10.5772/intechopen.90990
Edited by Venketeshwer Rao and Leticia Rao

Contributors
Jia-Ping Wu, Sergey Suchkov, Tahereh Seifi Salmi, Chyi-Huey Bai, Javad Alizargar, Ignacio Diez-Lopez, Belen Fernandez, Volkan Gelen, Abdulsamed Kükürt, Emin Şengül, Hacı Ahmet Deveci, Anca Mihaela Hâncu, Indu Saxena, Manoj Kumar, Suwarna Suman, Amarpreet Kaur, Abhilasha Abhilasha, Prasenjeet Mitra, Praveen Sharma, Alina Kurylowicz, Tauseef Ahmad, Pinky Kain, Shivam Kaushik, Shivangi Rawat, Saliha Sağnıç, Akikazu Takada, Fumiko Shimizu, Yukie Ishii, Mutsumi Ogawa, Tetsuya Takao, Ainhoa Sarasua Miranda, Isabel Lorente Blázquez

First published in London, United Kingdom, 2021 by IntechOpen
IntechOpen is the global imprint of INTECHOPEN LIMITED, registered in England and Wales, registration number: 11086078, 5 Princes Gate Court, London, SW7 2QJ, United Kingdom
Printed in Croatia

British Library Cataloguing-in-Publication Data
A catalogue record for this book is available from the British Library

Additional hard and PDF copies can be obtained from orders@intechopen.com

Role of Obesity in Human Health and Disease
Edited by Venketeshwer Rao and Leticia Rao
p. cm.
Print ISBN 978-1-83968-979-6
Online ISBN 978-1-83968-980-2
eBook (PDF) ISBN 978-1-83968-981-9

For EU product safety concerns:
IN TECH d.o.o., Prolaz Marije Krucifikse Kozulić 3, 51000 Rijeka, Croatia, info@intechopen.com or visit our website at intechopen.com.

Meet the editors

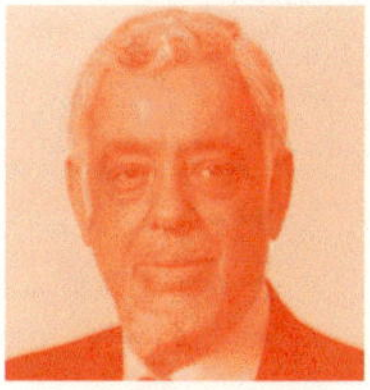

Dr. Rao, Professor Emeritus, Department of Nutritional Sciences, Faculty of Medicine, University of Toronto, has established a major focus in the area of diet and health. His research focuses on the role of oxidative stress and antioxidant phytochemicals in the causation and prevention of chronic diseases, with particular emphasis on the role of carotenoids and polyphenols. His research interests also include the role of prebiotics and probiotics in human health. He has more than 100 publications in scientific journals and several books and book chapters to his credit. He has a distinguished academic career spanning more than forty-five years. Dr. Rao is popularly sought by the international media to express his opinions about nutrition and health.

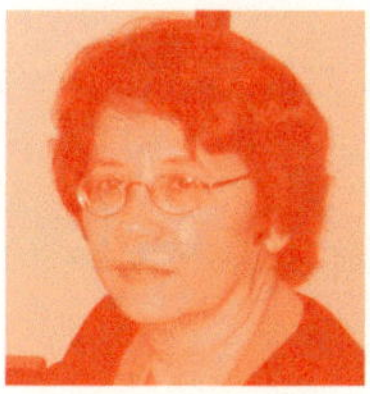

Dr. Leticia Rao is Professor Emeritus at the University of Toronto, Ontario, former director of the Calcium Research Laboratory, Department of Medicine, University of Toronto, and former staff scientist at St. Michael's Hospital, Toronto, Ontario. She has a BSc in Chemistry from the University of the Philippines, an MSc in Food Science from Oregon State University, and a Ph.D. in Biochemistry from the University of Toronto. Her expertise is in bone cell biology with a focus on preventing osteoporosis by studying bone cells in the laboratory and carrying out basic and clinical studies of drugs, nutritional supplements, and phytonutrients including carotenoids and polyphenols in postmenopausal women. Her research has been presented at national and international conferences and symposia and published extensively in peer-reviewed scientific journals. She co-authored The Bone-Building Solution and co-edited several books on phytochemicals and probiotics in human nutrition and health.

Contents

Preface

Obesity is considered one of the most important factors associated with overall health. There are several definitions for obesity, the most common being body mass index (BMI). Individuals with a BMI of 25 or more are considered overweight and those with a BMI of 30 or more are considered obese. There is convincing scientific evidence to indicate a positive association between obesity and several human health disorders such as cardiovascular diseases like heart disease and stroke, high blood pressure, type 2 diabetes, osteoarthritis, high cholesterol, and asthma and chronic obstructive pulmonary disease, among others. The good news is that obesity is a treatable health disorder. However, the bad news is that despite efforts by health professionals to regulate obesity, its prevalence has increased globally in the past two to three decades. Obesity was shown to be only behind high blood pressure, smoking, and high blood sugar in terms of number of deaths. A better understanding of the causes of obesity and mechanisms by which obesity increases the risk of human diseases can and will lead to developing effective strategies that could save lives. Studies have shown conclusively that genetic, environmental, and lifestyle factors, individually and collectively, influence the prevalence of obesity. Diet and exercise are among the important lifestyle factors.

Role of Obesity in Human Health and Disease contains chapters authored by international researchers that address some important aspects of the relationship between obesity and human health.

This book is organized into three sections. Section 1 "Obesity and Health," contains five chapters. The emphasis of Chapter 1 is on how food intake in various Japanese populations is correlated to BMI. Since BMI is an important indicator of obesity and health, this chapter provides an important understanding of how management of food intake can be a good strategy to control obesity and thereby health and quality of life. Chapter 2 provides a basic understanding of the causes and effects of endocrine disorders on obesity. This knowledge can be used effectively in the management of endocrine disorders and thereby obesity. Chapter 3, which is a review of the most recent research being carried out in the area of obesity and health, provides information about the nature of this research and the direction of future research. Chapter 4 addresses the relationship between obesity and endometrial cancer. The information provided in this chapter goes beyond the scope of cancer and provides insight into suggested mechanisms and management strategies that can be used to undertake research in other areas of health disorders as they relate to obesity. Chapter 5 looks at the recent popularity of a ketogenic diet and how it relates to sarcopenic obesity-related health issues. It provides some new guidelines regarding the role of diet in the management of obesity and health.

Section 2, "Causes of Obesity," contains two chapters. of Chapter 6 focuses on understanding the role of lifestyle factors on obesity and thereby overall health. Chapter 7 takes a broader approach to understanding the multiple causes of obesity. Both these chapters are important for understanding the causes of obesity, which can then be used to develop effective strategies to control obesity and improve the quality of human health.

Section 3, "Mechanisms by Which Obesity Influences Health Risks," contains three chapters. Chapter 8 looks at obesity in a pediatric patient and how basal metabolic profile might be an important influential factor. Chapter 9 presents information about leptin and its role in oxidative stress-induced apoptosis. Although it does not directly address obesity, it does deal with oxidative stress as a working mechanism perhaps for other human health disorders including obesity. Finally, Chapter 10 provides an interesting alternate model of *Drosophila* to study obesity by exploring the central taste circuits of fruit flies. It is possible that knowledge gained through this model may lead to applications for humans.

Overall, this book provides important information to health professionals, researchers, and other scientists that will be very useful in understanding the pathobiology of obesity, its causes, and mechanisms by which it can influence human health. The chapters provide thought-provoking ideas for future research in this important area of human health as well as for developing applicable and effective strategies to manage obesity and thereby improve human health and quality of life.

Dr. Venketeshwer Rao and Dr. Leticia Rao
University of Toronto,
Canada

Section 1

Obesity and Health

Chapter 1

Food Intakes and Correlations between Food Intakes and Body Mass Index (BMI) in Japanese Old Men, Women, and Male Medical Doctors

Akikazu Takada, Fumiko Shimizu, Yukie Ishii, Mutsumi Ogawa and Tetsuya Takao

Abstract

Objective; Obesity is an important health problem, leading to many metabolic diseases such as type2 diabetes mellitus, cardiovascular diseases, cancer. The are many diet proposals to combat obesity. Since obesity is relatively rare in Japan, we wante to know what kind of foods influence body mass index (BMI) in old Japanese people. METHODS; Healthy participants, old men and women and male medical doctors (MD) were given self-administered diet history questionnaires and described answers on each item by recollection of diets they took (7 days dietary recall). We used a brief-type self-administered diet history questionnaire (BDHQ) by using which the Japanese Ministry of Health, Labour and Welfare reports national Nutrition Surveys. From these questionnaires, we calculated the intakes of energy, carbohydrate, fat, protein or other foods. RESULTS; Me take more alcohol, salt fruit, beans than women. Intakes of major foods such as carbohydrate, lipid, and protein did not influence BMI in men and women. MD with higher BMI tend to take vegetables and fruits. MD may be more health concerned than lay people. CONCLUSION; within the range of foods intakes in Japan, no restriction of any food such as carbohydrate is not necessary for staying lean. Medical doctors seem to be very health concerned compared to lay people.

Keywords: carbohydrate, protein, lipid, cholesterol, DHA (docosahexaenoic acid), EPA (eicosapentaenoic acid), fish, glucose, insulin, BMI (body mass index),obesity

1. Introduction

A world wide obesity epidemic together with an increasing aging population threaten the health and functional independence of old adults [1]. Increase in obesity is reported in US or developing countries [2, 3].

In order to prevent an obesity epidemic, many weight-loss diets are proposed [4–6]. Low-carbohydrate, high-protein or high fat diets were compared with low-fat diets [7–11]. In fact, 4 weight-loss diets of low to high carbohydrate intake were compared [5]. Women assigned to follow the Atkins diet (high protein, low carbohydrate) showed a greater weight loss [5].

A Mediterranean diet (a moderate amount of fat and a high protein portion of monounsaturated fat) shows cardiovascular protective effects [12]. A recent review suggested that the Mediterranean diet was beneficial for weight loss [13, 14].

As stated later, the rate oof obese people is very low, in fact one of OECD countries with lowest obesity rate [15]. We have previously reported correlations between various foods intakes, plasma levels of amino acids or fatty acids in Japanese young and old men and women [16–19]. So it may be interesting to know what kinds of foods old Japanese men and women are taking and whether any kind of foods intake influence body mass index.

In the present article, we report about various foods intakes and their relationships to BMI in old Japanese men and women.

We also obtained data from od male medical doctors to know if there are changes in eating habits between lay people and men of a medical profession.

2. Ethics

This work has been approved by the Ethical committees of Showa Women's University and NPO (non-profit organization) "International projects on food and health" and has been carried out in accordance with The Code of Ethics of the World Medical Association (Declaration of Helsinki) for experiments.

3. Method

We asked male and female acquaintances older than 50 years old. Acquaintances mean that these participants are personal friends of our group member. We asked 1961 alumni of Keio University School of Medicine, who are class mates of one of the authors, A.Takada. The sample sizes and ages of participants are as follows. Acquaintances are older than 50 years old; men (n = 22, age; 61.8 ± 9.5) and women(n = 39, age; 67.4 ± 7.5) and medical doctors (MD) (n = 22, 79.6 ± 0.4). We did not ask premenopausal women to participate since data may be variable due to their hormonal influences so that sample sizes must be big to get statistically significant results. Dr. K. Matsuoka and K. Kato, who are internists, checked their health carefully and examined their blood samples then recruited them if there were no health problems such as diabetes, hypertension or not serious diseases experienced in the past. They did not smoke in the past. We also excluded people who took drugs for dyslipidemia, hyperglycemia, or hypertension. We collected blood samples early morning. Healthy participants were given self-administered diet history questionnaires and described answers on each item by recollection of diets they took (7 days dietary recall). We used a brief-type self-administered diet history questionnaire (BDHQ) by using which the Japanese Ministry of Health, Labour and Welfare reports national Nutrition Surveys. From these questionnaires, we calculated the intakes of energy, carbohydrate, fat, protein or other foods.

4. Statistics

The results are presented as means ± SEM. Statistical significance of the differences between groups was calculated according by one-way ANOVA. When ANOVA indicated a significant difference ($p < 0.05$) the mean values were compared using Tukey's least significant difference test at $p < 0.05$. Spearman's correlation tests were used to examine statistical significance.

5. Results

Table 1 shows that height, weight and BMI are smaller in old women than old men and MD. There was no difference in weight, height and BMI between lay men and MD.

Basic characteristics of participants and amounts of food intakes					
0		①old men)	②male MD	③old women	significance
		n = 22	n = 22	n = 39	p < 0.05
age		61.8 ± 9.5	79.6 ± 0.9	67.4 ± 7.5	①vs.②, ①vs.③, ②vs.③
height	cm	167.7 ± 6.7	165.3 ± 6.7	157.1 ± 5.8	①vs.③, ②vs.③
weight	kg	69.5 ± 12.8	65.4 ± 9.1	50.6 ± 6.8	①vs.③, ②vs.③
BMI	kg/m2	24.6 ± 3.7	23.9 ± 2.9	20.5 ± 2.5	①vs.③, ②vs.③
energy(kcal)	kcal/日	2247 ± 575	2282 ± 676	1941 ± 535	
protein	g/d	83.2 ± 29.1	89.2 ± 26.6	80.0 ± 27.3	
animal protein	g/d	48.8 ± 21.3	54.8 ± 22.8	47.4 ± 19.8	
vegetable protein	g/d	34.4 ± 10.2	34.4 ± 9.3	32.6 ± 10.9	
lipid	g/d	64.6 ± 20.7	68.2 ± 20.8	60.9 ± 20.9	
animal protein	g/d	31.0 ± 13.5	33.3 ± 13.5	29.0 ± 10.7	
vegetable lipid	g/d	33.6 ± 10.1	34.9 ± 9.9	31.9 ± 11.9	
carbohydrate	g/d	270.2 ± 70.6	281.7 ± 106.4	248.2 ± 76.9	
saturated fatty acid	g/d	16.8 ± 6.7	18.5 ± 6.3	16.3 ± 5.6	
monounsaturated fatty acid	g/d	23.4 ± 7.3	24.9 ± 8.0	21.6 ± 7.7	
poly unsaturated fatty acid	g/d	15.8 ± 4.8	15.5 ± 4.7	14.6 ± 5.3	
cholesterol	mg/d	459.3 ± 191.7	480.5 ± 178.2	440.4 ± 187.9	
soluble food fiber	g/d	3.5 ± 1.4	4.1 ± 1.4	4.0 ± 1.5	
insoluble food fiber	g/d	10.4 ± 4.1	11.9 ± 4.3	11.0 ± 4.1	
total food fiber	g/d	14.4 ± 5.6	16.6 ± 5.8	15.3 ± 5.7	
salt	g/d	13.1 ± 3.8	14.6 ± 4.4	11.5 ± 3.2	②vs.③
sucrose	g/d	17.0 ± 9.0	18.6 ± 12.7	15.1 ± 8.5	
alcohol	g/d	31.5 ± 27.5	24.5 ± 29.9	9.7 ± 16.5	①vs.③
n-3 fatty cid	g/d	3.3 ± 1.3	3.4 ± 1.3	3.1 ± 1.4	
n-6 fatty acid	g/d	12.4 ± 3.5	11.9 ± 3.6	11.4 ± 4.0	
grain	g/d	456.2 ± 161.8	368.0 ± 161.3	338.6 ± 171.6	①vs.③
potatoes	g/d	53.1 ± 44.0	73.7 ± 46.9	53.2 ± 41.3	
sucrose	g/d	7.6 ± 5.6	7.3 ± 6.1	5.1 ± 2.9	
beans	g/d	68.0 ± 51.0	50.1 ± 32.4	82.5 ± 59.3	
green, yellow vegetables	g/d	120.1 ± 91.0	175.8 ± 84.1	145.4 ± 75.7	
other vegetables	g/d	203.9 ± 105.6	241.9 ± 106.8	220.1 ± 117.5	
fruits	g/d	96.5 ± 73.2	221.6 ± 190.7	212.8 ± 115.9	①vs.②, ①vs.③
fish	g/d	97.1 ± 60.8	115.7 ± 66.4	94.0 ± 61.7	

meats	g/d	94.6 ± 45.7	96.8 ± 46.3	82.7 ± 34.1	
eggs	g/d	48.8 ± 35.8	41.7 ± 27.9	41.9 ± 27.1	
milk	g/d	123.1 ± 115.6	41.7 ± 27.9	169.7 ± 105.1	
oil	g/d	14.2 ± 5.3	11.4 ± 5.6	11.1 ± 5.8	
cakes	g/d	48.4 ± 31.6	67.1 ± 54.7	62.1 ± 43.1	
beverage	g/d	1005.4 ± 387.6	1082.5 ± 452.5	779.7 ± 429.9	②vs.③
spices	mg/d	313.4 ± 173.0	279.5 ± 156.5	222.0 ± 140.7	

Table 1.
Basic characteristics of participants and amounts of foods intakes.

Table 2 Correlations between foods intakes and BMI.

Men (lay or MD) take more salty foods than women. Also men drink more alcohol than women.

Table 2 shows that there was no correlation between energy, protein, carbohydrate, and lipid intakes and BMI.

Most interestingly, obese MD (high BMI) tend take vegetable protein, dietary fibers and green and yellow vegetables and fruits. Probably obese MD are more concerned about their health, So they intend to take more vegetables or fruits.

6. Discussion

The prevalence of overweight defined as body mass index (BMI) larger than 25 g/m^2 in adults increased from 21.5% in 1975 to 38.9% in 2016 [20]. Generally, people in the poor countries may be lacking nutritional foods, thus being less obese than people in the wealthier countries. However,,as national economic growth increases the prevalence of overweight and obesity shifted to people with lower personal wealth [21–23]. These shits result in increases in people suffering from cardiometabolic diseases and related conditions in poorer population.

Increase in the population of overweight or obesity in affluent countries such as USA have been suggested to be due to decreased physical activity and intakes of highly processed foods.

As stated above, many diet plans were proposed and examined. Among these, low carbohydrate-high protein diets and so called Mediterranean diet have been recommended [4–6].

Figure 1 shows comparisons of male and female BMI in various countries. As shown, People in wealthier countries do not necessarily have higher BMI. People in Tonga or Samoa in the pacific have unusually high BMI in men and women. Eating habits and genetics may count for this phenomenon. On the other hand people in North Korea or Nepar have very low BMI, possibly due to low intakes of nutritional foods.

Japan is one of the wealthiest countries, her GDP being third in the world. Never the less, Japanese men and women are very lean. BMI of men of Korea and China are in the same level with that of Japanese men, Chinese or Korean women have larger BMI compared with Japanese women.

Comparison of BMI among people in OECD countries, people in USA show one of the largest BMI. Countries of EU such as Germany, France, Checs show that BMI of people in these countries are between USA and most of Asian countries.

Our data indicate that changes in intakes of protein, carbohydrate or fata do not influence BMI. Thus within the range of eating habits no particular foods intakes being about obesity or slimness.

Correlation			
BMI vs. foods	**①old men (lay)**	**②old men(MD)**	**③old women**
	n = 22	n = 22	n = 39
energy	−0.097	0.268	0.125
protein	−0.070	0.251	0.158
animal protein	−0.040	0.081	0.125
vegetable protein	−0.116	0.517*	0.168
lipid	0.164	0.324	0.157
animal lipid	−0.001	0.235	0.066
vegetable lipid	0.338	0.361	0.216
carbohydrate	−0.141	0.243	0.073
saturated fatty acids	0.042	0.239	0.145
monounsaturated fatty acid	0.266	0.332	0.152
polyunsaturated fatty acids	0.172	0.361	0.190
cholesterol	0.230	0.247	−0.009
soluble dietary fiber	−0.066	0.621**	0.080
insoluble dietary fiber	−0.049	0.620**	0.161
total dietary fiber	−0.034	0.644**	0.136
salt	−0.088	0.366	0.203
sucrose	0.215	−0.121	0.022
alcohol	−0.179	−0.005	−0.024
n-3 fatty acids	0.038	0.197	0.196
n-6 fatty acids	0.218	0.379	0.181
grains	−0.205	0.073	−0.009
potatoes	−0.311	0.363	−0.047
sucrose	−0.258	−0.228	−0.037
beans	−0.261	0.272	0.289
green yellow vegetables	0.012	0.511*	0.095
other vegetables	0.082	0.481*	0.248
fruits	0.298	0.508*	−0.047
fish	−0.194	0.051	0.105
meats	0.119	0.183	0.125
eggs	0.356	0.365	−0.260
milk	−0.216	−0.270	0.082
oil	0.270	0.208	0.258
cakes	0.381	0.153	0.068
beverages	−0.111	0.124	0.130
seasonings, spices	−0.154	0.224	0.023

*,$p < 0.05$, **;$p < 0.01$.

Table 2.
Correlation between BMI vs. various foods intakes in men and women.

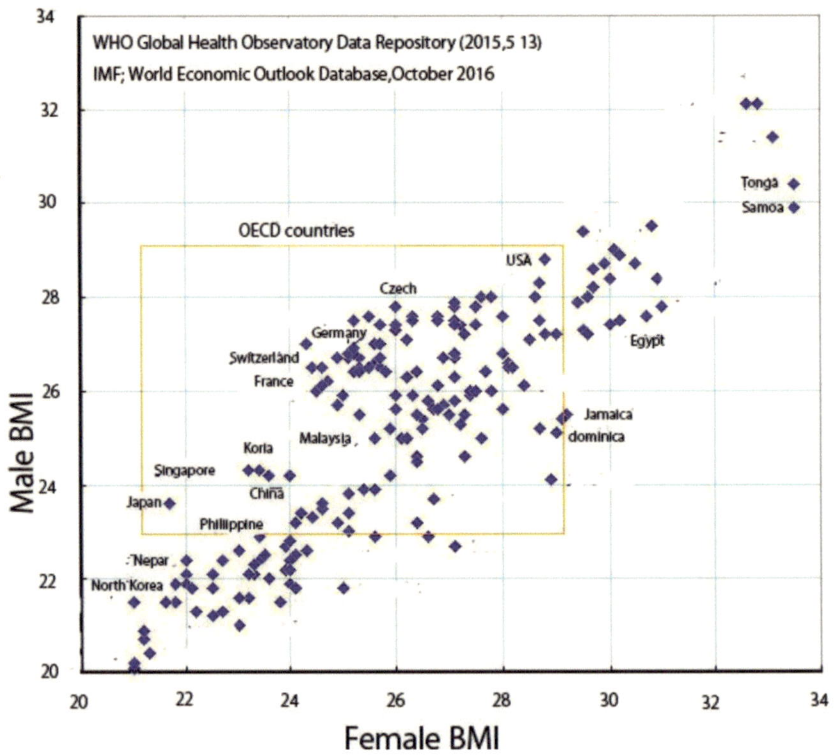

Figure 1.
BMI of male and female populations in various countries.

Japanese are very health concerned and are informed about various diet plans and their nutritional meanings by the media. So the amounts of foods taken by Japanese are in the range that a little change do not affect body weights.

There is a so-called Grant studies in which graduates of Harvard University were examined about their health, social status, or psychological or mental health for a long time [24]. We wanted to know whether medical doctors try to be healthier. As **Table 2** indicates there is no difference in weight, height or BMI between lay men and MD. In both groups, the amounts of energy, protein, lipid or carbohydrate taken did not affect BMI. However, MD, with higher BMI tend to take vegetables such as green-yellow vegetables or fruits. They may be quite concerned about keeping healthy.

We want to continue the study to know such differences are shown at the later age.

Acknowledgements

Experiments were designed and performed by all of the authors. AT wrote a manuscript. Statistical analyses were done by FS. All authors read the manuscript and approved the final version. All the authors had responsibilities for the final content. AT is a chairman of NPO "International Projects on Food and Health". The NPO is financially supported by people who agreed with the purpose of the organization and voluntarily donated for the project. Since no profit is obtained by the present research, there are no conflicts of interest, thus no conflicts of interest for any author. We are really grateful for 1961 alumni of Keio University School of Medicine for the contribution of the present works.

Financial support

This study was supported by grants by NPO "International Projects on Food and Health.

Author details

Akikazu Takada[1]*, Fumiko Shimizu[2], Yukie Ishii[2], Mutsumi Ogawa[2] and Tetsuya Takao[2]

1 International Projects on Food and Health (NPO), Tokyo, Japan

2 Faculty of Human and Environmental Sciences, Showa Women's University, Tokyo, Japan

*Address all correspondence to: takada-1a@kmd.biglobe.ne.jp

References

[1] Flegal KM, Kruszon-Moran D, Carroll MD, Fryar CD, Ogden CL. Trends in obesity among adults in the United States, 2005 to 2014. JAMA 2016;315:2284-2291.

[2] Ng M, Fleming T, Robinson M, Thomson B, Graetz N, Margono C, Mullany EC, Biryukov S, Abbafati C, Abera SF,, et al. Global, regional, and national prevalence of overweight and obesity in children and adults during 1980-2013: a systematic analysis for the Global Burden of Disease Study 2013. Lancet 2014;384:766-781.

[3] Amarya S, Singh K, Sabharwal M. Health consequences of obesity in the elderly. J Clin Gerontol Geriatr 2014;5: 63-67

[4] Obesity: preventing and managing the global epidemic: report of a WHO consultation. World Health Organ Tech Rep Ser 2000;894:1-253. 2. Kuczmarski RJ, Flegal KM, Campbell SM, Johnson CL. Increasing prevalence of overweight among US adults: the National Health and Nutrition Examination Surveys, 1960 to 1991. JAMA 1994;272:205-211.

[5] Poirier P, Giles TD, Bray GA, et al. Obesity and cardiovascular disease: pathophysiology, evaluation, and effect of weight loss: an update of the 1997 American Heart Association Scientific Statement on Obesity and Heart Disease from the Obesity Committee of the Council on Nutrition, Physical Activity, and Metabolism. Circulation 2006;113 :898-918

[6] Gardner CD, Kiazand A, Alhassan S, et al. Comparison of the Atkins, Zone, Ornish, and LEARN diets for change in weight and related risk factors among overweight premenopausal women: the A TO Z Weight Loss Study: a randomized trial. JAMA 2007;297: 969-977. [Erratum, JAMA 2007;298:178.]

[7] Brehm BJ, Seeley RJ, Daniels SR, D'Alessio DA. A randomized trial comparing a very low carbohydrate diet and a calorie-restricted low fat diet on body weight and cardiovascular risk factors in healthy women. J Clin Endocrinol Metab 2003;88:1617-1623.

[8] Foster GD, Wyatt HR, Hill JO, et al. A randomized trial of a low-carbohydrate diet for obesity. N Engl J Med 2003;348: 2082-2090.

[9] Stern L, Iqbal N, Seshadri P, et al. The effects of low-carbohydrate versus conventional weight loss diets in severely obese adults: one-year follow-up of a randomized trial. Ann Intern Med 2004;140: 778-785.

[10] Yancy WS Jr, Olsen MK, Guyton JR, Bakst RP, Westman EC. A low-carbohydrate, ketogenic diet versus a low-fat diet to treat obesity and hyperlipidemia: a randomized, controlled trial. Ann Intern Med 2004;140:769-777.

[11] Dansinger ML, Gleason JA, Griffith JL, Selker HP, Schaefer EJ. Comparison of the Atkins, Ornish, Weight Watchers, and Zone diets for weight loss and heart disease risk reduction: a randomized trial. JAMA 2005;293:43-53

[12] Covas MI, Nyyssönen K, Poulsen HE, et al. The effect of polyphenols in olive oil on heart disease risk factors: a randomized trial. Ann Intern Med 2006;145: 333-341.

[13] McManus K, Antinoro L, Sacks F. A randomized controlled trial of a moderate-fat, low-energy diet compared with a low fat, low-energy diet for weight loss in overweight adults.

Int J Obes Relat Metab Disord 2001;25:1503-1511.

[14] Esposito K, Marfella R, Ciotola M, et al. Effect of a Mediterranean-style diet on endothelial dysfunction and markers of vascular inflammation in the metabolic syndrome: a randomized trial. JAMA 2004;292:1440-446.

[15] WHO global Health Observatory Data Repository (2015,5.15), IMFWorld Economic Outlook Database, October, 2016.

[16] Shimizu F, Ogawa M, Takao T, Ishii Y, Takada A. Correlations among Various Foods Uptakes and Body Mass Index (BMI) or Plasma Parameters. Obes Open Access. 2016, 2(3): doi http://dx.doi.org/10.16966/2380-5528.123

[17] Ishii Y, Shimizu F., Ogawa M., Takao T., Takada A. (2016) Gender differences in foods uptakes, glycemic index, BMI, and various plasma parameters between young men and women in Japan. Integrated Foods, Nutrition and Metabolism 2016, 3: 427-430. doi: 10.15761/IFNM.1000163

[18] Shimizu F, Ishii Y, Ogawa M, Takao T. Matsuoka K., Kato K., Takada A., Relationship between Various Food Uptakes and Body Mass Index (BMI) in Japanese Young and Old Men and Women. J Clin Nutr Diet. 2017, 3:2. DOI: 10.4172/2472-1921.100046

[19] Shimizu F, Ishii Y, Ogawa M, Takao T, Matsuoka K., Kato K., Takada A. Age and Gender Influence Differently on Various Foods Intakes, Body Mass Index (BMI), and Levels of Various Plasma Parameters in Young and Old Men and Women in Japan. 2017;Obes Open Access 3(3): doi http://dx.doi.org/10.16966/2380-5528.134

[20] NCD Risk Factor Collaboration (NCD-RisC) Worldwide trends in body-mass index, underweight, overweight, and obesity from 1975 to 2016: a pooled analysis of 2416 population-based measurement studies in 128.9 million children, adolescents, and adults. Lancet. 2017; 390):2627-2642. https://doi.org/10.1016/S0140-6736(17)32129-3 PMID: 29029897

[21] Dinsa GD, Goryakin Y, Fumagalli E, Suhrcke M. Obesity and socioeconomic status in developing countries: a systematic review. Obesity reviews. 2012; 13:1067-1079. doi:10.1111/j.1467-789X.2012.01017.x PMID: 22764734

[22] Deuchert E, Cabus S, Tafreschi D. A short note on economic development and socioeconomic inequality in female body weight. Health economics. 2014; 23:861-869. https://doi.org/10.1002/hec.2968 PMID: 23873750

[23] Goryakin Y, Lobstein T, James WP, Suhrcke M. The impact of economic, political and social globalization on overweight and obesity in the 56 low and middle income countries. Social Science & Medicine. 2015; 133:67-76.

[24] Vaillant GE Triumphs of experiences. The men on the Harvard Grant study. The Belknap Press of Harvard University Press. Cambridge, Massachusetts, USA, 2012.

Chapter 2

Endocrine Disorders Accompanying Obesity - Effect or Cause?

Alina Kurylowicz

Abstract

Endocrine disorders including hypothyroidism and hypercortisolism are considered as causes of secondary obesity. However, several hormonal abnormalities can also be found in individuals with primary (simple) obesity. Part of them results from the adipose tissue dysfunction that, *via* secreted adipokines, modulates the function of endocrine organs and can be reversed with weight loss. However, part of them correspond to the real endocrine disorder and require appropriate treatment. Therefore in the management of obese patients, it is essential to distinguish between obesity-related abnormal results of hormonal tests and underlying endocrine disorder. This chapter presents pathophysiological concepts of obesity-related changes in the endocrine system and briefly reviews diagnostic algorithms helpful in distinguishing them from the co-existing endocrine disorders.

Keywords: obesity, endocrine disorders, hypothyroidism, hypercortisolism, hypogonadism, hyperandrogenism

1. Introduction

According to World Health Organization reports, the incidence of obesity has tripled in the last 30 years, and it is estimated that in 2025 obese individuals will constitute about 15% of the adult population [1]. Therefore, one can expect that obese patients would appear in the doctor's office more frequently, searching for medical assistance. In addition, undiagnosed and untreated hormonal disorders, such as hypothyroidism, hypercortisolism, and hypogonadism, can contribute to the development of secondary obesity, and their exclusion is sometimes necessary for the diagnosis of so-called "simple" or primary obesity. However, simple obesity itself may affect the function of the endocrine system, and adipose tissue dysfunction seems to play a pivotal role in this phenomenon. Excessive lipid accumulation leads to several changes in the adipocyte' metabolism, causing, among others, the dysfunction of the mitochondria and the associated endoplasmic reticulum stress [2]. These entail alternations of genes' expression, and thus – changes in the profile of substances secreted by adipose tissue (adipokines). These adipokines act in an endocrine manner and affect tissues and organs throughout the body, including the endocrine glands [3].

Therefore, in everyday medical practice, it is essential to understand the obesity-related changes in the endocrine system function to distinguish between the actual disease that requires treatment and changes secondary to obesity, where weight reduction is the best form of therapy. This chapter presents pathophysiological concepts of obesity-related changes in the functioning of the thyrotropic, adrenocorticotropic, and gonadotropic axes and briefly reviews diagnostic algorithms helpful in distinguishing them from the co-existing endocrine disorders.

2. The hypothalamic-pituitary-thyroid axis and obesity

The secretion of thyroid hormones (TH) is regulated by the hypothalamic–pituitary-thyroid (HPT) axis. The anterior pituitary lobe secretes thyroid-stimulating hormone (TSH, thyrotropin) upon the stimulation by thyrotropin-releasing hormone (TSH) produced by the hypothalamus. In turn, TH (triiodothyronine – T3 and thyroxine – T4) in a feedback inhibitory loop control both TRH and TSH release in order to ensure whole-body homeostasis. TH's pleiotropic actions include control of energy expenditure and body weight maintenance *via* regulation of a basal metabolic rate (BMR), adaptive thermogenesis, and appetite. Clinical studies suggest that thyroid status is associated with changes in body weight and adiposity. Even in euthyroid individuals, those with TSH levels in upper quintiles have higher body mass index (BMI) than those with TSH closer to the lower limit of the normal range, while variations of TH levels, even in the normal range, may promote weight gain or impair the effectiveness of weight-loss treatment [4, 5]. However, not all researcher managed to confirm this finding, that may mirror the fact that the metabolic effect of TH in target tissues is determined by variations in the activity of TH deiodinases, transporters, receptors, and availability of their corepressors and coactivators [4, 6]. Moreover, the relationship between thyroid and obesity is bidirectional since both TH and TSH affect adipose tissue metabolism, which in turn, *via* adipokines, may influence thyroid function and structure.

2.1 Influence of hypothyroidism on body mass and composition

Weight gain is a frequent complaint in hypothyroidism. Indeed, HT deficiency may increase body adiposity due to a decrease in BMR and thermogenesis. Moreover, water retention related to the accumulation of hyaluronic acid and a decreased renal flow and impaired peristalsis causing chronic constipation contributes to weight gain. However, according to observational studies, an increase in body weight related to hypothyroidism is usually of a limited extent. Moreover, supplementation with levothyroxine (LT4) leads only to a modest weight loss (usually of less than 10%) associated with excretion of excess body water, indicating that severe obesity is usually not secondary to hypothyroidism [7]. The American Thyroid Association (ATA) in the 2012 guidelines on hypothyroidism management underlines the fact that there is a lack of reliable scientific evidence in this field, and very few studies have directly assessed the association between hypothyroidism and obesity [8]. However, the European Society of Endocrinology (ESE) recommends testing routinely obese patients for hypothyroidism since HT deficiency contributes to an unfavorable lipid profile and thus potentiates their cardiovascular risk and the risk of metabolic syndrome. Of importance, untreated hypothyroidism reduces the effectiveness of weight loss therapies [5].

2.2 Obesity-related changes in thyroid function and structure

The majority of obese patients without diagnosed thyroid disease remain euthyroid [5, 9]. However, both overt hypothyroidism and subclinical hypothyroidism (characterized by elevated TSH level with free TH concentrations within normal limits) is observed more frequently in obese subjects, compared to the patients with normal body weight and is estimated at 14.0% and 14.6%, respectively [5, 9–14]. The pathogenesis of obesity-related changes in thyroid hormone levels is complex [15]. On the one hand, an increase in TSH level in obese individuals can be explained by the central resistance to locally-produced T3 and represents an adaptive process aimed to increase basal energy expenditure. On the other, increased TSH levels in obesity correlate with an excess of leptin, an adipokine produced by adipose tissue that can directly stimulate TRH and TSH secretion [16]. Moreover, leptin was found to activate deiodinases, enzymes responsible for the increase in free T4 (fT4) to free T3 (fT3) conversion, which is believed to constitute another mechanism that aims at the increase in BMR and energy expenditure [17]. Since elevated TSH level can be a form of adaptation of the central axis to obesity-related changes in metabolism in order to boost energy expenditure to prevent further weight gain, it has been proposed that hyperthyrotropinemia is an adequate term than subclinical hypothyroidism in this case [5, 18]. In addition, in subclinical hypothyroidism, fT4 and fT3 levels are usually low normal, while in most obese individuals, thyroid hormones are in the normal or high normal range, reflecting central hypothalamus-pituitary resistance [18].

Both ATA and ESE recommend the measurement of TSH as a screening test for thyroid dysfunction in obese individuals. Normal TSH enables to rule out primary hypothyroidism as a reason for secondary obesity; however, one should remember that decreased TSH level in an obese subject may suggest pituitary–hypothalamic dysfunction (representing less than 1% of cases of hypothyroidism). Therefore, the guidelines recommend measurement of fT4 only if TSH is elevated or if disorders other than primary hypothyroidism are suspected. In turn, routine measurement of fT3 in obese individuals with elevated TSH is not recommended [5, 19].

If TSH and fT4 levels in an obese patient suggest a diagnosis of subclinical hypothyroidism, the screening test for autoimmune thyroid disorder (AITD) should be performed. In this case, the determination of thyroid antibodies is helpful not only to diagnose AITD but also to identify individuals at risk of developing overt hypothyroidism. Therefore, the guidelines recommend the determination of thyroid peroxidase (TPO) antibodies and suggest that their level > 500 IU/ml indicates a high risk of progress [20]. From the pathophysiological point of view, obesity-associated dysfunction of the immune system (related to vitamin D deficiency, abnormal adipokine, and pro-inflammatory factors expression) can promote autoimmunity in obese individuals. Indeed, a recent meta-analysis showed the correlation between the presence of TPO antibodies and obesity [13]. However, despite the high sensitivity of modern assays, a consistent number of patients with primary hypothyroidism present negative tests for TPO antibodies, and the diagnosis of AITD is established based on a hypoechoic pattern of the thyroid gland in ultrasound examination (so-called seronegative AITD) [21].

Ultrasound-based diagnosis of AITD in obese patients can be challenging since obese individuals are more likely to present hypoechoic images of thyroid parenchyma. This finding is confirmed by the epidemiological studies, where the correlation of the ultrasound image with AITD was observed in only 20.9% of obese subjects compared to 85.7% in the normal-weight controls [22]. In turn, a hypoechoic pattern of the thyroid gland in ultrasound examination with an absence of antithyroid antibodies was observed in only 1.9% non-obese individuals *vs.* 64.8% in obese patients [22]. Thus, the hypoechoic thyroid picture in obese patients results from the increased permeability of thyroid blood vessels caused by the pro-inflammatory cytokines secreted by dysfunctional adipose tissue. As a result, plasma exudation and imbibition of parenchyma occur, which was confirmed by a fine-needle biopsy that did not show lymphocyte infiltrations ruling out Hashimoto disease as a cause of the hypoechoic pattern of the thyroid gland [22].

Given all the data presented above, a decision on the administration of TH to an obese patient with elevated TSH levels should be handled with caution. The ATA and ESE guidelines recommend treating LT4 in obese subjects with overt hypothyroidism and those with TSH ≥ 10mIU/l. The initial dose should depend on the clinical situation and be subsequently adjusted by regular assessment of TSH with the same target range as in the non-obese population [5, 19]. However, if elevated TSH (above the upper range but <10 mlU/L) is the only abnormality, without clinical symptoms, decreased fT4, thyroid antibodies, goiter, or associated thyroidal illness, it can be defined as obesity-associated hyperthyrotropinemia, and the treatment with LT4 to reduce body weight is not recommended [5, 23]. This approach seems to be justified since, until now, no randomized controlled trial nor systematic review was performed to evaluate the effectiveness of TH supplementation in obese adults with hyperthyrotropinemia.

However, some obese individuals with increased TSH level < 10 mlU/l who meet the diagnostic criteria for the mild subclinical hypothyroidism (e.g., showing clinical symptoms of hypothyroidism, TH levels in the low-normal range, present antithyroid antibodies) may benefit from LT4 supplementation. Furthermore, the same approach should be considered in women in the procreation period and pregnancy. On the contrary, age over 70 years and concurrent cardiovascular disease should direct the decision toward a follow-up strategy [5]. Especially since epidemiological studies suggest that LT4 replacement therapy for subclinical hypothyroidism does not improve health-related quality of life, survival, or decreased cardiovascular morbidity [12]. Also, administration of TH to euthyroid obese subjects to enhance weight loss is not recommended since it is associated with several adverse effects, including muscle wasting and weakness as well as cardiovascular complications [24].

Paradoxically, regardless of the method applied, the best treatment for obesity-related hyperthyreotropinemia is weight loss, leading to the reversal of the mechanisms causing central and peripheral resistance to TH. For instance, in an interventional study, after lifestyle interventions (diet combined with increased physical activity), the number of individuals with TSH level above the normal range decreased significantly after the intervention from 17.2% to 6.2%., while the mean TSH level in the whole group decreased from the mean 2.8 mU/l before the intervention to 2.2 mU/l) [25]. Similarly, regardless of the procedure, bariatric surgery results in the normalization of TSH in nearly all patients (reviewed in ref. [26]). These findings strongly suggest that obesity-associated hyperthyrotropinemia is transient and resolves after weight loss.

In summary, most obese individuals are euthyroid, even though their TSH levels usually exceed those observed in normal-weight individuals. The most common obesity-associated thyroid hormone abnormality is hyperthyrotropinemia that can be distinguished from the SH by the normal and/or high normal concentrations of thyroid hormones. In addition, obesity is associated with decreased thyroid echogenicity in ultrasound which does not mirror the presence of autoimmune thyroid disease. Independently, obesity increases the risk of thyroid autoimmunity. Patients with isolated hyperthyrotropinemia should not be treated with thyroid hormone replacement unless there are symptoms or other signs of thyroid disease. Indications for LT4 treatment in obese individuals are limited to overt hypothyroidism and some selected cases of its subclinical form. Administration of thyroid hormones to obese individuals without thyroid disease to induce weight reduction or improve metabolic profile is not justified and may lead to hyperthyroidism and its complications. Recommendations for testing for thyroid dysfunction in obese patients and their management are summarized in **Figure 1**.

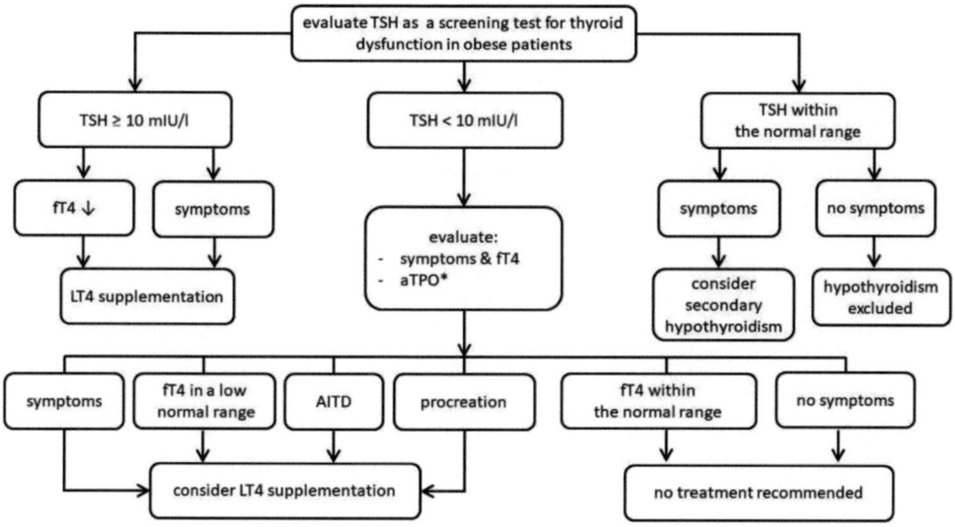

Figure 1.
*Testing for thyroid dysfunction and hypothyroidism treatment in obese patients (based on ref. [5]). AITD, autoimmune thyroid disorder; aTPO, thyroid peroxidase antibodies; fT4, free thyroxine; LT4, levothyroxine; TSH, thyroid-stimulating hormone; * If TSH and fT4 levels suggest subclinical hypothyroidism.*

Loss of weight leads to the normalization of TSH in most obese individuals; however, till now, no large-scale study showed how the echogenicity of the thyroid parenchyma changes after weight loss and whether there is a correlation with the ultrasound image and the incidence of autoimmune thyroid disease before and after weight loss.

3. The hypothalamic-pituitary-adrenal axis and obesity

Cortisol secretion is regulated by the hypothalamic–pituitary–adrenal (HPA) axis upon stimuli received from the central and peripheral nervous system and integrated into hypothalamic nuclei to counteract different types of stressors. Upon these stimuli, corticotropin-releasing hormone (CRH) and vasopressin are released by the paraventricular nucleus of the hypothalamus and stimulate the secretion of adrenocorticotropic hormone (ACTH, corticotropin). Subsequently, ACTH acts on the adrenal cortex to produce and release glucocorticoid hormones (mainly cortisol in humans). The HPA axis activity is controlled by cortisol in an inhibitory feedback loop *via* glucocorticoid receptors (GR), located mainly in the brain's hippocampus region. By interaction with GR, cortisol plays an essential role in the regulation of metabolism. In response to stress, cortisol, by mobilization of glucose, free fatty acids, and amino acids from endogenous resources, increases the availability of fuel substrates. In an emergency, these properties of cortisol assure the energy supply necessary to survive [27]. However, cortisol excess observed in patients with the Cushing's syndrome, caused either by the adrenal tumor (ACTH-independent hypercortisolism), tumors of the hypothalamic–pituitary system, or tumors outside the HPA axis that ectopically produce ACTH (ACTH-dependent hypercortisolism) or CRH, leads to the profound impairment of whole-body homeostasis [28].

3.1 Metabolic consequences of hypercortisolism

Even though proper cortisol secretion is vital for everyday existence, its excess intensifies catabolism, leading to decreased lean body mass and causing muscle atrophy. Moreover, to increase energy uptake, glucocorticoids stimulate appetite and food consumption contributing to the development of central obesity. Furthermore, by acting on the liver, muscle, adipose tissue, and pancreas, glucocorticoids increase gluconeogenesis, impair insulin sensitivity, and increase lipolysis and lipogenesis, leading to the development of the metabolic syndrome. Moreover, there is evidence from preclinical studies that glucocorticoids may interfere with the action of adipokines: by interference with the signaling system of the leptin receptor cortisol induces leptin resistance, characteristic for individuals with primary obesity [29]. Therefore the clinical picture of patients suffering from hypercortisolism resembles in many aspects primary obesity, and obesity is commonly listed among the different entities of so-called pseudo-Cushing states [30]. However, several issues in a clinical examination should be considered during the differential diagnosis.

Firstly, adipose tissue distribution in hypercortisolism concerns mainly the abdominal area, the neck, and the face, while the extremities remain lean due to muscle atrophy. Subjects with primary obesity usually have fat accumulation all over the body, including upper and lower extremities. Next, striae in obese individuals are usually pale, narrow, and their appearance is associated with pregnancy or rapid weight gain. On the contrary, striae related to cortisol excess are reddish or live red, wider than 1 cm, and appear suddenly without any identifiable cause. Moreover, patients with cortisol excess complain of unusual brushing, skin thinning, and facial plethora that are not specific symptoms in primary obesity. Excess of cortisol or co-secretion of androgens (by the adrenal tumor or ACTH-stimulated adrenal cortex) can result in typical features of hyperandrogenism that include acne, hirsutism, and alopecia. Furthermore, cortisol-induced osteolysis leads to osteoporosis that is rarely seen in obese subjects whose bones are protected by an endocrine activity of adipose tissue. Finally, hypercortisolism is associated with an increased frequency of non-metabolic complications that include, among others, thromboembolic incidents, severe infections, depressive and psychotic episodes resulting from the action of excess cortisol on other tissues and organs [30].

Apart from the clinical picture, the final diagnosis requires endocrine testing (described in detail elsewhere), especially in the case of individuals with so-called subclinical Cushing's syndrome [28]. This endocrine disorder is observed in individuals with incidentally found adrenal adenoma and ACTH-independent cortisol secretion that is not fully restrained by pituitary feedback. Even though patients with subclinical Cushing's syndrome do not present all clinical features of the full-blown disease (e.g., only 30–50% of them are obese) and hypercortisolism is of minimal intensity, it may eventually contribute to the development of metabolic and vascular complications [31]. The reason for unmasking endogenous hypercortisolism derives from its devastating complications affecting the quality of life and life expectancy unless adequately treated [5].

Therefore the question is if the diagnostic of Cushing's syndrome should be conducted in every obese patient. The epidemiological studies estimate the prevalence of Cushing's syndrome in obese individuals to be 0.9%, and in patients with type 2 diabetes with poor metabolic control, it rises to 2–3% [14]. The incidence of subclinical Cushing's syndrome has been more common in patients with obesity than in the general population, though the precise assessment of the disease frequency is difficult since the diagnostic criteria and treatment program have not been well established yet. Therefore, assuming the epidemic proportions of obesity and the low prevalence of hypercortisolism among patients with obesity, the ESE guidelines do not recommend routine screening of Cushing's syndrome in patients with obesity. However, such testing should be performed in patients who exhibit other specific features of hypercortisolism besides obesity, such as skin atrophy, osteoporosis, spontaneous ecchymoses, proximal myopathy, or wide purple striae.

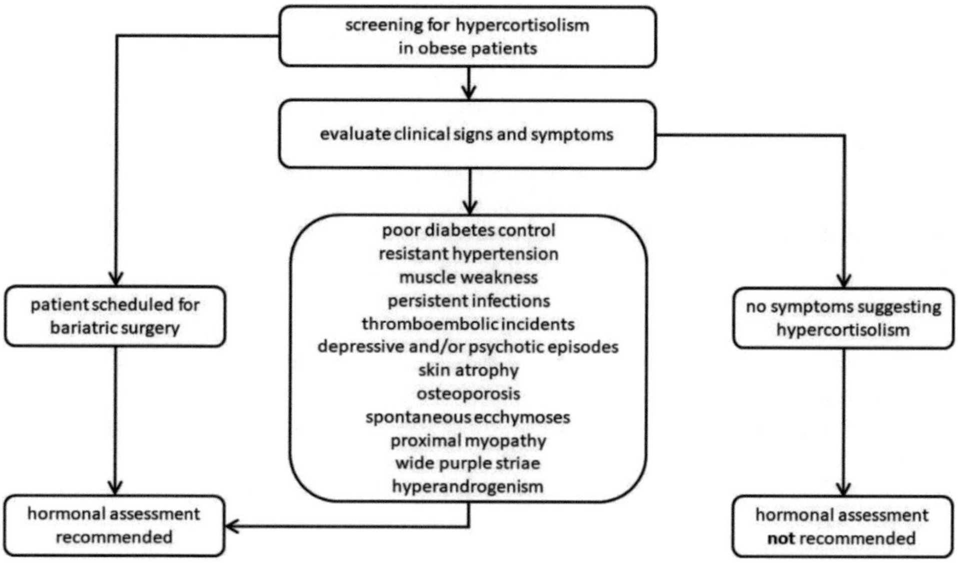

Figure 2.
Screening for hypercortisolism in obese patients (based on ref. [5]).

Moreover, given the high risk of surgical complications or adverse clinical outcomes following surgery, the screening for hypercortisolism should be considered in patients referred to bariatric surgery [5]. Recommendations for testing for hypercortisolism in obese patients are summarized in **Figure 2**.

3.2 Obesity-related HPA dysfunction

Obese patients constitute a heterogeneous population in terms of the HPA axis function [32]. Some of them have a normal circadian rhythm of cortisol secretion and its proper excretion in the urine. The remaining obese patients (especially those with abdominal obesity) present with the so-called functional hypercortisolism. This condition results both from the increased sensitivity of the HPA axis to stimuli, as well as from the increased peripheral cortisol synthesis (including the activation of 11β steroid dehydrogenase (11β-HSD) type 1, which converts cortisone into cortisol in adipose tissue) and the increased number of GR in peripheral tissues [33–36]. Clinically, in addition to some phenotypic features of Cushing's syndrome, these patients exhibit increased nocturnal ACTH and cortisol levels, increased urinary excretion of cortisol metabolites, and enlargement of adrenal glands in imaging studies [37]. The results of studies on the inhibition of cortisol secretion in the dexamethasone test (1 mg) in obese patients also indicate the existence of different phenotypes of obesity. While some patients show a normal response, in others, a low dose of dexamethasone does not inhibit the HPA axis [37, 38].

The type of HPA disturbances in obesity seems to depend not only on adipose tissue distribution (visceral *vs*. subcutaneous) but also on the individual pattern of a stress response. Individuals coping well with stress usually have normal HPA function with high morning and low evening cortisol values, a brisk response to feeding, and are sensitive to dexamethasone suppression. In contrast, patients vulnerable to stress have low variability in a circadian cortisol rhythm, a small feeding response, and do not inhibit cortisol secretion after administration of dexamethasone. This abnormal HPA axis function is associated with a worse metabolic profile, including higher waist-to-hip ratio (WHR), total and low-density lipoprotein cholesterol, and blood pressure. Moreover, due to the interactions with other central endocrine axes, HPA axis status may determine the function of other endocrine glands. Therefore, HPA axis overactivity inhibits the secretion of sex steroids, growth hormone, and TSH [32]. However, these two reaction patterns of the HPA axis are extremes, and between them are several intermediate forms. These include, for instance, a normal, basic HPA axis activity, with high variability, stimulated by perceived stress that can explain the described above diversity of findings. Other determinants of the heterogeneous responses of the HPA axis in obese individuals include, but are not limited to: differences in GR sensitivity which can be partially genetically determined, comorbidities such as depression, or lifestyle factors such as alcohol abuse [39].

In summary, abnormalities of HPA function are a common phenomenon among obese individuals; however, due to a variety of hormonal responses, several phenotypes can be distinguished that differ in metabolic risk and health consequences. In addition, the presence of overt hypercortisolism is relatively rare. Therefore, routine testing for Cushing's syndrome in obesity is not recommended unless some typical alerting clinical features are present.

While normalization of the HPT axis after weight-loss interventions is widely described, only single studies carried out on groups of about 30 individuals show that weight loss normalizes the excretion of cortisol and cortisone metabolites in the urine, which correlates with a decrease in the expression of 11 β-HSD type 1 in subcutaneous fat [40]. However, it is unclear which of the obesity-related disturbances in the HPA axis function are reversible and which sustain despite the weight reduction.

4. The hypothalamic-pituitary-gonadal axis and obesity

The secretion of sex hormones is regulated by the hypothalamic–pituitary-gonadal (HPG) axis. Briefly, gonadotropin-releasing hormone (GnRH) is secreted by the hypothalamus and stimulates the anterior pituitary lobe to release gonadotropins: luteinizing hormone (LH) and follicle-stimulating hormone (FSH), that subsequently stimulate gonads (ovaries and testes) to secrete estrogen and testosterone, as well as to control reproduction. While testosterone in a negative feedback loop inhibits GnRH and gonadotropins secretion, the regulation is more composed in the case of female sex steroids. In females, estrogen in a positive feedback loop stimulates LH secretion to prepare the reproductive organs for ovulation and implantation. In turn, after the ovulation, progesterone released by the corpus luteum inhibits proper cells in the hypothalamus and anterior pituitary lobe and stops the estrogen-LH positive feedback loop [41]. Since sex hormone receptors are spread all over the human body, apart from their pivotal role in the regulation of reproduction, sex steroids impact the function of several organs, including the adipose tissue. However, this relation is bidirectional since adipose tissue, *via* secretion of adipokines, modulates the HPG axis [42].

4.1 Metabolic consequences of hypogonadism

Sexual dimorphism of adipose tissue distribution appears in puberty, indicating the role of sex hormones in its development [43]. Estrogens drive fat accumulation in the gluteofemoral subcutaneous depot, and during puberty in girls, increasing circulating estrogens levels correlate with an increase in fat deposition in this area. In turn, a decline in estrogen concentration during menopause is associated in women with changes in adipose tissue distribution from gluteofemoral to visceral.

On the contrary, women who are on hormone replacement therapy do not display the characteristic abdominal weight gain pattern usually associated with menopause [44]. The ability of estrogens to affect body fat distribution is not limited to women. In males, loss of estrogen signaling or its pharmacological inhibition promotes adiposity and impairs glucose metabolism [45, 46]. Preclinical studies confirmed a significant role for estrogen in regulating adipose tissue distribution, metabolism, and inflammatory activity. Activation of estrogen receptors was found to inhibit adipocyte differentiation, lipid accumulation, and the expression of adipocyte-specific genes in primary human adipocytes [47]. Since estrogen influences adipose tissue amount and its metabolism, it may modulate the risk of obesity-related complications. In clinical studies, menopause is associated with a constant decline in insulin sensitivity parallel to an increase in serum inflammatory markers and unfavorable lipid profile [48]. In turn, transdermal administration of estradiol decreases the expression of genes encoding critical lipogenic enzymes in human adipose tissue that correlates with a decrease in plasma triglyceride levels [49].

Androgens also influence adipose tissue metabolism. By binding androgen receptors (AR) present in adipose tissue, especially in the visceral depot, testosterone up-regulates adrenergic receptors β that activate lipolysis. Moreover, androgens decrease in adipose tissue activity of lipoprotein lipase (LPL) responsible for the hydrolysis of circulating triglyceride-rich lipoproteins inhibiting in this way triglyceride uptake [50]. Androgen status, responsible, among others, for the muscle mass accrual in puberty, is crucial to acquire and maintain favorable body composition in men. Accordingly, several cross-sectional and longitudinal studies have reported an inverse correlation between serum testosterone level and indices of obesity and metabolic risk (reviewed in ref. [51]). In turn, interventional studies have shown a beneficial effect of testosterone replacement therapy on BMI, adipose tissue distribution, and body composition in hypogonadal men [14]. An essential voice in the discussion on the direction and causality of the relationship between adiposity and serum testosterone levels came from the genetic studies. The genetic risk for BMI was inversely associated with serum testosterone levels, while no association was observed between the genetic risk testosterone levels and BMI, suggesting that it is mainly adiposity affecting testosterone levels rather than the other way around [52].

4.2 Obesity-related gonadal dysfunction in men

Both in men and women, hypogonadism can be the cause but also the consequence of obesity. In a recent meta-analysis, the prevalence of hypogonadism in obese men in general, when measuring total testosterone (TT), was 43,8%, while in severely obese individuals referred to bariatric surgery – 75,0% [14]. Several underlying mechanisms are responsible for the development of obesity-related hypogonadism in men. Firstly, obesity is associated with increased aromatase cytochrome P450 activity in adipose tissue, resulting in the enhanced conversion of testosterone to estradiol. Subsequently, higher estradiol levels *via* stimulation of estrogen receptor β downregulate glucose transporter (GLUT) 4 induce insulin resistance [53]. In turn, insulin resistance leads to the decreased sex-hormone-binding globulin (SHBG) synthesis in the liver, which translates to a larger amount of TT available for conversion to estradiol in adipose tissue. In turn, high estrogen levels inhibit gonadotropin secretion from the pituitary gland. Therefore, obesity impairs sperm concentration, motility, and morphology, too [54]. Furthermore, the HPG axis is modulated by adipokines. For instance, elevated leptin levels inhibit the production of testosterone by Leydig cells, while low adiponectin concentrations contribute to hepatic insulin resistance in this way, further influencing SHBG synthesis [53, 55]. In addition, described above, obesity-associated dysfunction of the HPA axis resulting in functional hypercortisolism may contribute to the gonadotropin inhibition and, subsequently, reduced testosterone levels [56].

ESE does not recommend performing a routine hormonal screening for male hypogonadism in patients with obesity; however, testing should be considered when the clinical picture is suspicious. Then, TT plasma morning concentrations should be measured as an initial investigation, and when the result is low, the measurement should be repeated on two separate days in a fasting state. Since the equilibrium dialysis, which is the gold standard procedure to measure free testosterone, is hardly available, ESE suggests calculating bioavailable testosterone by using TT, SHBG, and albumin concentrations, when TT concentration is near the lower limit of the normal range [5, 57]. When low testosterone level is confirmed, the next step in the diagnostic algorithm includes measurement of FSH and LH to distinguish between primary and secondary hypogonadism [5]. Obesity-related hypogonadism in males is associated with low gonadotropin levels and sometimes with a predominance of FSH over LH, and its diagnosis requires exclusion of other causes of hypogonadotropic (secondary) hypogonadism [58]. When interpreting a testosterone measurement result, one should remember its level declines with age and can be affected by chronic diseases, drugs, lifestyle, and genetic predisposition [59]. Moreover, the assay technique used impacts the measurement result with the liquid chromatography–tandem mass spectrometry (LC–MS) method being a golden standard in sex steroids level determination [60]. The testosterone norms for obese individuals do not differ from the reference ranges accepted for the whole population; however, these vary between the countries [5]. In general, the diagnosis of male obesity-secondary hypogonadism should be based on a combination of low testosterone levels with clinical features of hypogonadism, including decreased sexual thoughts, erectile dysfunction, and reduced morning erections [61].

Since obesity can lead to functional male hypogonadism, which, in a vicious circle, can further promote obesity, the first-line therapy is focused on weight management. Unfortunately, non-invasive approaches focused on lifestyle modification aiming at 5% weight loss are frequently insufficient to normalize testosterone levels, and the best results can be achieved employing bariatric surgery [62]. In turn, due to the potential risks (e.g., those related to increased prothrombotic activity), testosterone replacement is not routinely recommended in obese individuals with functional male hypogonadism. However, it can be considered if testosterone levels and/or hypogonadism signs and symptoms do not improve [5].

In summary, low testosterone serum levels in obese men are frequent; however, it does not equate to androgen deficiency. Moreover, obesity-secondary hypogonadism in men is functional and can be reversed by proper weight management. The clinical assessment is of pivotal importance in assessing the causality of the relationship between body adiposity and hypogonadism. If the signs and symptoms of testosterone deficiency occurred first, before the weight gain – the diagnosis of hypogonadism as a cause of obesity can be established and testosterone replacement treatment administered. In the context of the metabolic risk, it is still unclear whether low testosterone levels in obesity are a marker or a risk factor for metabolic complications. The clinical approach to obesity-associated hypogonadism in men is summarized in **Figure 3**.

4.3 Obesity-related gonadal dysfunction in women

While obese men struggle with testosterone deficiency, the most common consequence of obesity in the context of HPG axis dysfunction in women is hyperandrogenism, frequently associated with hyperinsulinemia and infertility. The exact prevalence of biochemical hyperandrogenism in obese women is unknown

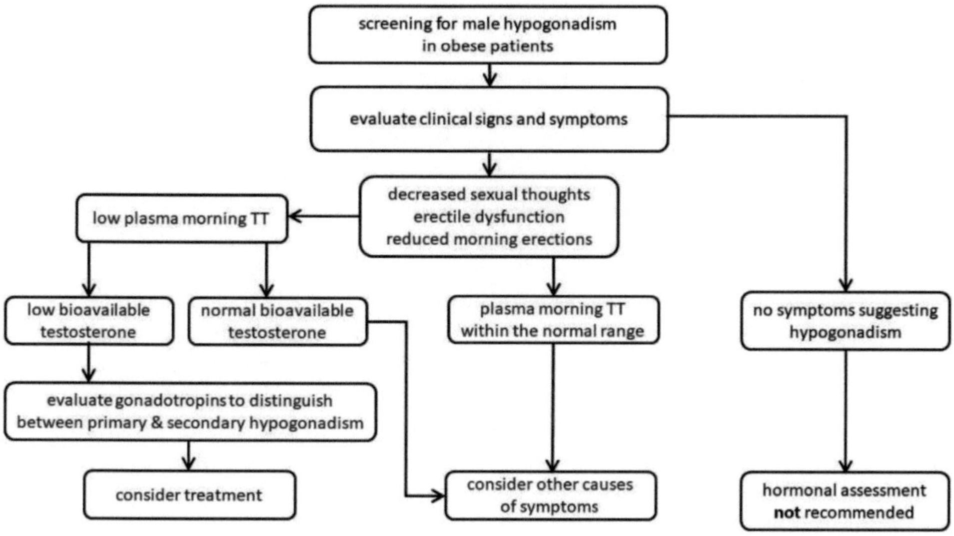

Figure 3.
The clinical approach to obesity-associated hypogonadism in men (based on ref. [5]). TT, total testosterone.

since most epidemiological studies were focused on the incidence of polycystic ovary syndrome (PCOS), which diagnosis can be established without the presence of clinical/biochemical androgen excess. However, the prevalence of PCOS in obese women is similar to the general population in reproductive age (25–29%) but increases with BMI [14].

In obese women, especially in those with visceral obesity, low SHBG levels lead to a relative increase in estrogens' concentration that stimulates the pulsatile LH secretion and subsequent steroidogenesis in the theca cell system. Similarly, high insulin and insulin-like growth factor I (IGF-I) levels stimulate 17α-hydroxylase activity in the theca cells, increasing the secretion of ovarian androgens [63]. In addition, obesity-related HPA axis dysfunction (described above) results in increased synthesis of adrenal androgens. In turn, adipose tissue of obese women is characterized by a higher activity of 5α-reductase, which transforms testosterone into a much more active androgen – dihydrotestosterone [64]. All these changes clinically manifest by hyperandrogenism (most often hirsutism) and menstrual and/or ovulation dysfunction. The cause of ovulation dysfunction in obese women may also be an increased concentration of leptin, which, by binding its receptors in the ovary, inhibits follicle maturation and steroidogenesis [65]. Furthermore, an obesity-associated increase in pro-inflammatory cytokines secretion from adipose tissue also contributes to the disturbing gonadotropin secretion in the pituitary [66]. Therefore, the percentage of ovulation cycles decreases with BMI, reaching only 12% in individuals with BMI ≥ 35 kg/m^2 and obese women, even when eumenorrheic, have reduced fecundity and worse outcomes of the *in vitro* fertilization (IVF) [67]. Apart from the HPG dysfunction, obesity negatively influences the oocyte and the embryo development that manifests by disrupted meiotic spindle formation and mitochondrial function. Moreover, obesity-associated low-grade inflammation has a toxic effect on the reproductive tissues, including the endometrium, characterized by impaired stromal decidualization that leads to impaired receptivity and placental abnormalities. In addition, chronic inflammation and the altered adipokines secretion impairs steroidogenesis and can directly affect the embryo. All these factors contribute to the higher rates of miscarriage, stillbirth, and preeclampsia in obese women [68].

Studies in women with PCOS show that weight loss achieved by a lifestyle intervention may reduce hyperinsulinemia and thus break the vicious cycle of excessive androgen synthesis [69]. Similar changes occur in obese women who experience weight loss as a result of bariatric procedures. In a recent meta-analysis, resolution of PCOS was found in 96% of affected women after bariatric surgery, which was associated with an increase in SHBG level and a decrease in serum estradiol and TT. These changes in sex hormone levels in 53% of individuals resulted in the resolution of hirsutism and 96% – in the resolution of menstrual dysfunction [70]. However, most studies on the assessment of androgen concentrations in obese women were based on measurements performed with immunoassays, which are characterized by a high percentage of false-positive results, and as it was mentioned above, currently the reference method in the measurement of androgen concentrations is LC–MS [71]. In the context of infertility, in obese women, successful weight loss improves ovulation rates and menstrual irregularity, increasing the chances of pregnancy due to natural conception and IVF. According to meta-analyses, there appears to be no significant difference between the patients after weight-loss interventions and never obese controls concerning rates of miscarriage and IVF conceptions [67]. However, there is still a lack of randomized controlled trials that would assess, for instance, the effect of weight loss on numbers of oocytes retrieved for IVF and time to conception.

ESE guidelines do not recommend routine testing for gonadal dysfunction in female obese patients unless clinical symptoms (e.g., acne, hirsutism, androgenic alopecia, acanthosis nigricans, menstrual abnormalities, oligo-anovulation, infertility) occur. When there is a clinical suspicion of PCOS, the diagnostic procedures should include hormonal testing and ovarian ultrasound. If the diagnosis of PCOS is excluded, other diseases leading to hyperandrogenism and infertility should be considered, e.g., hyperprolactinemia, thyroid dysfunction, congenital adrenal hyperplasia, and hypercortisolism. If PCOS is diagnosed, additional testing toward glucose intolerance should be performed [5].

In summary, hyperandrogenism and infertility seem to be the main manifestation of obesity-related HPG axis dysfunction in women, and in both, weight management should be considered first-line therapy. However, if the HPG axis dysfunction sustains despite the successful weight loss or if the patient presents signs and/or symptoms suggesting an underlying disease not related to obesity, the causative treatment should be undertaken.

5. Conclusions and further directions

The increasing incidence of obesity translates to the increased number of obese individuals referred to endocrinologists, either because of clinical suspicion of an underlying endocrine disease-causing weight gain or concern that obesity may have caused endocrine dysfunction. As described above, the relationship between obesity and endocrine dysfunction is bidirectional and complex and concerns all main hormonal axes. Based on the meta-analyses of observational and interventional studies, endocrine sociates proposed clinical guidelines to facilitate the management of obese individuals in everyday practice. In most cases, those guidelines advise a cautious approach and limit the diagnostics to the cases with a clear clinical picture. Apart from the TSH measurement, no other hormonal assessment is recommended to an asymptomatic obese individual unless he or she is referred to bariatric surgery when a screening toward hypercortisolism should be performed.

Since most obesity-related hormonal disturbances are reversible in the case of HPT and HPG axes, weight management should be the first-line strategy, and treatment considered if the abnormalities sustain despite the weight loss. However, given the diversity of changes in the HPA axis that occur in obese individuals, the influence of weight management on cortisol secretion requires further investigation.

Acknowledgements

This work was supported by the National Science Centre Poland grant 2018/31/B/NZ5/01556.

Conflict of interest

The author declares no conflict of interest.

Author details

Alina Kurylowicz
Mossakowski Medical Research Centre, Polish Academy of Sciences, Warsaw, Poland

*Address all correspondence to: akurylowicz@imdik.pan.pl

References

[1] Global Obesity Observatory. Available from: www.worldobesity.org [Accessed: 2021-06-03]

[2] Woo CY, Jang JE, Lee SE, Koh EH, Lee KU. Mitochondrial Dysfunction in Adipocytes as a Primary Cause of Adipose Tissue Inflammation. Diabetes Metab J. 2019;43:247-256. DOI: 10.4093/dmj.2018.0221

[3] Pasquali R, Vicennati V, Gambineri A. Adrenal and gonadal function in obesity. J Endocrinol Invest. 2002;25:893-898. DOI: 10.1007/BF03344053

[4] Mullur R, Liu YY, Brent GA. Thyroid hormone regulation of metabolism. Physiol Rev. 2014;94:355-382. DOI: 10.1152/physrev.00030.2013

[5] Pasquali R, Casanueva F, Haluzik M, van Hulsteijn L, Ledoux S, Monteiro MP, Salvador J, Santini F, Toplak H, Dekkers OM. European Society of Endocrinology Clinical Practice Guideline: Endocrine work-up in obesity. Eur J Endocrinol. 2020;182:G1-G32. DOI: 10.1530/EJE-19-0893

[6] Ríos-Prego M, Anibarro L, Sánchez-Sobrino P. Relationship between thyroid dysfunction and body weight: a not so evident paradigm. Int J Gen Med. 2019;12:299-304. DOI: 10.2147/IJGM.S206983

[7] Karmisholt J, Andersen S, Laurberg P. Weight loss after therapy of hypothyroidism is mainly caused by excretion of excess body water associated with myxoedema. J Clin Endocrinol Metab. 2011;96:E99-103. DOI: 10.1210/jc.2010-1521

[8] Garber JR, Cobin RH, Gharib H, Hennessey JV, Klein I, Mechanick JI, Pessah-Pollack R, Singer PA, Woeber KA; American Association of Clinical Endocrinologists and American Thyroid Association Taskforce on Hypothyroidism in Adults. Clinical practice guidelines for hypothyroidism in adults: cosponsored by the American Association of Clinical Endocrinologists and the American Thyroid Association. Endocr Pract. 2012;18:988-1028. DOI: 10.4158/EP12280.GL

[9] Reinehr T. Obesity and thyroid function. Mol Cell Endocrinol. 2010;316:165-171. DOI: 10.1016/j.mce.2009.06.005

[10] Knudsen N, Laurberg P, Rasmussen LB, Bülow I, Perrild H, Ovesen L, Jørgensen T. Small differences in thyroid function may be important for body mass index and the occurrence of obesity in the population. J Clin Endocrinol Metab. 2005;90:4019-4024. DOI: 10.1210/jc.2004-2225

[11] Chikunguwo S, Brethauer S, Nirujogi V, Pitt T, Udomsawaengsup S, Chand B, Schauer P. Influence of obesity and surgical weight loss on thyroid hormone levels. Surg Obes Relat Dis. 2007;3:631-636. DOI: 10.1016/j.soard.2007.07.011

[12] Villar HC, Saconato H, Valente O, Atallah AN. Thyroid hormone replacement for subclinical hypothyroidism. Cochrane Database Syst Rev. 2007;3:CD003419. DOI: 10.1002/14651858.CD003419.pub2

[13] Song RH, Wang B, Yao QM, Li Q, Jia X, Zhang JA. The Impact of Obesity on Thyroid Autoimmunity and Dysfunction: A Systematic Review and Meta-Analysis. Front Immunol. 2019;10:2349. DOI: 10.3389/fimmu.2019.02349

[14] van Hulsteijn LT, Pasquali R, Casanueva F, Haluzik M, Ledoux S, Monteiro MP, Salvador J, Santini F, Toplak H, Dekkers OM. Prevalence of endocrine disorders in obese patients:

systematic review and meta-analysis. Eur J Endocrinol. 2020;182:11-21. DOI: 10.1530/EJE-19-0666

[15] García-Solís P, García OP, Hernández-Puga G, Sánchez-Tusie AA, Sáenz-Luna CE, Hernández-Montiel HL, Solis-S JC. Thyroid hormones and obesity: a known but poorly understood relationship. Endokrynol Pol. 2018;69:292-303. DOI: 10.5603/EP.2018.0032

[16] Ortiga-Carvalho TM, Oliveira KJ, Soares BA, Pazos-Moura CC. The role of leptin in the regulation of TSH secretion in the fed state: in vivo and in vitro studies. J Endocrinol. 2002; 174:121-125. DOI: 10.1677/joe.0.1740121

[17] Zimmermann-Belsing T, Brabant G, Holst JJ, Feldt-Rasmussen U. Circulating leptin and thyroid dysfunction. Eur J Endocrinol. 2003;149:257-271. DOI: 10.1530/eje.0.1490257

[18] Janssen IM, Homan J, Schijns W, Betzel B, Aarts EO, Berends FJ, de Boer H. Subclinical hypothyroidism and its relation to obesity in patients before and after Roux-en-Y gastric bypass. Surg Obes Relat Dis. 2015;11:1257-1263. DOI: 10.1016/j.soard.2015.02.021

[19] LeFevre ML; U.S. Preventive Services Task Force. Screening for thyroid dysfunction: U.S. Preventive Services Task Force recommendation statement. Ann Intern Med. 2015;162:641-650. DOI: 10.7326/M15-0483

[20] Marzullo P, Minocci A, Tagliaferri MA, Guzzaloni G, Di Blasio A, De Medici C, Aimaretti G, Liuzzi A. Investigations of thyroid hormones and antibodies in obesity: leptin levels are associated with thyroid autoimmunity independent of bioanthropometric, hormonal, and weight-related determinants. J Clin Endocrinol Metab. 2010;95:3965-3972. DOI: 10.1210/jc.2009-2798

[21] Rotondi M, de Martinis L, Coperchini F, Pignatti P, Pirali B, Ghilotti S, Fonte R, Magri F, Chiovato L. Serum negative autoimmune thyroiditis displays a milder clinical picture compared with classic Hashimoto's thyroiditis. Eur J Endocrinol. 2014;171:31-36. DOI: 10.1530/EJE-14-0147

[22] Rotondi M, Cappelli C, Leporati P, Chytiris S, Zerbini F, Fonte R, Magri F, Castellano M, Chiovato L. A hypoechoic pattern of the thyroid at ultrasound does not indicate autoimmune thyroid diseases in patients with morbid obesity. Eur J Endocrinol. 2010;163:105-1099. DOI: 10.1530/EJE-10-0288

[23] Pearce SH, Brabant G, Duntas LH, Monzani F, Peeters RP, Razvi S, Wemeau JL. 2013 ETA Guideline: Management of Subclinical Hypothyroidism. Eur Thyroid J. 2013;2:215-228. DOI: 10.1159/000356507

[24] Kaptein EM, Beale E, Chan LS. Thyroid hormone therapy for obesity and nonthyroidal illnesses: a systematic review. J Clin Endocrinol Metab. 2009;94:3663-3675. DOI: 10.1210/jc.2009-0899

[25] Radetti G, Longhi S, Baiocchi M, Cassar W, Buzi F. Changes in lifestyle improve body composition, thyroid function, and structure in obese children. J Endocrinol Invest. 2012;35:281-285. DOI: 10.3275/7763

[26] Gajda SN, Kuryłowicz A, Żach M, Bednarczuk T, Wyleżoł M. Diagnosis and treatment of thyroid disorders in obese patients - what do we know? Endokrynol Pol. 2019;70:271-276. DOI: 10.5603/EP.a2018.0089

[27] Arlt W, Stewart PM. Adrenal corticosteroid biosynthesis, metabolism, and action. Endocrinol Metab Clin North Am. 2005;34:293-313. DOI: 10.1016/j.ecl.2005.01.002

[28] Pappachan JM, Hariman C, Edavalath M, Waldron J, Hanna FW. Cushing's syndrome: a practical approach to diagnosis and differential diagnoses. J Clin Pathol. 2017;70:350-359. DOI: 10.1136/jclinpath-2016-203933

[29] Aschbacher K, Rodriguez-Fernandez M, van Wietmarschen H, Tomiyama AJ, Jain S, Epel E, Doyle FJ 3rd, van der Greef J. The hypothalamic-pituitary-adrenal-leptin axis and metabolic health: a systems approach to resilience, robustness and control. Interface Focus. 2014;4:20140020. DOI: 10.1098/rsfs.2014.0020

[30] Ferraù F, Korbonits M. Metabolic Syndrome in Cushing's Syndrome Patients. Front Horm Res. 2018;49:85-103. DOI: 10.1159/000486002

[31] Terzolo M, Pia A, Reimondo G. Subclinical Cushing's syndrome: definition and management. Clin Endocrinol (Oxf). 2012;76:12-18. DOI: 10.1111/j.1365-2265.2011.04253.x

[32] Björntorp P, Rosmond R. Obesity and cortisol. Nutrition. 2000;16:924-936. DOI: 10.1016/s0899-9007(00)00422-6

[33] Pasquali R. Is the hypothalamic-pituitary-adrenal axis really hyperactivated in visceral obesity? J Endocrinol Invest. 1998;21:268-271. DOI: 10.1007/BF03347314

[34] Vicennati V, Ceroni L, Gagliardi L, Gambineri A, Pasquali R. Comment: response of the hypothalamic-pituitary-adrenocortical axis to high-protein/fat and high-carbohydrate meals in women with different obesity phenotypes. J Clin Endocrinol Metab. 2002;87:3984-3988. DOI: 10.1210/jcem.87.8.8718

[35] Jessop DS, Dallman MF, Fleming D, Lightman SL. Resistance to glucocorticoid feedback in obesity. J Clin Endocrinol Metab. 2001;86:4109-4114. DOI: 10.1210/jcem.86.9.7826

[36] Rask E, Olsson T, Söderberg S, Andrew R, Livingstone DE, Johnson O, Walker BR. Tissue-specific dysregulation of cortisol metabolism in human obesity. J Clin Endocrinol Metab. 2001;86:1418-1421. DOI: 10.1210/jcem.86.3.7453

[37] Pasquali R, Vicennati V, Gambineri A. Adrenal and gonadal function in obesity. J Endocrinol Invest. 2002;25:893-898. DOI: 10.1007/BF03344053

[38] Rosmond R, Björntorp P. The interactions between hypothalamic-pituitary-adrenal axis activity, testosterone, insulin-like growth factor I and abdominal obesity with metabolism and blood pressure in men. Int J Obes Relat Metab Disord. 1998;22:1184-1196. DOI: 10.1038/sj.ijo.0800745

[39] Björntorp P, Rosmond R. The metabolic syndrome--a neuroendocrine disorder? Br J Nutr. 2000;83:S49-S57. DOI: 10.1017/s0007114500000957

[40] Rask E, Simonyte K, Lönn L, Axelson M. Cortisol metabolism after weight loss: associations with 11 β-HSD type 1 and markers of obesity in women. Clin Endocrinol (Oxf). 2013;78:700-705. DOI: 10.1111/j.1365-2265.2012.04333.x

[41] Klein CE. The Hypothalamic-Pituitary-Gonadal Axis. In: Kufe DW, Pollock RE, Weichselbaum RR, et al., editors. Holland-Frei Cancer Medicine. 6th ed. Hamilton (ON): BC Decker; 2003. Available from: https://www.ncbi.nlm.nih.gov/books/NBK13386/

[42] Tsatsanis C, Dermitzaki E, Avgoustinaki P, Malliaraki N, Mytaras V, Margioris AN. The impact of adipose tissue-derived factors on the hypothalamic-pituitary-gonadal (HPG) axis. Hormones (Athens). 2015;14:549-562. DOI:10.14310/horm.2002.1649.

[43] Jeffery E, Wing A, Holtrup B, Sebo Z, Kaplan JL, Saavedra-Peña R,

Church CD, Colman L, Berry R, Rodeheffer MS. The Adipose Tissue Microenvironment Regulates Depot-Specific Adipogenesis in Obesity. Cell Metab. 2016;24:142-150. DOI: 10.1016/j.cmet.2016.05.012

[44] Gambacciani M, Ciaponi M, Cappagli B, Piaggesi L, De Simone L, Orlandi R, Genazzani AR. Body weight, body fat distribution, and hormonal replacement therapy in early postmenopausal women. J Clin Endocrinol Metab. 1997;82:414-417. DOI: 10.1210/jcem.82.2.3735

[45] Simpson ER. Genetic mutations resulting in estrogen insufficiency in the male. Mol Cell Endocrinol. 1998;145:55-59. DOI: 10.1016/s0303-7207(98)00169-5

[46] Chao J, Rubinow KB, Kratz M, Amory JK, Matsumoto AM, Page ST. Short-Term Estrogen Withdrawal Increases Adiposity in Healthy Men. J Clin Endocrinol Metab. 2016;101:3724-3731. DOI: 10.1210/jc.2016-1482

[47] Park HJ, Della-Fera MA, Hausman DB, Rayalam S, Ambati S, Baile CA. Genistein inhibits differentiation of primary human adipocytes. J Nutr Biochem. 2009;20:140-148. DOI: 10.1016/j.jnutbio.2008.01.006

[48] Carr MC. The emergence of the metabolic syndrome with menopause. J Clin Endocrinol Metab. 2003;88:2404-2411. DOI: 10.1210/jc.2003-030242

[49] Lundholm L, Zang H, Hirschberg AL, Gustafsson JA, Arner P, Dahlman-Wright K. Key lipogenic gene expression can be decreased by estrogen in human adipose tissue. Fertil Steril. 2008;90:44-48. DOI: 10.1016/j.fertnstert.2007.06.011

[50] Lee HK, Lee JK, Cho B. The role of androgen in the adipose tissue of males. World J Mens Health. 2013;31:136-140. DOI: 10.5534/wjmh.2013.31.2.136

[51] Lapauw B, Kaufman JM. MANAGEMENT OF ENDOCRINE DISEASE: Rationale and current evidence for testosterone therapy in the management of obesity and its complications. Eur J Endocrinol. 2020;183:R167-R183. DOI: 10.1530/EJE-20-0394

[52] Eriksson J, Haring R, Grarup N, Vandenput L, Wallaschofski H, Lorentzen E, Hansen T, Mellström D, Pedersen O, Nauck M, Lorentzon M, Nystrup Husemoen LL, Völzke H, Karlsson M, Baumeister SE, Linneberg A, Ohlsson C. Causal relationship between obesity and serum testosterone status in men: A bi-directional mendelian randomization analysis. PLoS One. 2017;12:e0176277. DOI: 10.1371/journal.pone.0176277

[53] Cohen PG. Obesity in men: the hypogonadal-estrogen receptor relationship and its effect on glucose homeostasis. Med Hypotheses. 2008;70:358-360. DOI: 10.1016/j.mehy.2007.05.020

[54] Liu Y, Ding Z. Obesity, a serious etiologic factor for male subfertility in modern society. Reproduction. 2017;154:R123-R131. DOI: 10.1530/REP-17-0161

[55] Baldelli R, Dieguez C, Casanueva FF. The role of leptin in reproduction: experimental and clinical aspects. Ann Med. 2002;34:5-18. DOI: 10.1080/078538902317338599.

[56] Unuane D, Tournaye H, Velkeniers B, Poppe K. Endocrine disorders & female infertility. Best Pract Res Clin Endocrinol Metab. 2011;25:861-873. DOI: 10.1016/j.beem.2011.08.001

[57] Bhasin S, Brito JP, Cunningham GR, Hayes FJ, Hodis HN, Matsumoto AM, Snyder PJ, Swerdloff RS, Wu FC, Yialamas MA. Testosterone Therapy in Men With Hypogonadism: An Endocrine Society Clinical Practice

Guideline. J Clin Endocrinol Metab. 2018;103:1715-1744. DOI: 10.1210/jc.2018-00229

[58] Calderón B, Gómez-Martín JM, Vega-Piñero B, Martín-Hidalgo A, Galindo J, Luque-Ramírez M, Escobar-Morreale HF, Botella-Carretero JI. Prevalence of male secondary hypogonadism in moderate to severe obesity and its relationship with insulin resistance and excess body weight. Andrology. 2016;4:62-67. DOI: 10.1111/andr.12135

[59] Trost LW, Mulhall JP. Challenges in Testosterone Measurement, Data Interpretation, and Methodological Appraisal of Interventional Trials. J Sex Med. 2016;13:1029-1046. DOI: 10.1016/j.jsxm.2016.04.068

[60] Wang C, Catlin DH, Demers LM, Starcevic B, Swerdloff RS. Measurement of total serum testosterone in adult men: comparison of current laboratory methods versus liquid chromatography-tandem mass spectrometry. J Clin Endocrinol Metab. 2004;89:534-543. DOI: 10.1210/jc.2003-031287

[61] De Lorenzo A, Noce A, Moriconi E, Rampello T, Marrone G, Di Daniele N, Rovella V. MOSH Syndrome (Male Obesity Secondary Hypogonadism): Clinical Assessment and Possible Therapeutic Approaches. Nutrients. 2018;10:474. DOI: 10.3390/nu10040474

[62] Pellitero S, Olaizola I, Alastrue A, Martínez E, Granada ML, Balibrea JM, Moreno P, Serra A, Navarro-Díaz M, Romero R, Puig-Domingo M. Hypogonadotropic hypogonadism in morbidly obese males is reversed after bariatric surgery. Obes Surg. 2012;22:1835-1842. DOI: 10.1007/s11695-012-0734-9

[63] Pasquali R, Gambineri A, Pagotto U. The impact of obesity on reproduction in women with polycystic ovary syndrome. BJOG. 2006;113:1148-1159. DOI: 10.1111/j.1471-0528.2006.00990.x

[64] Fassnacht M, Schlenz N, Schneider SB, Wudy SA, Allolio B, Arlt W. Beyond adrenal and ovarian androgen generation: Increased peripheral 5 alpha-reductase activity in women with polycystic ovary syndrome. J Clin Endocrinol Metab. 2003;88:2760-2766. DOI: 10.1210/jc.2002-021875

[65] Childs GV, Odle AK, MacNicol MC, MacNicol AM. The Importance of Leptin to Reproduction. Endocrinology. 2021;162:bqaa204. DOI: 10.1210/endocr/bqaa204

[66] González F. Inflammation in Polycystic Ovary Syndrome: underpinning of insulin resistance and ovarian dysfunction. Steroids. 2012;77:300-305. DOI: 10.1016/j.steroids.2011.12.003

[67] Best D, Avenell A, Bhattacharya S. How effective are weight-loss interventions for improving fertility in women and men who are overweight or obese? A systematic review and meta-analysis of the evidence. Hum Reprod Update. 2017;23:681-705. doi: 10.1093/humupd/dmx027

[68] Broughton DE, Moley KH. Obesity and female infertility: potential mediators of obesity's impact. Fertil Steril. 2017;107:840-847. DOI: 10.1016/j.fertnstert.2017.01.017

[69] Moran LJ, Tassone EC, Boyle J, Brennan L, Harrison CL, Hirschberg AL, Lim S, Marsh K, Misso ML, Redman L, Thondan M, Wijeyaratne C, Garad R, Stepto NK, Teede HJ. Evidence summaries and recommendations from the international evidence-based guideline for the assessment and management of polycystic ovary syndrome: Lifestyle management. Obes Rev. 2020;21:e13046. DOI: 10.1111/obr.13046

[70] Escobar-Morreale HF, Santacruz E, Luque-Ramírez M, Botella Carretero JI. Prevalence of 'obesity-associated gonadal dysfunction' in severely obese men and women and its resolution after bariatric surgery: a systematic review and meta-analysis. Hum Reprod Update. 2017;23:390-408. DOI: 10.1093/humupd/dmx012

[71] Fanelli F, Gambineri A, Mezzullo M, Vicennati V, Pelusi C, Pasquali R, Pagotto U. Revisiting hyper- and hypo-androgenism by tandem mass spectrometry. Rev Endocr Metab Disord. 2013;14:185-205. DOI: 10.1007/s11154-013-9243-y

Chapter 3

Top 100 Most Cited Studies in Obesity Research: A Bibliometric Analysis

Tauseef Ahmad

Abstract

Obesity represents a major global public health problem. In the past few decades the prevalence of obesity has increased worldwide. In 2016, an estimated 1.9 billion adults were overweight; of these more than 650 million were obese. There is an urgent need for potential solutions and deeper understanding of the risk factors responsible for obesity. A bibliometric analysis study was designed to provide a comprehensive overview of top 100 most cited studies on obesity indexed in Web of Science database. The online search was conducted on June 6, 2021 using the keywords "Obesity" OR "Obese" OR "Overweight" in title filed with no limitations on document types or languages. The top 100 cited studies were selected in descending order based on number of citations. The obtained data were imported in to Microsoft Excel 2019 to extract the basic information such as title, authors name, journal name, year of publication and total citations. In addition, the data were also imported in to HistCite™ for further citation analysis, and VOSviewer software for windows to plot the data for network visualization mapping. The initial search retrieved a total of 167,553 documents on obesity. Of the total retrieved documents, only top 100 most cited studies on obesity were included for further analysis. These studies were published from 1982 to 2017 in English language. Most of the studies were published as an article (n = 84). The highly cited study on obesity was "Establishing a standard definition for child overweight and obesity worldwide: international survey" published in BMJ-British Medical Journal (Impact Factor 39.890, Incites Journal Citation Reports, 2021) in 2000 cited 10,543 times. The average number of citations per study was 2,947.22 (ranging from 1,566 to 10,543 citations). Two studies had more than 10,000 citations. A total of 2,272 authors from 111 countries were involved. The most prolific author was Flegal KM authored 14 studies with 53,558 citations. The highly active country in obesity research was United States of America. The included studies were published in 33 journals. The most attractive journal was JAMA-Journal of the American Medical Association (Impact Factor 56.272) published 17 studies and cited globally 51,853 times. The most frequently used keywords were obesity (n = 87) and overweight (n = 22). The countries with highest total link strength was United States of America (n = 155), followed by England (n = 140), and Scotland (n = 130). Our results show that most number of highly cited studies were published in developed countries. The findings of this study can serve as a standard benchmark for researchers to provide the quality bibliographic references and insights into the future research trends and scientific cooperation in obesity research.

Keywords: Obesity, Overweight, bibliometric analysis

1. Introduction

Obesity represents a major public health challenge, in the past few decades the prevalence of obesity has increased worldwide and associated with serious adverse health outcomes [1, 2]. According to the statistics of World Health Organization, in 2016, an estimated 1.9 billion adults (18 years and older) were overweight, of these more than 650 million were obese. In 2019, 38 million children (under age of 5 years) were overweight or obese [3].

Obesity associated comorbidities including certain cancer, depression, fatty liver disease, hepatic steatosis, hyperlipidemia, hypertension, obstructive sleep apnea, orthopedic conditions, type 2 diabetes mellitus and social isolation [1, 4, 5]. There is an urgent need for potential solutions and deeper understanding of the risk factors responsible for obesity.

Bibliometric type studies are of great interest, conducted not only to present an overall overview of the published scientific literature but also critical and subjective summarization of the most influential scientific studies [6–8].

2. Aim

This study aimed to provide a comprehensive overview of top 100 most cited studies on obesity. The finding can serve as a standard benchmark for researchers and to provide the quality bibliographic references.

3. Methods

3.1 Study design

Bibliometric citation analysis study.

3.2 Searching strategy and database

On June 6, 2021 the online search was conducted on Web of Science, Core Collection database (Philadelphia, Pennsylvania, United State of America). The search keywords used were "Obesity" OR "Obese" OR "Overweight" in title filed with no limitations on documents types or languages. The top 100 cited studies were selected in descending order based on number of citations.

3.3 Data extraction

The obtained studies were imported in to Microsoft Excel 2019 to extract the basic information such as title, authors name, journal name, year of publication and total citations. In addition, the downloaded dataset were imported in to HistCite™ for further citation analysis.

3.4 Visualization network

Visualization network co-authorship countries and co-occurrence all keywords were plotted by using VOSviewer software version 1.6.15 (https://www.vosviewer.com/) for windows.

4. Ethical approval

This study did not involve any human or animal subjects, thus, ethical approval was not required.

5. Results

The initial search retrieved a total of 167,553 documents on obesity indexed in Web of Science database. Of the total retrieved documents, only top 100 most studies on obesity were included in this study. The included studies were published in English language. Most of the studies were published as an article (n = 84) followed by review (n = 14) and letter (n = 1). The average number of citations per study was 2,947.22, ranging from 1,566 to 10,543 citations.

The most cited study on obesity was "Establishing a standard definition for child overweight and obesity worldwide: international survey" published in BMJ-British Medical Journal in 2000 cited 10,543 times. Another study "Positional cloning of the mouse obese gene and its human homolog" published in Nature in 1994 was cited 10,214 times. A total of 10 studies were cited more than 5,000 times. Furthermore, 52 studies were cited at least 2,000 times, while the remaining studies were cited more than 1,500 times. The top 100 studies on obesity is presented in **Table 1**.

5.1 Most prolific authors

A total of 2,272 authors contributed to top 100 most cited studies. The most prolific author was Flegal KM authored 14 studies with 53,558 citations, followed by followed by Carroll MD (n = 10, citations = 36,950), and Ogden CL (n = 9, citations = 34,784). Only nine authors authored at least five studies as shown in **Table 2**. In addition, only 22 authors contributed in at least three studies.

5.2 Most active countries

A total 111 countries were involved in top 100 most cited studies on obesity. The most active country was United States of America (studies contributed: 75, citations: 217,788), followed by United Kingdom (studies contributed: 18, citations: 57,015), Canada (studies contributed: 9, citations: 17,920), Japan (studies contributed: 9, citations: 26,695), France (studies contributed: 8, citations: 21,228), Sweden (studies contributed: 8, citations: 20,632), and Netherlands (studies contributed: 7, citations: 13,018) as shown in **Table 3**. Only 21 countries were involved at least in four studies.

5.3 Journals

The top 100 most cited studies were published in 33 journals. The most attractive journal was JAMA-Journal of the American Medical Association published 17 studies and cited globally 51,853 times as shown in **Table 4**. Only seven journals published at least 4 studies, six journals published two studies each, while the remaining journals published a single study each.

5.4 Commonly used keywords

A total of 366 keywords were used in the top 100 most cited studies. The most widely used keywords were obesity (n = 87) and overweight (n = 22) as shown in **Table 5**.

Rank	Study reference	LCS	LCS/t	GCS	GCS/t
1	Cole et al. [9]	5	0.28	10543	585.72
2	Zhang et al. [10]	14	0.58	10218	425.75
3	Alberti et al. [11]	0	0.00	7170	796.67
4	Ogden et al. [12]	7	0.58	6501	541.75
5	Weisberg et al. [13]	9	0.60	6360	424.00
6	Turnbaugh et al. [14]	9	0.75	6237	519.75
7	Ng et al. [15]	2	0.50	6092	1523.00
8	Turner et al. [16]	1	0.05	5585	279.25
9	Ogden et al. [17]	2	0.50	5530	1382.50
10	Hotamisligil et al. [18]	12	0.48	5305	212.20
11	Calle et al. [19]	2	0.13	4927	328.47
12	Considine et al. [20]	1	0.05	4888	222.18
13	Ley et al. [21]	4	0.33	4624	385.33
14	Flegal et al. [22]	9	0.56	4575	285.94
15	Flegal et al. [23]	5	0.63	4510	563.75
16	Xu et al. [24]	5	0.33	4501	300.07
17	Turnbaugh et al. [25]	2	0.22	4499	499.89
18	Pi-Sunyer et al. [26]	0	0.00	4046	202.30
19	Halaas et al. [27]	8	0.35	3846	167.22
20	DeFronzo et al. [28]	0	0.00	3653	135.30
21	Flegal et al. [29]	3	0.50	3653	608.83
22	Pelleymounter et al. [30]	7	0.30	3611	157.00
23	Yamauchi et al. [31]	3	0.18	3603	211.94
24	Arita et al. [32]	4	0.21	3588	188.84
25	Ley et al. [33]	7	0.54	3439	264.54
26	Steppan et al. [34]	4	0.24	3335	196.18
27	Furukawa et al. [35]	1	0.07	3314	236.71
28	Cani et al. [36]	3	0.27	3183	289.36
29	Must et al. [37]	3	0.16	3081	162.16
30	Hedley et al. [38]	8	0.57	3077	219.79
31	Kopelman [39]	3	0.17	3001	166.72
32	Maffei et al. [40]	3	0.13	2989	129.96
33	Black et al. [41]	1	0.20	2937	587.40
34	Sjostrom et al. [42]	0	0.00	2910	264.55
35	Hubert et al. [43]	6	0.17	2908	83.09
36	Frayling et al. [44]	0	0.00	2908	264.36
37	Haslam and James [45]	1	0.08	2900	223.08
38	Mokdad et al. [46]	2	0.13	2816	187.73
39	Whitaker et al. [47]	2	0.10	2766	131.71
40	Barlow [48]	0	0.00	2764	251.27
41	Lumeng et al. [49]	0	0.00	2762	251.09

Rank	Study reference	LCS	LCS/t	GCS	GCS/t
42	Kahn et al. [50]	1	0.08	2747	228.92
43	Ogden et al. [51]	1	0.17	2704	450.67
44	Weyer et al. [52]	0	0.00	2694	158.47
45	Christakis and Fowler [53]	1	0.09	2687	244.27
46	Ogden et al. [54]	5	0.31	2660	166.25
47	Ozcan et al. [55]	1	0.07	2602	185.86
48	Despres and Lemieux [56]	0	0.00	2581	215.08
49	Hotamisligil et al. [57]	7	0.30	2580	112.17
50	Cani et al. [58]	2	0.20	2516	251.60
51	Hirosumi et al. [59]	2	0.13	2304	144.00
52	Huszar et al. [60]	1	0.05	2295	109.29
53	Calle and Kaaks [61]	0	0.00	2286	163.29
54	Swinburn et al. [62]	4	0.57	2196	313.71
55	Weiss et al. [63]	0	0.00	2178	155.57
56	Flegal et al. [64]	7	0.35	2166	108.30
57	Kuczmarski et al. [65]	11	0.46	2137	89.04
58	Montague et al. [66]	5	0.24	2081	99.10
59	Ezzati et al. [67]	0	0.00	2073	2073.00
60	Kahn and Flier [68]	3	0.17	2068	114.89
61	Gregor and Hotamisligil [69]	0	0.00	2026	289.43
62	Flegal et al. [70]	2	0.40	2021	404.20
63	Locke et al. [71]	0	0.00	1967	655.67
64	Luppino et al. [72]	0	0.00	1951	243.88
65	Wortsman et al. [73]	0	0.00	1934	107.44
66	Hotamisligil et al. [74]	5	0.23	1933	87.86
67	Flegal et al. [75]	2	0.15	1907	146.69
68	Yudkin et al. [76]	2	0.11	1873	98.58
69	Mokdad et al. [77]	2	0.12	1861	109.47
70	Popkin et al. [78]	1	0.17	1856	309.33
71	Yusuf et al. [79]	1	0.08	1841	141.62
72	Guh et al. [80]	0	0.00	1836	204.00
73	Everard et al. [81]	0	0.00	1836	367.20
74	Wang and Lobstein [82]	1	0.08	1832	152.67
75	Ebbeling et al. [83]	0	0.00	1823	113.94
76	Wang and Beydoun [84]	1	0.09	1821	165.55
77	Ridaura et al. [85]	0	0.00	1799	359.80
78	Kenchaiah et al. [86]	4	0.25	1725	107.81
79	Afshin et al. [87]	0	0.00	1703	1703.00
80	Elchebly et al. [88]	0	0.00	1702	89.58
81	Dietz [89]	1	0.05	1701	85.05
82	Poirier et al. [90]	1	0.08	1687	140.58

Rank	Study reference	LCS	LCS/t	GCS	GCS/t
83	Van Gaal et al. [91]	0	0.00	1682	140.17
84	Newgard et al. [92]	1	0.11	1682	186.89
85	Turnbaugh et al. [93]	2	0.20	1674	167.40
86	Spiegelman and Flier [94]	2	0.12	1663	97.82
87	Kanda et al. [95]	3	0.25	1661	138.42
88	Uysal et al. [96]	7	0.33	1660	79.05
89	Hu et al. [97]	3	0.14	1659	75.41
90	Finkelstein et al. [98]	1	0.11	1645	182.78
91	Mozaffarian [99]	0	0.00	1640	820.00
92	Larsson et al. [100]	1	0.03	1633	48.03
93	Mokdad et al. [101]	2	0.11	1631	85.84
94	Visser et al. [102]	1	0.05	1615	85.00
95	Kissebah et al. [103]	1	0.03	1612	44.78
96	Wang et al. [104]	3	0.43	1610	230.00
97	Clement et al. [105]	1	0.05	1588	79.40
98	Puhl and Heuer [106]	0	0.00	1582	175.78
99	Flegal et al. [107]	0	0.00	1574	787.00
100	Turek et al. [108]	0	0.00	1566	120.46

Note: LCS: Local citation score; LCS/t: Local citation score per year; GCS: Global citation score; GCS/t: Global citation score per year.

Table 1.
Top 100 most cited studies on obesity.

S. No.	Author	Studies	LCS	LCS/t	GCS	GCS/t
1	Flegal KM	14	67	5.461386	53558	6340.429
2	Carroll MD	10	47	4.171429	36950	5114.773
3	Ogden CL	9	40	3.821429	34784	5006.473
4	Hotamisligil GS	7	34	1.541382	18410	1110.571
5	Dietz WH	6	15	0.819507	22538	1238.22
6	Gordon JI	6	24	2.044017	22272	2196.711
7	Johnson CL	5	40	2.254762	14615	869.3149
8	Mokdad AH	5	8	0.856244	14103	3609.046
9	Spiegelman BM	5	29	1.265631	13140	585.4702
10	Kengne AP	4	2	0.5	11941	7372
11	Khang YH	4	2	0.5	11941	7372
12	Kit BK	4	8	1.566667	13908	2846.2
13	Ley RE	4	22	1.844017	18799	1669.511
14	Turnbaugh PJ	4	17	1.505556	17034	1572.372

Note: LCS: Local citation score; LCS/t: Local citation score per year; GCS: Global citation score; GCS/t: Global citation score per year.

Table 2.
Authors with at least 4 studies.

S. No.	Country	Number of studies	LCS	GCS
1	United States of America	75	207	217788
2	United Kingdom	18	32	57015
3	Canada	9	7	17920
4	Japan	9	13	26695
5	France	8	11	21228
6	Sweden	8	12	20632
7	Netherlands	7	3	13018
8	Belgium	6	5	12993
9	Finland	6	2	16579
10	Australia	5	6	14031
11	Italy	5	2	15488
12	Pakistan	5	3	14772
13	Switzerland	5	3	11196
14	Brazil	4	3	12805
15	Estonia	4	2	11835
16	Germany	4	2	11835
17	Norway	4	2	11835
18	Peoples Republic of China	4	2	11835
19	Saudi Arabia	4	2	11835
20	South Korea	4	2	11835

Note: LCS: Local citation score; GCS: Global citation score.

Table 3.
Country with at least 3 studies.

Journal name	Number of studies	LCS	LCS/t	GCS	GCS/t
JAMA-Journal of the American Medical Association (IF: 56.272, Q1)	17	65	5.400378	51853	6276.611
Nature (IF: 49.962, Q1)	14	52	3.120612	48524	3834.997
Lancet (IF: 79.321, Q1)	9	13	1.903846	27057	5484.994
Science (IF: 47.728, Q1)	9	33	1.430875	25272	1644.342
New England Journal of Medicine (IF: 91.245, Q1)	8	10	0.614935	23784	3157.565
Journal of Clinical Investigation (IF: 14.808, Q1)	7	28	1.725776	23246	1577.351
Circulation (IF: 29.690, Q1)	4	7	0.254762	13405	1840.336

Note: IF: Impact Factor, Incites Journal Citation Reports, 2021; Q: Quartile; LCS: Local citation score; LCS/t: Local citation score per year; GCS: Global citation score; GCS/t: Global citation score per year.

Table 4.
Journals published at least 4 studies.

5.5 Year of publication

The top 100 most cited on obesity were published from 1982 to 2017 as shown in **Figure 1**. The highest number of studies were published in 2006 (n = 9, citations = 29,552) and 2007 (n = 7, citations = 19,035) as presented in **Figures 1** and **2**.

S. No.	Word	Occurrence	LCS	GCS
1	Obesity	87	205	245145
2	Overweight	22	58	73740
3	Insulin	17	55	45751
4	Resistance	16	54	43149
5	Prevalence	12	62	46421
6	Adults	11	41	38279
7	Diabetes	10	13	32966
8	Trends	10	34	27357

Note: LCS: Local citation score; GCS: Global citation score.

Table 5.
The keywords used at least ten times.

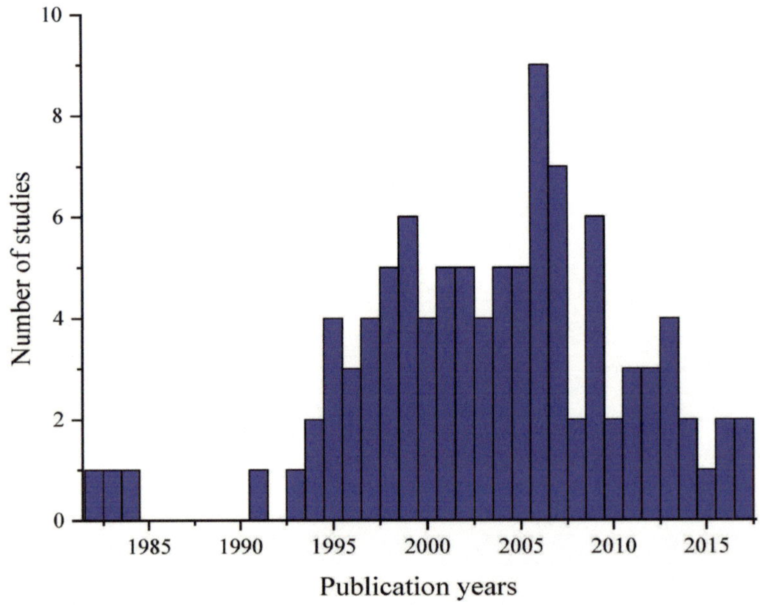

Figure 1.
Publication years of top 100 most cited studies in obesity research.

5.6 Co-authorship countries network visualization

The minimum number of studies for a country was fixed at 3. Of the total countries, only 38 countries were plotted based on total link strength (TLS) as shown in **Figure 3**. The countries with highest TLS were United States of America (155), England (140), and Scotland (130).

5.7 Co-occurrence all keywords network visualization

Of the total keywords, only 69 were plotted as shown in **Figure 4**. The keyword body-mass index has the highest TLS 117, followed by overweight (65), adipose-tissue (56), prevalence (53), weight (52), and obesity (49).

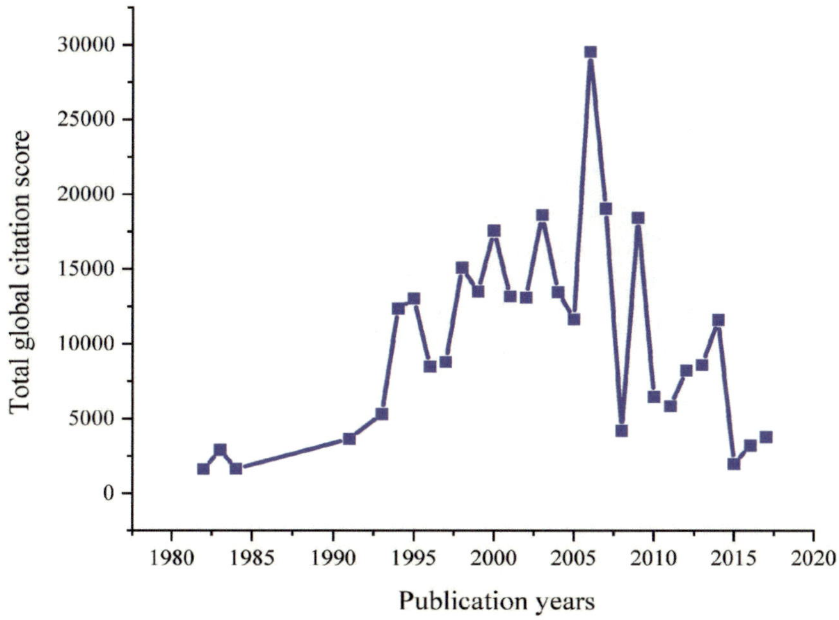

Figure 2.
Total global citation score per year of top 100 most cited studies in obesity research.

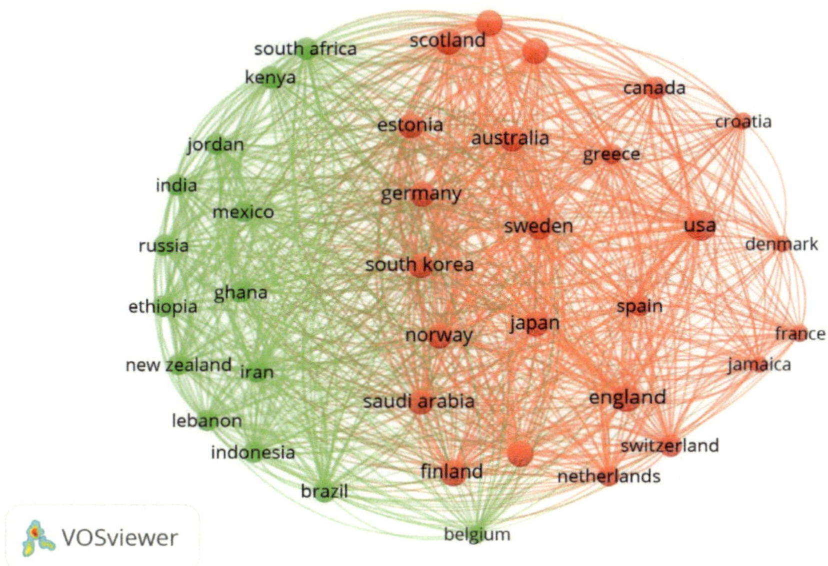

Figure 3.
Co-authorship countries network visualization. Two clusters are formed; red color represents cluster 1 (24 items), and green color represents cluster 2 (14 items).

6. Discussion

In recent years, bibliometric type studies have been increased significantly, these studies not only recognize the most influential studies in certain area but also determine the research shift and other important insights into the bibliometric parameters.

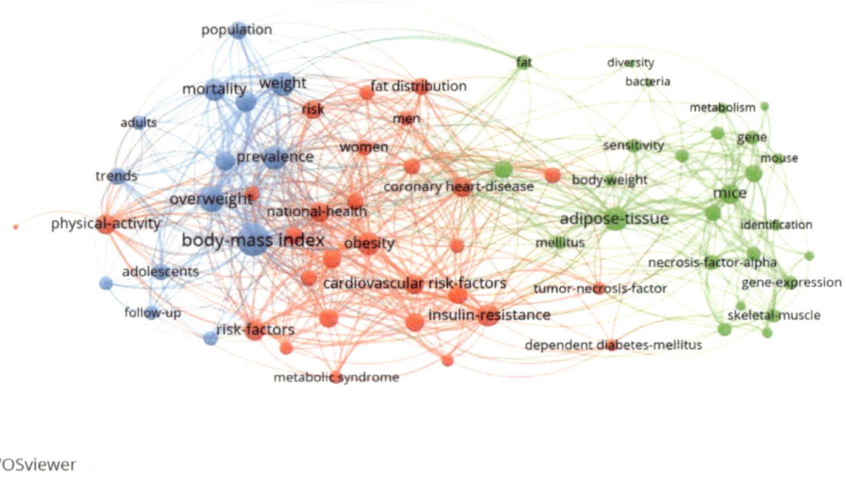

Figure 4.
Co-occurrence all keywords network visualization. Three clusters are formed; red color represents cluster 1 (29 items), green color represents cluster 2 (26 items), and blue color represents cluster 3 (14 items).

Globally, obesity is a major public health problem and the prevalence has increased in the past few decades. Therefore, this study was undertaken to recognize the most influential studies in obesity research and provide essential bibliographic information. To the best of our knowledge this is the first bibliometric analysis on top 100 most cited studies on obesity indexed in Web of Science database. The highly cited study in obesity research received a total of 10,543 citations. The study published in a highly rated journal in medicine had an impact factor of 39.890 and placed in quartile 1 (Q1) category. The study entitled "Establishing a standard definition for child overweight and obesity worldwide: international survey" provides cut off points for body mass index in childhood of six large nationally representative cross sectional growth studies [9].

Another study received a total of 10,218 citations. The study titled "Positional cloning of the mouse obese gene and its human homologue" discusses the potential role of obese gene and these genes may function as part of a signaling pathway from adipose tissue that acts to regulate the size of the body fat depot [10].

The top 100 most cited were published in 33 journals. The most attractive and core journals in obesity research were JAMA-Journal of the American Medical Association (n = 17), and Nature (n = 14) had an impact factor of 56.272, and 49.962 respectively. A total of 31 studies were published in these two journals with a total citations of 100,377, thus representing the quality of work and aiming of the authors for high impact factor journals. Influential studies on obesity were published in higher impact factor journals. Furthermore, studies published in higher impact factor journals are more likely to be cited by the scientific community. The impact factor shows importance and quality of a journal [109]. The top three authors based on number of studies in obesity research were Flegal KM (n = 14, citations = 53,558), followed by Carroll MD (n = 10, citations = 36,950), and Ogden CL (n = 9, citations = 34,784). In our study, the leading country was United States of America contributed in a total of 75 studies with a total citations of 217,788. The finding is in line with studies in other research areas [110–113].

7. Conclusion

This study provides a comprehensive information of the most cited studies in obesity research. Majority of the most cited studies were published by developed countries in higher impact factor journals. The current study might be helpful to researchers for insights into the future research trends and scientific cooperation.

Author details

Tauseef Ahmad
Department of Epidemiology and Health Statistics, School of Public Health, Southeast University, Nanjing, China

*Address all correspondence to: hamdard_hu@yahoo.com; tahmad@seu.edu.cn

References

[1] Blüher M. Obesity: global epidemiology and pathogenesis. Nat Rev Endocrinol. 2019 May;15(5):288-298. doi: 10.1038/s41574-019-0176-8. PMID: 30814686.

[2] Hajri T, Angamarca-Armijos V, Caceres L. Prevalence of stunting and obesity in Ecuador: a systematic review. Public Health Nutr. 2021 Jun;24(8):2259-2272. doi: 10.1017/S1368980020002049. Epub 2020 Jul 29. PMID: 32723419.

[3] World Health Organization. Obesity and overweight. World Health Organization, 2020. Available from: https://www.who.int/news-room/fact-sheets/detail/obesity-and-overweight (accessed on: June 6, 2021).

[4] Güngör NK. Overweight and obesity in children and adolescents. J Clin Res Pediatr Endocrinol. 2014 Sep;6(3):129-43. doi: 10.4274/Jcrpe.1471. PMID: 25241606; PMCID: PMC4293641.

[5] Albrecht NM, Iyengar BS. Pediatric Obesity: An Economic Perspective. Front Public Health. 2021 Jan 8;8:619647. doi: 10.3389/fpubh.2020.619647. PMID: 33490029; PMCID: PMC7820704.

[6] Corsini F, Certomà C, Dyer M, Frey M. Participatory energy: Research, imaginaries and practices on people' contribute to energy systems in the smart city. Technol Forecast Soc Change. 2018;142:322-332. https://doi.org/10.1016/j.techfore.2018.07.028.

[7] Fabregat-Aibar L, Barberà-Mariné MG, Terceño A, Pié L. A bibliometric and visualization analysis of socially responsible funds. Sustainability. 2019;11(9):2526. doi: 10.3390/su11092526.

[8] Ahmad T, Murad MA, Baig M, Hui J. Research trends in COVI-19 vaccie: a bibliometric analysis. Hum Vaccin Immunother. 2021. doi: 10.1080/21645515.2021.1886806. Epub ahead of print.

[9] Cole TJ, Bellizzi MC, Flegal KM, Dietz WH. Establishing a standard definition for child overweight and obesity worldwide: international survey. BMJ-British Medical Journal. 2000b; 320 (7244): 1240-1243.

[10] Zhang YY, Proenca R, Maffei M, Barone M, Leopold L, et al. Positional cloning of the mouse obese gene and its human homolog. Nature. 1994b; 372 (6505): 425-432.

[11] Alberti KGMM, Eckel RH, Grundy SM, Zimmet PZ, Cleeman JI, et al. Harmonizing the Metabolic Syndrome A Joint Interim Statement of the International Diabetes Federation Task Force on Epidemiology and Prevention; National Heart, Lung, and Blood Institute; American Heart Association; World Heart Federation; International Atherosclerosis Society; and International Association for the Study of Obesity. Circulation. 2009; 120 (16): 1640-1645.

[12] Ogden CL, Carroll MD, Curtin LR, McDowell MA, Tabak CJ, et al. Prevalence of overweight and obesity in the United States, 1999-2004. JAMA-Journal of the American Medical Association. 2006; 295 (13): 1549-1555.

[13] Weisberg SP, McCann D, Desai M, Rosenbaum M, Leibel RL, et al. Obesity is associated with macrophage accumulation in adipose tissue. Journal of Clinical Investigation. 2003; 112 (12): 1796-1808.

[14] Turnbaugh PJ, Ley RE, Mahowald MA, Magrini V, Mardis ER, et al. An obesity-associated gut microbiome with increased capacity for energy harvest. Nature. 2006; 444 (7122): 1027-1031.

[15] Ng M, Fleming T, Robinson M, Thomson B, Graetz N, et al. Global, regional, and national prevalence of overweight and obesity in children and adults during 1980-2013: a systematic analysis for the Global Burden of Disease Study 2013. Lancet. 2014; 384 (9945): 766-781.

[16] Turner RC, Holman RR, Stratton IM, Cull CA, Matthews DR, et al. Effect of intensive blood-glucose control with metformin on complications in overweight patients with type 2 diabetes (UKPDS 34). Lancet. 1998; 352 (9131): 854-865.

[17] Ogden CL, Carroll MD, Kit BK, Flegal KM. Prevalence of Childhood and Adult Obesity in the United States, 2011-2012. JAMA-Journal of the American Medical Association. 2014; 311 (8): 806-814.

[18] Hotamisligil GS, Shargill NS, Spiegelman BM. Adipose expression of tumor-necrosis-factor-alpha - direct role in obesity-linked insulin resistance. Science. 1993; 259 (5091): 87-91.

[19] Calle EE, Rodriguez C, Walker-Thurmond K, Thun MJ. Overweight, obesity, and mortality from cancer in a prospectively studied cohort of US adults. New England Journal of Medicine. 2003; 348 (17): 1625-1638.

[20] Considine RV, Sinha MK, Heiman ML, Kriauciunas A, Stephens TW, et al. Serum immunoreactive leptin concentrations in normal-weight and obese humans. New England Journal of Medicine. 1996; 334 (5): 292-295.

[21] Ley RE, Turnbaugh PJ, Klein S, Gordon JI. Microbial ecology - Human gut microbes associated with obesity. Nature. 2006; 444 (7122): 1022-1023.

[22] Flegal KM, Carroll MD, Ogden CL, Johnson CL. Prevalence and trends in obesity among US adults, 1999-2000. JAMA-Journal of the American Medical Association. 2002; 288 (14): 1723-1727.

[23] Flegal KM, Carroll MD, Ogden CL, Curtin LR. Prevalence and Trends in Obesity Among US Adults, 1999-2008. JAMA-Journal of the American Medical Association. 2010; 303 (3): 235-241.

[24] Xu HY, Barnes GT, Yang Q, Tan Q, Yang DS, et al. Chronic inflammation in fat plays a crucial role in the development of obesity-related insulin resistance. Journal of Clinical Investigation. 2003; 112 (12): 1821-1830.

[25] Turnbaugh PJ, Hamady M, Yatsunenko T, Cantarel BL, Duncan A, et al. A core gut microbiome in obese and lean twins. Nature. 2009; 457 (7228): 480-485.

[26] Pi-Sunyer FX. NHLBI Obesity Education Initiative Expert Panel on the identification, evaluation, and treatment of overweight and obesity in adults - The evidence report. Obesity Research. 1998; 6: 51S-209S.

[27] Halaas JL, Gajiwala KS, Maffei M, Cohen SL, Chait BT, et al. Weight-reducing effects of the plasma-protein encoded by the obese gene. Science. 1995; 269 (5223): 543-546.

[28] DeFronzo RA, Ferrannini E. Insulin resistance. A multifaceted syndrome responsible for NIDDM, obesity, hypertension, dyslipidemia, and atherosclerotic cardiovascular disease. Diabetes Care. 1991;14(3):173-194.

[29] Flegal KM, Carroll MD, Kit BK, Ogden CL. Prevalence of Obesity and Trends in the Distribution of Body Mass Index Among US Adults, 1999-2010. JAMA-Journal of the American Medical Association. 2012; 307 (5): 491-497.

[30] Pelleymounter MA, Cullen MJ, Baker MB, Hecht R, Winters D, et al. Effects of the obese gene-product on

body-weight regulation in OB/OB mice. Science. 1995; 269 (5223): 540-543.

[31] Yamauchi T, Kamon J, Waki H, Terauchi Y, Kubota N, et al. The fat-derived hormone adiponectin reverses insulin resistance associated with both lipoatrophy and obesity. Nature Medicine. 2001; 7 (8): 941-946.

[32] Arita Y, Kihara S, Ouchi N, Takahashi M, Maeda K, et al. Paradoxical decrease of an adipose-specific protein, adiponectin, in obesity. Biochemical and Biophysical Research Communications. 1999; 257 (1): 79-83.

[33] Ley RE, Backhed F, Turnbaugh P, Lozupone CA, Knight RD, et al. Obesity alters gut microbial ecology. Proceedings of the National Academy of Sciences of the United States of America. 2005; 102 (31): 11070-11075.

[34] Steppan CM, Bailey ST, Bhat S, Brown EJ, Banerjee RR, et al. The hormone resistin links obesity to diabetes. Nature. 2001; 409 (6818): 307-312.

[35] Furukawa S, Fujita T, Shimabukuro M, Iwaki M, Yamada Y, et al. Increased oxidative stress in obesity and its impact on metabolic syndrome. Journal of Clinical Investigation. 2004; 114 (12): 1752-1761.

[36] Cani PD, Amar J, Iglesias MA, Poggi M, Knauf C, et al. Metabolic endotoxemia initiates obesity and insulin resistance. Diabetes. 2007; 56 (7): 1761-1772.

[37] Must A, Spadano J, Coakley EH, Field AE, Colditz G, et al. The disease burden associated with overweight and obesity. JAMA-Journal of the American Medical Association. 1999; 282 (16): 1523-1529.

[38] Hedley AA, Ogden CL, Johnson CL, Carroll MD, Curtin LR, et al. Prevalence of overweight and obesity among US children, adolescents, and adults, 1999-2002. JAMA-Journal of the American Medical Association. 2004; 291 (23): 2847-2850.

[39] Kopelman PG. Obesity as a medical problem. Nature. 2000; 404 (6778): 635-643.

[40] Maffei M, Halaas J, Ravussin E, Pratley RE, Lee GH, et al. Leptin levels in human and rodent - measurement of plasma leptin and OB RNA in obese and weight-reduced subjects. Nature Medicine. 1995; 1 (11): 1155-1161.

[41] Black RE, Victora CG, Walker SP, Bhutta ZA, Christian P, et al. Maternal and child undernutrition and overweight in low-income and middle-income countries. Lancet. 2013; 382 (9890): 427-451.

[42] Sjostrom L, Narbro K, Sjostrom D, Karason K, Larsson B, et al. Effects of bariatric surgery on mortality in Swedish obese subjects. New England Journal of Medicine. 2007; 357 (8): 741-752.

[43] Hubert HB, Feinleib M, Mcnamara PM, Castelli WP. Obesity as an independent risk factor for cardiovascular-disease - a 26-year follow-up of participants in the Framingham heart-study. Circulation. 1983; 67 (5): 968-977.

[44] Frayling TM, Timpson NJ, Weedon MN, Zeggini E, Freathy RM, et al. A common variant in the FTO gene is associated with body mass index and predisposes to childhood and adult obesity. Science. 2007; 316 (5826): 889-894.

[45] Haslam DW, James WPT. Obesity. Lancet. 2005; 366 (9492): 1197-1209.

[46] Mokdad AH, Ford ES, Bowman BA, Dietz WH, Vinicor F, et al. Prevalence of obesity, diabetes, and obesity-related health risk factors, 2001. JAMA-Journal

of the American Medical Association. 2003; 289 (1): 76-79.

[47] Whitaker RC, Wright JA, Pepe MS, Seidel KD, Dietz WH. Predicting obesity in young adulthood from childhood and parental obesity. New England Journal of Medicine. 1997; 337 (13): 869-873.

[48] Barlow SE. Expert committee recommendations regarding the prevention, assessment, and treatment of child and adolescent overweight and obesity: Summary report. Pediatrics. 2007; 120: S164-S192.

[49] Lumeng CN, Bodzin JL, Saltiel AR. Obesity induces a phenotypic switch in adipose tissue macrophage polarization. Journal of Clinical Investigation. 2007; 117 (1): 175-184.

[50] Kahn SE, Hull RL, Utzschneider KM. Mechanisms linking obesity to insulin resistance and type 2 diabetes. Nature. 2006; 444 (7121): 840-846.

[51] Ogden CL, Carroll MD, Kit BK, Flegal KM. Prevalence of obesity and trends in Body Mass Index among US children and adolescents, 1999-2010. Jama-Journal of the American Medical Association. 2012; 307 (5): 483-490.

[52] Weyer C, Funahashi T, Tanaka S, Hotta K, Matsuzawa Y, et al. Hypoadiponectinemia in obesity and type 2 diabetes: Close association with insulin resistance and hyperinsulinemia. Journal of Clinical Endocrinology & Metabolism. 2001; 86 (5): 1930-1935.

[53] Christakis NA, Fowler JH. The spread of obesity in a large social network over 32 years. New England Journal of Medicine. 2007; 357 (4): 370-379.

[54] Ogden CL, Flegal KM, Carroll MD, Johnson CL. Prevalence and trends in overweight among US children and adolescents, 1999-2000. JAMA-Journal of the American Medical Association. 2002; 288 (14): 1728-1732.

[55] Ozcan U, Cao Q, Yilmaz E, Lee AH, Iwakoshi NN, et al. Endoplasmic reticulum stress links obesity, insulin action, and type 2 diabetes. Science. 2004; 306 (5695): 457-461.

[56] Despres JP, Lemieux I. Abdominal obesity and metabolic syndrome. Nature. 2006; 444 (7121): 881-887.

[57] Hotamisligil GS, Arner P, Caro JF, Atkinson RL, Spiegelman BM. Increased adipose-tissue expression of tumor-necrosis-factor-alpha in human obesity and insulin-resistance. Journal of Clinical Investigation. 1995; 95 (5): 2409-2415.

[58] Cani PD, Bibiloni R, Knauf C, Neyrinck AM, Neyrinck AM, et al. Changes in gut microbiota control metabolic endotoxemia-induced inflammation in high-fat diet-induced obesity and diabetes in mice. Diabetes. 2008; 57 (6): 1470-1481.

[59] Hirosumi J, Tuncman G, Chang LF, Gorgun CZ, Uysal KT, et al. A central role for JNK in obesity and insulin resistance. Nature. 2002; 420 (6913): 333-336.

[60] Huszar D, Lynch CA, FairchildHuntress V, Dunmore JH, Fang Q, et al. Targeted disruption of the melanocortin-4 receptor results in obesity in mice. Cell. 1997; 88 (1): 131-141

[61] Calle EE, Kaaks R. Overweight, obesity and cancer: Epidemiological evidence and proposed mechanisms. Nature Reviews Cancer. 2004; 4 (8): 579-591.

[62] Swinburn BA, Sacks G, Hall KD, McPherson K, Finegood DT, et al. Obesity 1 The global obesity pandemic: shaped by global drivers and local

environments. Lancet. 2011; 378 (9793): 804-814.

[63] Weiss R, Dziura J, Burgert TS, Tamborlane WV, Taksali SE, et al. Obesity and the metabolic syndrome in children and adolescents. New England Journal of Medicine. 2004; 350 (23): 2362-2374.

[64] Flegal KM, Carroll MD, Kuczmarski RJ, Johnson CL. Overweight and obesity in the United States: prevalence and trends, 1960-1994. International Journal of Obesity. 1998; 22 (1): 39-47.

[65] Kuczmarski RJ, Flegal KM, Campbell SM, Johnson CL. Increasing prevalence of overweight among US adults - the national-health and nutrition examination surveys, 1960 to 1991. JAMA-Journal of the American Medical Association. 1994; 272 (3): 205-211.

[66] Montague CT, Farooqi IS, Whitehead JP, Soos MA, Rau H, et al. Congenital leptin deficiency is associated with severe early-onset obesity in humans. Nature. 1997; 387 (6636): 903-908.

[67] Ezzati M, Bentham J, Di Cesare M, Bilano V, Bixby H, et al. Worldwide trends in body-mass index, underweight, overweight, and obesity from 1975 to 2016: a pooled analysis of 2416 population-based measurement studies in 128.9 million children, adolescents, and adults. Lancet. 2017; 390 (10113): 2627-2642.

[68] Kahn BB, Flier JS. Obesity and insulin resistance. Journal of Clinical Investigation. 2000; 106 (4): 473-481.

[69] Gregor MF, Hotamisligil GS. Inflammatory mechanisms in obesity. Annual Review Of Immunology. 2011; 29: 415-445.

[70] Flegal KM, Kit BK, Orpana H, Graubard BI. Association of all-cause mortality with overweight and obesity using standard Body Mass Index categories: A systematic review and meta-analysis. JAMA-Journal of the American Medical Association. 2013; 309 (1): 71-82.

[71] Locke AE, Kahali B, Berndt SI, Justice AE, Pers TH, et al. Genetic studies of body mass index yield new insights for obesity biology. Nature. 2015; 518 (7538): 197-206.

[72] Luppino FS, de Wit LM, Bouvy PF, Stijnen T, Cuijpers P, et al. Overweight, obesity, and depression: A systematic review and meta-analysis of longitudinal studies. Archives of General Psychiatry. 2010; 67 (3): 220-229.

[73] Wortsman J, Matsuoka LY, Chen TC, Lu ZR, Holick MF. Decreased bioavailability of vitamin D in obesity. American Journal of Clinical Nutrition. 2000; 72 (3): 690-693.

[74] Hotamisligil GS, Peraldi P, Budavari A, Ellis R, White MF, et al. IRS-1-mediated inhibition of insulin receptor tyrosine kinase activity in TNF-alpha- and obesity-induced insulin resistance. Science. 1996; 271 (5249): 665-668.

[75] Flegal KM, Graubard BI, Williamson DF, Gail MH. Excess deaths associated with underweight, overweight, and obesity. JAMA-Journal of the American Medical Association. 2005; 293 (15): 1861-1867.

[76] Yudkin JS, Stehouwer CDA, Emeis JJ, Coppack SW. C-reactive protein in wealthy subjects: Associations with obesity, insulin resistance, and endothelial dysfunction - a potential role for cytokines originating from adipose tissue? Arteriosclerosis Thrombosis and Vascular Biology. 1999; 19 (4): 972-978.

[77] Mokdad AH, Bowman BA, Ford ES, Vinicor F, Marks JS, et al. The

continuing epidemics of obesity and diabetes in the United States. JAMA-Journal of the American Medical Association. 2001 SEP 12; 286 (10): 1195-1200.

[78] Popkin BM, Adair LS, Ng SW. Global nutrition transition and the pandemic of obesity in developing countries. Nutrition Reviews. 2012; 70 (1): 3-21.

[79] Yusuf S, Hawken S, Ounpuu S, Bautista L, Franzosi MG, et al. Obesity and the risk of myocardial infarction in 27,000 participants from 52 countries: A case-control study. Lancet. 2005; 366 (9497): 1640-1649.

[80] Guh DP, Zhang W, Bansback N, Amarsi Z, Birmingham CL, et al. The incidence of co-morbidities related to obesity and overweight: A systematic review and meta-analysis. BMC Public Health. 2009; 9: 88.

[81] Everard A, Belzer C, Geurts L, Ouwerkerk JP, Druart C, et al. Cross-talk between Akkermansia muciniphila and intestinal epithelium controls diet-induced obesity. Proceedings of the National Academy of Sciences of the United States of America. 2013; 110 (22): 9066-9071.

[82] Wang Y, Lobstein T. Worldwide trends in childhood overweight and obesity. International Journal Of Pediatric Obesity. 2006; 1 (1): 11-25.

[83] Ebbeling CB, Pawlak DB, Ludwig DS. Childhood obesity: public-health crisis, common sense cure. Lancet. 2002; 360 (9331): 473-482.

[84] Wang Y, Beydoun MA. The obesity epidemic in the United States - Gender, age, socioeconomic, Racial/Ethnic, and geographic characteristics: A systematic review and meta-regression analysis. Epidemiologic Reviews. 2007; 29: 6-28.

[85] Ridaura VK, Faith JJ, Rey FE, Cheng JY, Duncan AE, et al. Gut Microbiota from Twins Discordant for Obesity Modulate Metabolism in Mice. Science. 2013; 341(6150):1241214.

[86] Kenchaiah S, Evans JC, Levy D, Wilson PWF, Benjamin EJ, et al. Obesity and the risk of heart failure. New England Journal of Medicine. 2002; 347 (5): 305-313.

[87] Afshin A, Forouzanfar MH, Reitsma MB, Sur P, Estep K, et al. Health effects of overweight and obesity in 195 countries over 25 years. New England Journal Of Medicine. 2017; 377 (1): 13-27.

[88] Elchebly M, Payette P, Michaliszyn E, Cromlish W, Collins S, et al. Increased insulin sensitivity and obesity resistance in mice lacking the protein tyrosine phosphatase-1B gene. Science. 1999; 283 (5407): 1544-1548.

[89] Dietz WH. Health consequences of obesity in youth: Childhood predictors of adult disease. Pediatrics. 1998; 101 (3): 518-525.

[90] Poirier P, Giles TD, Bray GA, Hong YL, Stern JS, et al. Obesity and cardiovascular disease: Pathophysiology, evaluation, and effect of weight loss - An update of the 1997 American Heart Association Scientific Statement on obesity and heart disease from the Obesity Committee of the Council on Nutrition, Physical Activity, and Metabolism. Circulation. 2006; 113 (6): 898-918.

[91] Van Gaal LF, Mertens IL, De Block CE. Mechanisms linking obesity with cardiovascular disease. Nature. 2006; 444 (7121): 875-880.

[92] Newgard CB, An J, Bain JR, Muehlbauer MJ, Stevens RD, et al. A branched-chain amino acid-related metabolic signature that differentiates obese and lean humans and contributes to insulin resistance. Cell Metabolism. 2009; 9 (4): 311-326.

[93] Turnbaugh PJ, Baeckhed F, Fulton L, Gordon JI. Diet-induced obesity is linked to marked but reversible alterations in the mouse distal gut microbiome. Cell Host & Microbe. 2008; 3 (4): 213-223.

[94] Spiegelman BM, Flier JS. Obesity and the regulation of energy balance. Cell. 2001; 104 (4): 531-543.

[95] Kanda H, Tateya S, Tamori Y, Kotani K, Hiasa KI, et al. MCP-1 contributes to macrophage infiltration into adipose tissue, insulin resistance, and hepatic steatosis in obesity. Journal of Clinical Investigation. 2006; 116 (6): 1494-1505.

[96] Uysal KT, Wiesbrock SM, Marino MW, Hotamisligil GS. Protection from obesity-induced insulin resistance in mice lacking TNF-alpha function. Nature. 1997; 389 (6651): 610-614.

[97] Hu E, Liang P, Spiegelman BM. AdipoQ is a novel adipose-specific gene dysregulated in obesity. Journal of Biological Chemistry. 1996; 271 (18): 10697-10703.

[98] Finkelstein EA, Trogdon JG, Cohen JW, Dietz W. Annual medical spending attributable to obesity: Payer- and service-specific estimates. Health Affairs. 2009; 28 (5): W822-W831.

[99] Mozaffarian D. Dietary and policy priorities for cardiovascular disease, diabetes, and obesity: A comprehensive review. Circulation. 2016; 133 (2): 187-225.

[100] Larsson B, Svardsudd K, Welin L, Wilhelmsen L, Bjorntorp P, et al. Abdominal adipose-tissue distribution, obesity, and risk of cardiovascular-disease and death - 13 year follow up of participants in the study of men born in 1913. British Medical Journal. 1984; 288 (6428): 1401-1404.

[101] Mokdad AH, Serdula MK, Dietz WH, Bowman BA, Marks JS, et al. The spread of the obesity epidemic in the United States, 1991-1998. JAMA-Journal of the American Medical Association. 1999; 282 (16): 1519-1522.

[102] Visser M, Bouter LM, McQuillan GM, Wener MH, Harris TB. Elevated C-reactive protein levels in overweight and obese adults. JAMA-Journal of the American Medical Association. 1999; 282 (22): 2131-2135.

[103] Kissebah AH, Vydelingum N, Murray R, Evans Dj, Hartz AJ, et al. Relation of body-fat distribution to metabolic complications of obesity. Journal of Clinical Endocrinology & Metabolism. 1982; 54 (2): 254-260.

[104] Wang YC, McPherson K, Marsh T, Gortmaker SL, Brown M. Health and economic burden of the projected obesity trends in the USA and the UK. Lancet. 2011; 378 (9793): 815-825.

[105] Clement K, Vaisse C, Lahlou N, Cabrol S, Pelloux V, et al. A mutation in the human leptin receptor gene causes obesity and pituitary dysfunction. Nature. 1998; 392 (6674): 398-401.

[106] Puhl RM, Heuer CA. The Stigma of Obesity: A Review and Update. Obesity. 2009; 17 (5): 941-964.

[107] Flegal KM, Kruszon-Moran D, Carroll MD, Fryar CD, Ogden CL. Trends in obesity among adults in the United States, 2005 to 2014. JAMA-Journal of the American Medical Association. 2016; 315 (21): 2284-2291.

[108] Turek FW, Joshu C, Kohsaka A, Lin E, Ivanova G, et al. Obesity and metabolic syndrome in circadian Clock mutant mice. Science. 2005; 308 (5724): 1043-1045.

[109] Seglen PO. Citations and journal impact factors: questionable indicators of research quality. Allergy. 1997

Nov;52(11):1050-1056. doi: 10.1111/j.1398-9995.1997.tb00175.x. PMID: 9404555.

[110] Jin B, Wu XA, Du SD. Top 100 most frequently cited papers in liver cancer: a bibliometric analysis. ANZ J Surg. 2020 Jan;90(1-2):21-26. doi: 10.1111/ans.15414. Epub 2019 Sep 3. PMID: 31480098.

[111] Liu C, Yuan Q, Mao Z, Hu P, Chi K, Geng X, Hong Q, Sun X. The top 100 most cited articles on rhabdomyolysis: A bibliometric analysis. Am J Emerg Med. 2020 Sep;38(9):1754-1759. doi: 10.1016/j.ajem.2020.05.031. Epub 2020 May 17. PMID: 32739844.

[112] Elarjani T, Almutairi OT, Alhussinan M, Alzhrani G, Alotaibi FE, Bafaquh M, Orz Y, AlYamany M, Alturki AY. Bibliometric Analysis of the Top 100 Most Cited Articles on Cerebral Vasospasm. World Neurosurg. 2021 Jan;145:e68-e82. doi: 10.1016/j.wneu.2020.09.099. Epub 2020 Sep 25. PMID: 32980568.

[113] Shi S, Gao Y, Liu M, Bu Y, Wu J, Tian J, Zhang J. Top 100 most-cited articles on exosomes in the field of cancer: a bibliometric analysis and evidence mapping. Clin Exp Med. 2021 May;21(2):181-194. doi: 10.1007/s10238-020-00624-5. Epub 2020 Apr 7. PMID: 32266495.

Chapter 4

Obesity and Endometrial Cancer

Saliha Sağnıç

Abstract

Obesity is a very common health problem in almost all societies. Although obesity is a problem especially in high-income or upper-middle-income countries, it is predicted that obesity will increase rapidly in the future in developing countries. Excess body weight is associated with an increased risk for many malignancies and its impact on cancer incidence and mortality is well established. The role of obesity in the pathogenesis of endometrial cancer has been proved. The incidence of endometrial cancer is increasing due to an increasing prevalence of obesity. Approximately 57% of endometrial cancers in the United States are thought to be attributable to being overweight and obese. The mechanisms underlying the relationship between obesity and endometrial cancer have not been fully defined, however adipokines are known to stimulate cell proliferation in endometrial carcinoma. By preventing obesity and reducing its prevalence, deaths from endometrial cancer can be reduced.

Keywords: endometrial cancer, obesity, global epidemic, prevention

1. Introduction

Obesity is a very common health problem in almost all societies. Although obesity is a problem especially in high-income or upper-middle-income countries, it is predicted that obesity will increase rapidly in the future in developing countries. The worldwide prevalence of obesity has more than doubled among women and tripled among men over the past four decades [1]. Excess body weight is associated with an increased risk for many malignancies and its impact on cancer incidence and mortality is well established [2]. This makes obesity an important public health problem. Despite clear evidence linking endometrial cancer and obesity, public awareness is poor [3, 4]. Weight, weight gain, and obesity account for about 20% of all cancer cases. Although the role of obesity in the pathogenesis of endometrial cancer has been proved, its importance in the esophagus, thyroid, colon, kidney, liver, melanoma, multiple myeloma, rectum, gallbladder, leukemia, lymphoma, and prostate in men and breast cancer in postmenopausal women is also demonstrated [5, 6].

Endometrial cancer is the most common female genital tract malignancy in high-income countries and the second most common gynecological cancer in low-middle-income countries. Endometrial carcinoma is a histological diagnosis based on characteristic findings in an endometrial biopsy, curettage, or hysterectomy specimen. A woman's lifetime risk of endometrial cancer in the general population is 3%. The incidence peaks between the ages of 60 and 70, but less than 5% of cases emerge before age of 40. The incidence of endometrial cancer is increasing due to an increasing prevalence of obesity, decreased use of menopausal hormone therapy with progestins, increased prevalence of diabetes, and changes in reproductive behavior (eg, nulliparity) [7, 8]. Most patients are diagnosed at an early stage and therefore have a five-year survival rate of more than 90%. Unfortunately, approximately 30% of women have stage III or IV disease, with 5-year survival rates significantly worse than in early-stage patients, 60% and 20%, respectively [9].

The primary complaint is abnormal uterine bleeding in 70% to 90% of endometrial carcinoma cases [10]. Premenopausal patients with abnormal uterine bleeding have a lower risk of cancer than postmenopausal women with the same complaint. In patients younger than 45 years of age, abnormal uterine bleeding tends to be persistent and is more likely to occur if there is a history of unopposed estrogen exposure (eg. obesity, chronic anovulation). The emergence of endometrial carcinoma in postmenopausal women requires evaluation of endogenous and exogenous estrogen sources because unopposed estrogen (estrogen therapy, obesity, selective estrogenic receptor modulators, some herbs, sex cord-stromal tumors) is a risk factor for the disease.

Endometrial carcinoma is sometimes discovered incidentally when a hysterectomy is performed for benign disease. To minimize this coincidence and optimize the surgical procedure performed, patients with abnormal uterine bleeding should always undergo endometrial sampling before performing a hysterectomy, and the results should be evaluated to determine the extent of surgery before the operation. Occult uterine cancer risk is significantly associated with race/ethnicity, obesity, comorbidity, personal history of malignancy, and cause of hysterectomy [11].

Typically, a pelvic examination is usually normal in patients with early-stage endometrial carcinoma. In women with more advanced disease, the uterus can be palpated as larger and fixed for the age of the patient. With blind endometrial sampling, the sensitivity is 90% or higher. History of colorectal cancer, endometrial polyps, and morbid obesity are risk factors for false-negative endometrial sampling [12]. In case of high clinical suspicion, hysteroscopy and targeted lesion-directed biopsy can be performed to reduce the false-negative rate. It is important to repeat endometrial sampling to exclude endometrial hyperplasia or carcinoma, especially in patients with risk factors for malignancy (eg. obesity, chronic anovulation).

More than 90% of uterine cancers originate from the endometrium, with most of the remainder originating from the myometrial muscle or less frequently from the endometrial stroma [13]. Adenocarcinoma of the endometrium is the most common histological type. The prognosis of endometrial carcinoma is primarily determined by the stage, grade, and histology of the disease. Most patients have a favorable prognosis as the majority of the histological type is the endometrioid type and presents with early-stage disease. Serous and clear cell types and other uterine cancers are associated with poor prognosis. Most women with low-risk endometrial cancer die from another cause, and cardiovascular disease is the leading cause of death among endometrial cancer patients [14]. The endometrioid type is the subtype predominantly associated with obesity; however, more aggressive subtypes (such as serous, clear cell, and carcinosarcoma) have recently been stated to increase with obesity [15].

Endometrial carcinomas are divided into two categories that differ in incidence, response to hormones, clinicopathological features, and risk factors [16, 17]. However, this approach does not adequately address the complexity of these neoplasms. Because 25% of high-grade endometrioid carcinomas progress like serous carcinomas [18].

Type 1: It accounts for about 80 percent of endometrial carcinomas. Includes tumors with grade 1 or 2 endometrioid histology; It may result from intraepithelial neoplasm (atypical and/or complex endometrial hyperplasia), typically has a favorable prognosis, is estrogen-induced, and responsive to progestins on therapy. While estrogen excess is important in its etiology, unexposure to progesterone is probably equally important. The increasing prevalence of obesity, decreased use of menopausal hormone therapy with progestins, and decreased propensity to delivery in women explain the increasing prevalence of type 1 endometrial carcinoma.

Type 2: Accounts for 10 to 20 percent of endometrial carcinomas. Includes grade 3 endometrioid tumors as well as histological types of non-endometrioid types: serous, clear cell, mucinous, squamous, transitional cell, mesonephric, and undifferentiated. These patients generally have lower body mass indexes and are older than type 1 patients. These neoplasms are insensitive to estrogen, often occur in the atrophic endometrium, and have a poor prognosis. The reason for the increased incidence of type 2 neoplasms is unknown.

The Cancer Genome Atlas (TCGA) Research Network has significantly improved our understanding of the molecular level of endometrial cancer and introduced not two but four molecular subtypes [18];

1. POLE (ultra mutated) tumors,

2. Microsatellite unstable tumors,

3. Tumors with high copy number, mostly with TP53 mutations,

4. The group remaining without these changes.

2. Risk factors for endometrial cancer

The main risk factor for type I (endometrioid) endometrial carcinoma is an excess of endogenous or exogenous estrogen that is not adequately opposed with progestin [19]. In a woman with a uterus, oral, transdermal, and vaginal systemic estrogen therapy without the administration of progestin results in a marked increased risk of developing endometrial premalignant lesions and endometrial carcinoma. Unopposed estrogen increases the risk of endometrial cancer by 2–10 times [20]. Studies have reported an increased risk of endometrial cancer in patients using estrogen alone, depending on the dose and duration of use [21–23]. The risk of endometrial cancer in postmenopausal patients is estimated to be approximately 1 in 1000; therefore, studies have shown that patients receiving unopposed estrogen have an increased absolute risk of up to 1 in 100 [24]. Other risk factors include tamoxifen therapy, chronic anovulation, obesity, nulliparity, early menarche, late menopause, ovarian granulosa cell tumor, Cowden syndrome, having a first-degree relative with endometrial cancer, history of pelvic radiotherapy, diabetes mellitus and hypertension, and Lynch syndrome. A history of breast cancer is a risk factor for the development of endometrial cancer, partly because of the use of tamoxifen in the treatment of breast cancer, the increased risk of breast cancer in conditions such as obesity, and Cowden syndrome. As patients with hypertension and diabetes mellitus are generally obese, much of the risk these two comorbid conditions have in developing endometrial cancer may be attributable to obesity [25]. However, there are also studies stating that each has an independent risk factor [26, 27].

3. Obesity

Obesity is a chronic disease that is considered a global epidemic today. Obesity is defined by the World Health Organization (WHO) as excessive accumulation of fat in the body to the extent that it impairs health. According to WHO estimates, 39% of adults worldwide were overweight and 13% were obese in 2016. Obesity is defined as an excess weight rather than excess fat, as it is impractical to determine body fat percentage. Based on the body mass index (BMI) of the definition and grading of obesity, it is evaluated with the formula (BMI=Weight (kg)/Height (m^2)). BMI provides a better estimate of total body fat compared to bodyweight alone [28]. According to the World Health Organization (WHO) standards, someone with a body mass index (BMI) >30 kg/m^2 is classified as obese. Obesity classification according to body mass index in adults is demostrated in **Table 1** [29–31]. According to the World Food Security and Nutrition Status 2019, obesity rates are increasing day by day in almost every country and the global adult obesity rate has reached 13.2% [32]. Today, overweight and obesity are considered to increase the overall health burden more than smoking. Obesity is associated with a significant increase in morbidity (including diabetes mellitus, hypertension, dyslipidemia, cardiovascular diseases, cerebrovascular accident, sleep apnea, and cancer) and mortality [33]. Weight loss reduces obesity-related morbidity. Due to the potential stigma risk of obesity, routine screening, diagnosis, and management are rare, and there is insufficient awareness of the health problems caused by obesity in the population.

The type of obesity with increased waist circumference or waist/hip ratio is called central (abdominal, visceral, android, or male-type obesity) obesity. According to WHO, a waist circumference of 88 cm or more in women and 102 cm or more in men indicates the presence of central obesity. Patients with central obesity have higher mortality rates [34] because these patients are at high risk for heart disease, diabetes, hypertension, dyslipidemia, and non-alcoholic fatty liver disease [34, 35]. Central obesity is a component of metabolic syndrome. The association of metabolic syndrome with endometrial cancer has also been reported [36, 37]. However, there is no data to suggest that outcomes can be improved with more effective management of associated medical conditions. In the Prospective Studies Collaboration analysis, in the upper BMI range (25 to 50 kg/m^2), every 5 kg/m^2 increase in BMI is associated with coronary heart disease (CHD), stroke, diabetes, chronic kidney disease, and cancer (liver, kidney, breast, endometrial, prostate and colon) have been demonstrated to result in a significant increase in deaths [38].

Most cases of obesity are related to behaviors such as a sedentary lifestyle and increased calorie intake. Obesity develops with excessive fat accumulation in the body secondary to high energy intake. Energy homeostasis is impaired due to an increase in energy intake or a decrease in energy expenditure [39]. Interactions between genetic/epigenetic factors and behavioral/social factors and chronic stress regulate energy balance. High-calorie diet, physical inactivity, sedentary lifestyle, and in addition, eating disorders accelerate the development of obesity. In addition, hypertrophy, hyperplasia and inflammation in adipocytes cause many changes in the structure of adipose tissue and the secretion of adipokines such as leptin, interleukin-6, and

Underweight	BMI <18.5 kg/m^2
Normal weight	BMI ≥18.5 to 24.9 kg/m^2
Overweight	BMI ≥25 to 29.9 kg/m^2
Obesity	BMI ≥30 kg/m^2
Obesity class 1	BMI 30 to 34.9 kg/m^2
Obesity class 2	BMI 35 to 39.9 kg/m^2
Obesity class 3	BMI ≥40 kg/m^2 (also referred to as severe, extreme, or massive obesity)

BMI, body mass index.

Table 1.
Classification of body mass index.

tumor necrosis factor-a. With the increasing prevalence of obesity, there is a growing awareness of its impact on cancers. Obesity has been defined as a risk factor affecting the severity of the disease and mortality in people with cancer.

4. The relationship between endometrial cancer and obesity

Obesity is known to increase the risk of endometrial cancer in women [40, 41]. Approximately 57% of endometrial cancers in the United States are thought to be attributable to being overweight and obese. The incidence of endometrial cancer increases as body mass index (BMI) increases [42]. More importantly, obesity and overweight can increase the likelihood of dying from cancer. A review of the literature states that most of the associations between adiposity indices and endometrial cancer are supported by strong or highly suggestive evidence. A review (IARC) from a comprehensive meta-analysis of weight, physical activity, and cancer incidence by the International Agency for Research on Cancer demonstrated that it is the cause of 39% of endometrial cancer cases [43].

The cause and effect relationship between obesity and endometrial cancer can be explained by 3 mechanisms; first; in obese patients, the adrenal glands secrete more androgen precursors for conversion to estrogen in peripheral tissues. An androgen, androstenedione, (A) is converted to estrone (E1) mainly in peripheral adipose tissue, and this conversion is increased in adipose tissue of obese patients. Plasma SHBG levels that bind estradiol (E2) are reduced in obese subjects and therefore higher-than-normal amounts of serum estradiol are present in the circulation, thereby increasing the estrogenic stimulus in target tissues [44]. Proinflammatory cytokines such as tumor necrosis factor-a in obesity are associated with low plasma SHBG levels [45]. Obese patients also have changes in the concentration of insulin-like growth factors and their binding proteins and insulin resistance, all of which may contribute to an increased risk of endometrial cancer in these patients [46]. The triad of obesity, insulin resistance, and adipokine aberrations is linked to cancer [47], since adipokines impair insulin signaling and contribute to insulin resistance [48]. Other mechanisms in pathophysiology are subclinical chronic low-grade inflammation, oxidative stress, and sex hormone biosynthesis [6]. Adipokine-mediated chronic inflammation and cellular stress cause genetic instability and DNA damage [42]. All of these mechanisms lead to endometrial hyperplasia and cancer. Despite all these conditions, obese patients who do not have metabolic problems seem to have an increased risk of endometrial cancer [49].

The mechanisms underlying the relationship between obesity and endometrial cancer have not been fully defined. However, estrogens and proinflammatory adipokines are known to stimulate cell proliferation in endometrial carcinoma. In addition to stimulating cell proliferation, estrogen also has mutagenic properties. Genotoxic metabolites of estrogen react with DNA and contribute to DNA breaks and genetic instability [50]. Although the role of estrogen metabolites in the pathogenesis of breast cancer is well defined, their role in the context of endometrial cancer has not been fully understood. However, defects in DNA mismatch repair genes were detected in one-third of endometrial cancer cases. Visceral fat is a complex endocrine organ composed of adipocytes, preadipocytes, macrophages, stromal, nerve, and stem cells [42]. Adipokines secreted by these cells increase endometrial proliferation and promote tumor formation [51], even mesenchymal stem cells support tumor growth and progression [52, 53].

Cyclic secretion of ovarian estrogen and estrogen-induced cyclic secretion of insulin-like growth factor 1 (IGF1) in premenopausal women stimulates endometrial proliferation [54, 55]. In postmenopausal women, especially adipose tissue is the main site of estrogen synthesis [56]. Aromatase enzyme, which provides estrogen synthesis from androgens, is mainly found in adipose tissue [57]. As body adiposity increases, the amount and activity of aromatase increases [58]. Steroid hormone synthesis from cholesterol and estrogen synthesis from androgens by aromatase enzyme is shown in **Figure 1**.

In a pooled analysis of individual patient data from 10 cohort and 14 case–control studies, including more than 14,000 endometrial cancer cases and more than 35,000 controls, for type I endometrial cancer, by body mass index (BMI): overweight (BMI) 25.0 to <30.0 kg/m^2) OR 1.5, OR 2.5 (30.0 to <35.0 kg/m^2) for class 1 obesity, OR 4.5 for class 2 obesity (35.0 to 39.9 kg/m^2) and calculated as 7.1 for class 3 obesity (≥40.0 kg/m^2). For type 2 endometrial cancer, the ORs were calculated as 1.2 for overweight, 1.7 for class 1 obesity, 2.2 for class 2 obesity, and 3.1 for class 3 obesity [59]. Higher BMI is associated with the development of endometrial cancer at a younger age (<45 years old) [60]. In another meta-analysis, body mass index and waist-to-hip ratio were associated with increased cancer risk in premenopausal women (RR 1.49 per 5 kg/m^2; CI 1.39–1.61) and for total endometrial cancer (RR 1.21 per 0.1 unit; CI 1.13–1.29), respectively [61].

Severely obese patients (BMI ≥40 kg/m^2) who develop endometrial cancer are more likely to have a less aggressive histological subtype (endometrioid 87% vs. serous or clear cell 75%) compared to patients with BMI <30 kg/m^2 [62]. Therefore, patients with severe obesity are more likely to present with stage I disease (77 versus 61%) or low-grade histology (44% vs. 24%), but severe obesity is associated with an increased risk of death in endometrial cancer patients [63, 64]. After being diagnosed with endometrial cancer, being obese indicates worse outcomes. Obesity has a negative effect on all-cause mortality. A retrospective study found that morbidly obese women with early-stage disease had higher mortality rates compared with women with a normal body mass index, accounting for 67% of these deaths. It has been determined that there are obesity-related causes unrelated to cancer [65]. Increased mortality may be due to sustained stimulation of metastatic cells by endogenous estrogen or may result from obesity-related conditions such as diabetes or cardiovascular disease [66, 67].

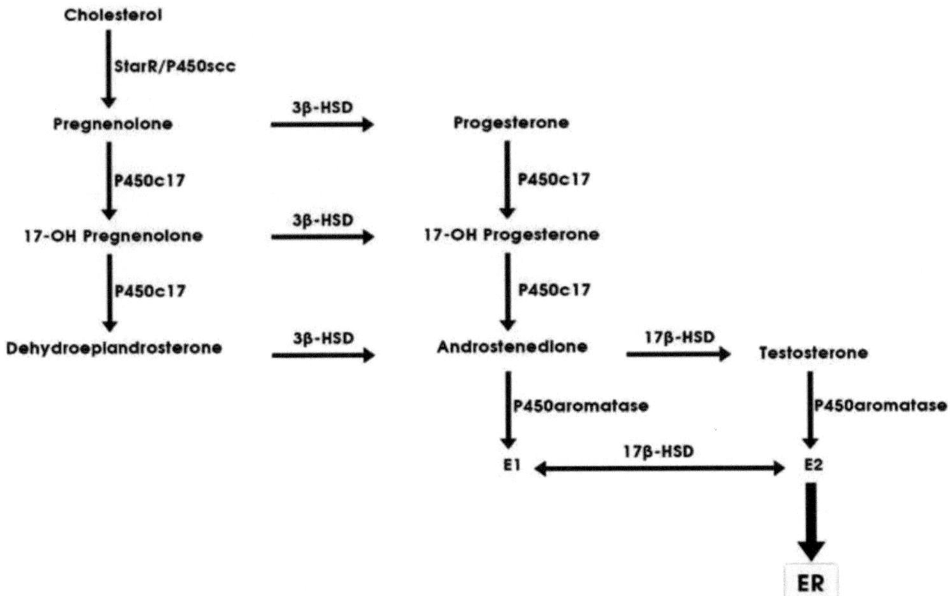

Figure 1.
Steroid hormone synthesis.

After obese women are diagnosed with endometrial cancer, clinical management strategies can be complex. As the operations of obese patients are technically more difficult it takes a longer time than normal-weight individuals. Since these patients also have many co-morbid medical problems, both perioperative and postoperative complication rates are increased. Even though the patients have early-stage cancer, they may not be able to be operated on due to concomitant systemic diseases such as cardiovascular and diabetes mellitus, and they may have to undergo primary radiotherapy. Robotic surgery may provide an advantage over conventional laparoscopy in such patients [68, 69].

Meta-analyses show that increased physical activity reduces the risk of endometrial cancer [70–72]. Exercise may provide moderate protection against endometrial cancer [73]. Physical activity benefits by reducing obesity and making positive changes in immune function, endogenous sexual and metabolic hormone levels, and growth factors [74]. Losing weight through lifestyle changes such as diet and physical activity or bariatric surgery can reduce obesity. Bariatric surgery has been associated with a 50% to 80% reduction in the occurrence of endometrial cancer in a meta-analysis of controlled trials [75, 76]. Obesity-related hormonal and metabolic disorders and drugs aimed at correcting insulin resistance can also be used as a prevention strategy. Losing weight has health benefits beyond protecting the endometrium. Preventing or treating obesity can provide significant lifelong health benefits. Public health interventions may be beneficial to reduce the incidence of endometrial cancer in the community. Obese patients should receive counseling about health risks, lifestyle changes, obesity treatment options, and risk factor reduction.

5. Conclusion

By preventing obesity and reducing its prevalence, deaths from endometrial cancer can be reduced. Prevention strategies should focus on changing the environmental and lifestyle risk factors that cause endometrial cancer. General lifestyle recommendations include being physically active and maintaining a healthy weight. Healthy weight is considered a risk reducer and has a positive effect on blood pressure, glucose metabolism, cardiac and vascular function. Therefore, reducing obesity reduces morbidity and mortality from endometrial cancer. More public awareness is needed regarding the cause and effect relationship between obesity and endometrial cancer. Public health education including obesity prevention is of great importance.

Author details

Saliha Sağnıç
Division of Gynecologic Oncology, Department of Gynecology Obstetrics, Akdeniz University, Antalya, Turkey

*Address all correspondence to: drsalihasagnic@hotmail.com

References

[1] Trends in adult body-mass index in 200 countries from 1975 to 2014: a pooled analysis of 1698 population-based measurement studies with 19•2 million participants. Lancet, 2016. 387(10026): p. 1377-1396.

[2] Lauby-Secretan, B., et al., Body Fatness and Cancer--Viewpoint of the IARC Working Group. N Engl J Med, 2016. 375(8): p. 794-8.

[3] Soliman, P.T., et al., Limited public knowledge of obesity and endometrial cancer risk: what women know. Obstet Gynecol, 2008. 112(4): p. 835-42.

[4] Beavis, A.L., et al., Almost half of women with endometrial cancer or hyperplasia do not know that obesity affects their cancer risk. Gynecol Oncol Rep, 2015. 13: p. 71-5.

[5] Wolin, K.Y., K. Carson, and G.A. Colditz, Obesity and cancer. Oncologist, 2010. 15(6): p. 556-65.

[6] Avgerinos, K.I., et al., Obesity and cancer risk: Emerging biological mechanisms and perspectives. Metabolism, 2019. 92: p. 121-135.

[7] Constantine, G.D., et al., Increased Incidence of Endometrial Cancer Following the Women's Health Initiative: An Assessment of Risk Factors. J Womens Health (Larchmt), 2019. 28(2): p. 237-243.

[8] Cote, M.L., et al., The Growing Burden of Endometrial Cancer: A Major Racial Disparity Affecting Black Women. Cancer Epidemiol Biomarkers Prev, 2015. 24(9): p. 1407-15.

[9] McDonald, M.E. and D.P. Bender, Endometrial Cancer: Obesity, Genetics, and Targeted Agents. Obstet Gynecol Clin North Am, 2019. 46(1): p. 89-105.

[10] ACOG practice bulletin, clinical management guidelines for obstetrician-gynecologists, number 65, August 2005: management of endometrial cancer. Obstet Gynecol, 2005. 106(2): p. 413-25.

[11] Desai, V.B., et al., Prevalence, characteristics, and risk factors of occult uterine cancer in presumed benign hysterectomy. Am J Obstet Gynecol, 2019. 221(1): p. 39.e1-39.e14.

[12] Torres, M.L., et al., Risk factors for developing endometrial cancer after benign endometrial sampling. Obstet Gynecol, 2012. 120(5): p. 998-1004.

[13] https://www.cancer.net/cancer-types/uterine-cancer/statistics.

[14] Ward, K.K., et al., Cardiovascular disease is the leading cause of death among endometrial cancer patients. Gynecol Oncol, 2012. 126(2): p. 176-9.

[15] McCullough, M.L., et al., Body mass and endometrial cancer risk by hormone replacement therapy and cancer subtype. Cancer Epidemiol Biomarkers Prev, 2008. 17(1): p. 73-9.

[16] Bokhman, J.V., Two pathogenetic types of endometrial carcinoma. Gynecol Oncol, 1983. 15(1): p. 10-7.

[17] Felix, A.S., et al., Factors associated with Type I and Type II endometrial cancer. Cancer Causes Control, 2010. 21(11): p. 1851-6.

[18] Colombo, N., et al., ESMO-ESGO-ESTRO Consensus Conference on Endometrial Cancer: diagnosis, treatment and follow-up. Ann Oncol, 2016. 27(1): p. 16-41.

[19] Lukanova, A., et al., Circulating levels of sex steroid hormones and risk of endometrial cancer in postmenopausal women. Int J Cancer, 2004. 108(3): p. 425-32.

[20] Brinton, L.A. and A.S. Felix, Menopausal hormone therapy and risk of endometrial cancer. J Steroid Biochem Mol Biol, 2014. 142: p. 83-9.

[21] Weiderpass, E., et al., Risk of endometrial cancer following estrogen replacement with and without progestins. J Natl Cancer Inst, 1999. 91(13): p. 1131-7.

[22] Strom, B.L., et al., Case-control study of postmenopausal hormone replacement therapy and endometrial cancer. Am J Epidemiol, 2006. 164(8): p. 775-86.

[23] Furness, S., et al., Hormone therapy in postmenopausal women and risk of endometrial hyperplasia. Cochrane Database Syst Rev, 2009(2): p. Cd000402.

[24] Henderson, B.E., The cancer question: an overview of recent epidemiologic and retrospective data. Am J Obstet Gynecol, 1989. 161(6 Pt 2): p. 1859-64.

[25] Lindemann, K., et al., Body mass, diabetes and smoking, and endometrial cancer risk: a follow-up study. Br J Cancer, 2008. 98(9): p. 1582-5.

[26] Friberg, E., C.S. Mantzoros, and A. Wolk, Diabetes and risk of endometrial cancer: a population-based prospective cohort study. Cancer Epidemiol Biomarkers Prev, 2007. 16(2): p. 276-80.

[27] Weiderpass, E., et al., Body size in different periods of life, diabetes mellitus, hypertension, and risk of postmenopausal endometrial cancer (Sweden). Cancer Causes Control, 2000. 11(2): p. 185-92.

[28] Mei, Z., et al., Validity of body mass index compared with other body-composition screening indexes for the assessment of body fatness in children and adolescents. Am J Clin Nutr, 2002. 75(6): p. 978-85.

[29] Appropriate body-mass index for Asian populations and its implications for policy and intervention strategies. Lancet, 2004. 363(9403): p. 157-63.

[30] Obesity: preventing and managing the global epidemic. Report of a WHO consultation. World Health Organ Tech Rep Ser, 2000. 894: p. i-xii, 1-253.

[31] Clinical Guidelines on the Identification, Evaluation, and Treatment of Overweight and Obesity in Adults--The Evidence Report. National Institutes of Health. Obes Res, 1998. 6 Suppl 2: p. 51s-209s.

[32] FAO, The state of food security and nutrition in the World. 2019.

[33] Mayoral, L.P., et al., Obesity subtypes, related biomarkers & heterogeneity. Indian J Med Res, 2020. 151(1): p. 11-21.

[34] Jacobs, E.J., et al., Waist circumference and all-cause mortality in a large US cohort. Arch Intern Med, 2010. 170(15): p. 1293-301.

[35] Tsai, A.G. and T.A. Wadden, In the clinic: obesity. Ann Intern Med, 2013. 159(5): p. ITC3-1-ITC3-15; quiz ITC3-16.

[36] Bjørge, T., et al., Metabolic syndrome and endometrial carcinoma. Am J Epidemiol, 2010. 171(8): p. 892-902.

[37] Rosato, V., et al., Metabolic syndrome and endometrial cancer risk. Ann Oncol, 2011. 22(4): p. 884-889.

[38] Whitlock, G., et al., Body-mass index and cause-specific mortality in 900 000 adults: collaborative analyses of 57 prospective studies. Lancet, 2009. 373(9669): p. 1083-96.

[39] Tchang, B.G., K.H. Saunders, and L.I. Igel, Best Practices in the Management of Overweight and Obesity. Med Clin North Am, 2021. 105(1): p. 149-174.

[40] Donkers, H., et al., Obesity and visceral fat: Survival impact in high-grade endometrial cancer. Eur J Obstet Gynecol Reprod Biol, 2021. 256: p. 425-432.

[41] Rodriguez, A.M., et al., Factors associated with endometrial cancer and hyperplasia among middle-aged and older Hispanics. Gynecol Oncol, 2021. 160(1): p. 16-23.

[42] Onstad, M.A., R.E. Schmandt, and K.H. Lu, Addressing the Role of Obesity in Endometrial Cancer Risk, Prevention, and Treatment. J Clin Oncol, 2016. 34(35): p. 4225-4230.

[43] Weight Control and Physical Activity in International Agency for Research on Cancer. 2002: Lyon. p. 1-315.

[44] Siiteri, P.K., Adipose tissue as a source of hormones. Am J Clin Nutr, 1987. 45(1 Suppl): p. 277-82.

[45] Simó, R., et al., Molecular Mechanism of TNFα-Induced Down-Regulation of SHBG Expression. Mol Endocrinol, 2012. 26(3): p. 438-46.

[46] Amant, F., et al., Endometrial cancer. Lancet, 2005. 366(9484): p. 491-505.

[47] Dimou, N.L., et al., Circulating adipokine concentrations and risk of five obesity-related cancers: A Mendelian randomization study. Int J Cancer, 2021. 148(7): p. 1625-1636.

[48] Mu, N., et al., Insulin resistance: a significant risk factor of endometrial cancer. Gynecol Oncol, 2012. 125(3): p. 751-7.

[49] Cao, Z., et al., Association of obesity status and metabolic syndrome with site-specific cancers: a population-based cohort study. Br J Cancer, 2020. 123(8): p. 1336-1344.

[50] Cavalieri, E.L. and E.G. Rogan, Depurinating estrogen-DNA adducts, generators of cancer initiation: their minimization leads to cancer prevention. Clin Transl Med, 2016. 5(1): p. 12.

[51] Renehan, A.G., M. Zwahlen, and M. Egger, Adiposity and cancer risk: new mechanistic insights from epidemiology. Nat Rev Cancer, 2015. 15(8): p. 484-98.

[52] Klopp, A.H., et al., Omental adipose tissue-derived stromal cells promote vascularization and growth of endometrial tumors. Clin Cancer Res, 2012. 18(3): p. 771-82.

[53] Pope, B.D., et al., Microenvironmental Control of Adipocyte Fate and Function. Trends Cell Biol, 2016. 26(10): p. 745-755.

[54] Mihm, M., S. Gangooly, and S. Muttukrishna, The normal menstrual cycle in women. Anim Reprod Sci, 2011. 124(3-4): p. 229-36.

[55] McCampbell, A.S., et al., Developmental reprogramming of IGF signaling and susceptibility to endometrial hyperplasia in the rat. Lab Invest, 2008. 88(6): p. 615-26.

[56] Davis, S.R., et al., Menopause. Nat Rev Dis Primers, 2015. 1: p. 15004.

[57] Blakemore, J. and F. Naftolin, Aromatase: Contributions to Physiology and Disease in Women and Men. Physiology (Bethesda), 2016. 31(4): p. 258-69.

[58] Bulun, S.E. and E.R. Simpson, Regulation of aromatase expression in human tissues. Breast Cancer Res Treat, 1994. 30(1): p. 19-29.

[59] Setiawan, V.W., et al., Type I and II endometrial cancers: have they different risk factors? J Clin Oncol, 2013. 31(20): p. 2607-18.

[60] Pellerin, G.P. and M.A. Finan, Endometrial cancer in women 45 years of age or younger: a clinicopathological analysis. Am J Obstet Gynecol, 2005. 193(5): p. 1640-4.

[61] Raglan, O., et al., Risk factors for endometrial cancer: An umbrella review of the literature. Int J Cancer, 2019. 145(7): p. 1719-1730.

[62] Everett, E., et al., The effect of body mass index on clinical/pathologic features, surgical morbidity, and outcome in patients with endometrial cancer. Gynecol Oncol, 2003. 90(1): p. 150-7.

[63] Fader, A.N., et al., Endometrial cancer and obesity: epidemiology, biomarkers, prevention and survivorship. Gynecol Oncol, 2009. 114(1): p. 121-7.

[64] Calle, E.E., et al., Overweight, obesity, and mortality from cancer in a prospectively studied cohort of U.S. adults. N Engl J Med, 2003. 348(17): p. 1625-38.

[65] von Gruenigen, V.E., et al., Treatment effects, disease recurrence, and survival in obese women with early endometrial carcinoma: a Gynecologic Oncology Group study. Cancer, 2006. 107(12): p. 2786-91.

[66] Abu-Abid, S., A. Szold, and J. Klausner, Obesity and cancer. J Med, 2002. 33(1-4): p. 73-86.

[67] Schouten, L.J., R.A. Goldbohm, and P.A. van den Brandt, Anthropometry, physical activity, and endometrial cancer risk: results from the Netherlands Cohort Study. J Natl Cancer Inst, 2004. 96(21): p. 1635-8.

[68] Gehrig, P.A., et al., What is the optimal minimally invasive surgical procedure for endometrial cancer staging in the obese and morbidly obese woman? Gynecol Oncol, 2008. 111(1): p. 41-5.

[69] Kawai, E., et al., Impact of obesity on surgical and oncologic outcomes in patients with endometrial cancer treated with a robotic approach. J Obstet Gynaecol Res, 2021. 47(1): p. 128-136.

[70] Schmid, D., et al., A systematic review and meta-analysis of physical activity and endometrial cancer risk. Eur J Epidemiol, 2015. 30(5): p. 397-412.

[71] Moore, S.C., et al., Physical activity, sedentary behaviours, and the prevention of endometrial cancer. Br J Cancer, 2010. 103(7): p. 933-8.

[72] Friedenreich, C.M., C. Ryder-Burbidge, and J. McNeil, Physical activity, obesity and sedentary behavior in cancer etiology: epidemiologic evidence and biologic mechanisms. Mol Oncol, 2021. 15(3): p. 790-800.

[73] Kyu, H.H., et al., Physical activity and risk of breast cancer, colon cancer, diabetes, ischemic heart disease, and ischemic stroke events: systematic review and dose-response meta-analysis for the Global Burden of Disease Study 2013. Bmj, 2016. 354: p. i3857.

[74] Friedenreich, C.M. and M.R. Orenstein, Physical activity and cancer prevention: etiologic evidence and biological mechanisms. J Nutr, 2002. 132(11 Suppl): p. 3456s-3464s.

[75] Schauer, D.P., et al., Bariatric Surgery and the Risk of Cancer in a Large Multisite Cohort. Ann Surg, 2019. 269(1): p. 95-101.

[76] Zhang, X., et al., Intentional weight loss, weight cycling, and endometrial cancer risk: a systematic review and meta-analysis. Int J Gynecol Cancer, 2019. 29(9): p. 1361-1371.

Chapter 5

Ketogenic Diet Is Good for Aging-Related Sarcopenic Obesity

Sergey Suchkov, Tahereh Seifi Salmi, Chyi-Huey Bai, Javad Alizargar and Jia-Ping Wu

Abstract

Sarcopenic obesity is a skeletal muscle weight loss disease. It has happened at an elderly age. A ketogenic diet is a low-carbohydrate (5%), moderate protein (15%), and a higher-fat diet (80%) can help sarcopenic obese patients burn their fat more effectively. It has many benefits for muscle and fat weight loss. A ketogenic diet can be especially useful for losing excess body fat without hunger and for improving type 2 diabetes. That is because of only a few carbohydrates in the diet, the liver converts fat into fatty acids and ketones. Ketone bodies can replace higher ATP energy. This diet forces the human body to burn fat. This is a good way to lose fat weight without restriction.

Keywords: sarcopenic obesity, ketogenic diet, fat, muscle, type 2 diabetes

1. Introduction

The ketogenic diet is a mixed diet containing low carbohydrates, consisting primarily of proteins and fat [1, 2]. Some healthy foods are eaten on a ketogenic diet, for example, seafood, low-carb vegetables, cheese, eggs, meat, poultry, coffee, and tea. The importance of high fat in aging-related sarcopenic obesity reducing regimens on different metabolic models are shown by comparing the effects of four different types of ketogenic dietary regimens [3, 4]. Standard ketogenic diet (SKD): This typically contains a very low, only 5% carbohydrate, 15% moderate proteins, 80% high fat diet. This classic SKD contains a 3:1 ratio to combined protein and carbohydrate. High protein ketogenic diet (HPKD): This contains 5% carbohydrate, 35% protein, and 60% fat. This type is similar to a standard ketogenic diet, but includes more protein [5]. Cyclical ketogenic diet (CKD): This ketogenic diet involves 5 periods of ketogenic days followed by 2 high carbohydrate days [6]. Targeted ketogenic diet (TKD): This ketogenic diet allows you to add carbohydrate around workouts. Although this ketogenic diet is usually safe for weight loss, diabetes, epilepsy, and aging-related sarcopenic obesity, there maybe have some initial side effects while your body adapts [7–9]. Ketogenic diets forces to burn fats rather than carbohydrates. A ketogenic diet, a high fat, in food is converted triglyceride (TG). The liver convers triacylglycerol (TAG) into fatty acid and ketone bodies [10]. Elevated ketone bodies in the blood eventually lowers the aging-related sarcopenic obesity. We hoped to obtain the benefits of ketone dietary therapy that could be maintained indefinitely. Ketone bodies were produced β-hydroxybutyrate,

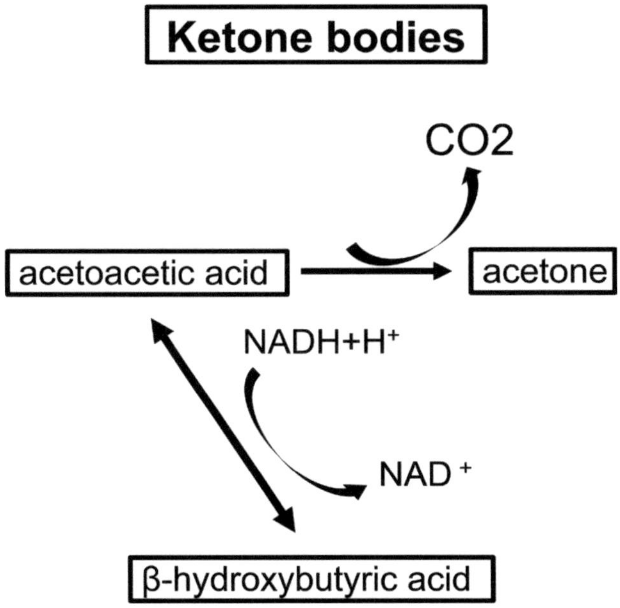

Figure 1.
Ketone bodies. Interrelationships of these three substances. Under certain a high rate of fatty acid oxidation, the liver products collectively of β-hydroxybutyrate, acetoacetate and acetone.

acetoacetate, and acetone by the liver in they consumed a very low-carbohydrate, and excess high-fat diet (**Figure 1**) [11, 12].

2. Ketogenic diet is good for aging-related sarcopenic obesity

Sarcopenic obesity is caused reduced skeletal muscle mass and strength in order adults. Sarcopenic obesity is most commonly caused by a combination of age and excessive food energy intake, not exercising enough, smoking or heavy alcohol use, although a few caused by genes [13]. Inflammation with aging is known to be a major contributor to sarcopenia [14]. Therefore, sarcopenic obesity has been defined as the loss of skeletal muscle mass and overweight in the older age. As sarcopenic obesity grow older, up to half of the muscle is lost and skeletal muscle is often replaced with fat tissue, particularly in sarcopenic obesity [15]. This is an importance of sarcopenic obesity in the health care for older people. Sarcopenia obesity starts at approximately 40 years of age and there is an estimated muscle mass loss of about 3 ~ 8% per decade, stretching process speeds up until the age of 70 years; after that age, a 15% loss ensues per decade [16]. This group proposed that sarcopenic obesity is diagnosed based on over whole-body weight combination with poor physical functioning [17].

The production of ketone bodies is from the liver. The reverse situation occurs in extrahepatic tissue. Responsible for ketone body formation are associated mainly with the mitochondria. Acetoacetate was formed from the terminal four carbons of a fatty acid upon oxidation. The liver is equipped with the production of aceto-acetate from acetoacetyl-CoA (**Figure 2**). This accounts for the net production of ketone bodies by the liver. Sarcopenic obesity is a newly recognized geriatric syn-drome by age-related decline of low skeletal muscle plus a combined approach of overweight body mass that occurs with advancing age [18]. There are several factors contributing to the disorder. Chronic low-grade inflammation has been identified as the initiator in the early stages of many disorders such as physical disability, poor

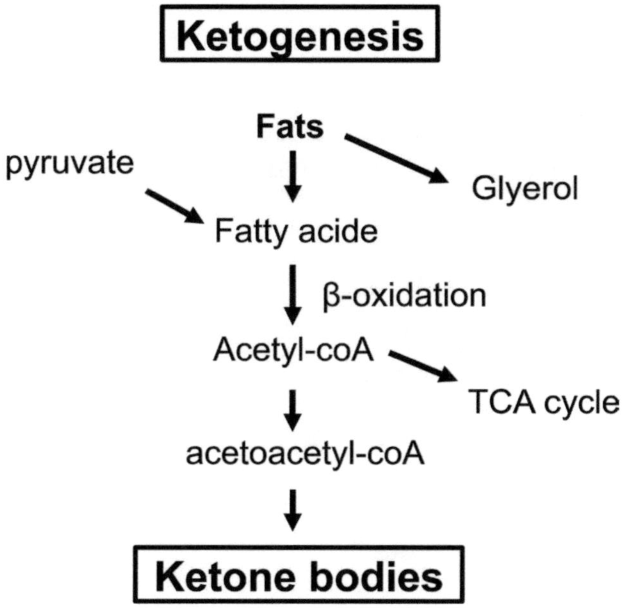

Figure 2.
Ketogenesis.

nutrition, and smoking [19, 20]. However, a widely accepted definition of sarcopenic obesity or obese sarcopenia suitable for use in research and clinical practice is still lacking. Sarcopenic obesity is increases the risk of aging-related type 2 diabetes susceptibility to obesity, and it can be the cause of functional dependence and disability in the elderly population [21]. Sarcopenic obesity was significantly associated with greater odds of sarcopenia, overfat, and sarcopenic obesity in women, but not in men [22]. Among older adult sarcopenic obesity characteristics, reduced lean mass at its extreme termed sarcopenia and excess body fatness are predictors of poor health outcomes in the general population. Sarcopenic obesity is at its extreme referred to as ketogenic diet of theorized compound these individual risks [23]. On average, by 20–40% for both men and women in sarcopenic obesity-induced muscles loss and overweight. Overall prevalence of sarcopenia was 26.7% in women and 73.3% in men, which increased with age. Prevalence of obesity was 74.6% in women and 67.1% in men [24]. Thus, defining sarcopenic obesity only in terms of muscle mass is too narrow maybe of limited clinical value that becomes more common in people over the age of 65. Sarcopenic obesity factor seropositivity, and a lack of current treatment with disease-modifying anti-sarcopenic obesity drugs were significantly associated with abnormal body composition such as increasing joint deformity, disability scores and C-reactive protein levels [25]. After middle age, adults lose 3% of their muscle strength every year, on average, to perform many routine activities [26]. These factors contribute to sarcopenic obesity to the characteristic skeletal muscle atrophy and weakness. Sarcopenic obesity also shortens life expectancy in those it affects, compared to individuals with normal muscle strength. Aging-related-sarcopenic obesity is caused by an imbalance between signals for muscle cell growth and signals for teardown [27]. Skeletal muscle cell growth processes are called "muscle anabolism," and fat cell teardown processes are called "fat catabolism" (**Figure 3**). Ketogenic diet acts with protein-destroying enzymes to keep muscle steady through a cycle of growth, stress or injury, destruction, and then healing. However, during aging your body becomes resistant to the growth signals, tipping the balance toward catabolism and muscle loss [28].

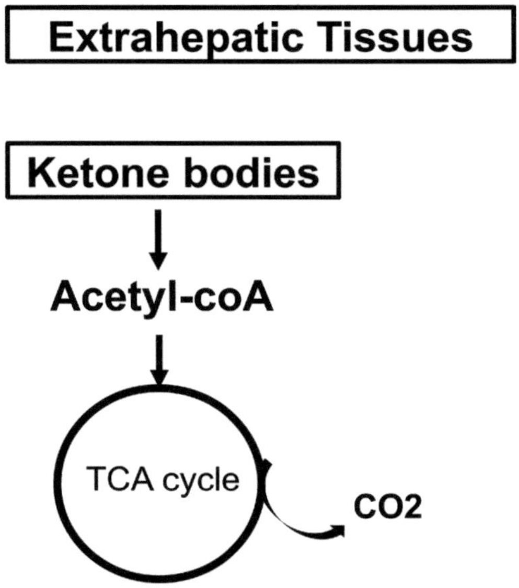

Figure 3.
The ketone bodies use. Extrahepatic tissues utilize them as respiratory substrates. The ketone bodies from the liver to the extrahepatic tissues coupled with very low activity of enzymes responsible for their utilization. Ketone bodies serve as a fuel for extrahepatic tissues.

The Older women with sarcopenic obesity have an increased all-cause mortality risk independent of obesity [29]. Sarcopenic obesity with obesity and aging, loss of muscle mass as a primary event, and this loss is a major contributor to fat gain, which in turn reinforces the muscle loss. Markedly elevated acetoacetic acid and β-hydroxybutyric acid production in the liver sarcopenic obesity. The various etiologic factors of sarcopenia in aging all lead to loss of muscle [30]. With the increase ketone body in skeletal muscle, acetoacetic acid and β-hydroxybutyric acid secretion are increased, and both lead to sarcopenic obesity resistance, which reduces the fat mass in sarcopenic obesity skeletal muscle and normal anabolic effect of insulin on amino acid transport in muscle [30, 31]. In addition, there is some evidence that acetoacetic acid and β-hydroxybutyric acid reduces fat mass secretion, suppressing another major anabolic stimulus. In addition, higher acetoacetic acid and β-hydroxybutyric acid levels may exert direct catabolic effects on muscle [32] (**Figure 4**).

Sarcopenic obesity in older adults is associated with skeletal poorer performance and strength parameters. Despite β-hydroxybutyric acid in clinical use as a therapy for sarcopenic obesity for several years, the ketogenic diet remains a therapy in search of an explanation [33]. The action of the ketogenic diet is the optimal indications for its clinical use are incompletely defined. We defined the abnormalities in body composition and abdominal fat that occur in sarcopenic obesity is associated with the aging-related presence of skeletal muscle dysfunction. Some features of clinical experience have been replicated in animal models, including the role of ketosis, elevation of triglyceride, total cholesterol, HMG CoA reductase, testosterone. Sarcopenic obesity by both classic ketogenic and β-hydroxybutyric acid diets are better effective at younger ages, and rapid reversal of the sarcopenic obesity effect when the diet is discontinued [34]. Sarcopenic obesity have been implicated in muscle atrophy and dysfunction due to denervation, muscular dystrophy, and disuse. A ketogenic diet plays key roles in sarcopenic obesity in muscle atrophy and the potential of the ketogenic diet for the treatment of sarcopenic obesity in regulating metabolism in skeletal muscle. Several β-hydroxybutyric acid isoforms are potential targets for intervention in sarcopenic obesity. Supplementary of

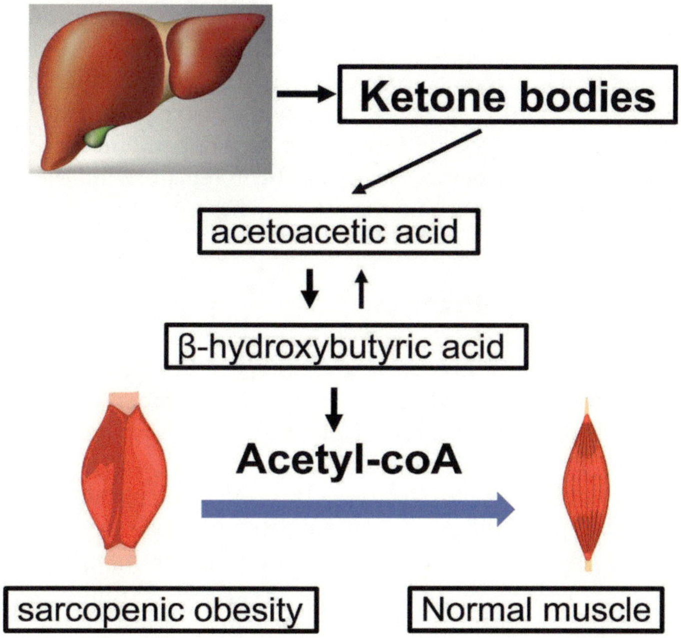

Figure 4.
A ketogenic diet can rebuild skeletal muscle. A ketogenic diet can help you lose fat in the skeletal muscle from sarcopenic obesity. β-hydroxybutyric acid provides the main fuel for moderate and high-intensity exercise.

acetoacetic acid and β-hydroxybutyric acid prevents muscle atrophy due to nutrient deprivation [35]. A ketogenic diet regulates metabolism in skeletal muscle and may inhibit oxidative metabolism during aging. Both of acetoacetic acid and β-hydroxybutyric acid have been implicated in muscle atrophy due to skeletal muscle denervation, a process implicated in sarcopenic obesity. Acetoacetic acid or β-hydroxybutyric acid is already in use in the clinic, and there is promise in targeting skeletal muscle for the treatment of sarcopenic obesity [36]. As in the clinical arena, there has been a recent resurgence of interest in pursuing basic questions related to the ketogenic diet. There have been very few animal studies of the ketogenic diet, and those that have been performed are difficult to compare because of wide discrepancies in experimental methods [37]. Earlier models concentrated on the effect of the ketogenic diet on sarcopenic obesity. The effects on the ketogenic diet and satiety, weight loss, and nitrogen balance are discussed as well as influences on electrolytes and the sympathetic system [38]. Hormonal changes of the ketogenic diet regimens and the impact on mood and subjective acceptance are compared. Experimental approaches such as brain metabolic pathways and histological techniques hold much promise in the effort to understand this intriguing alternative to standard ketogenic diet [39]. Though no recommendation for a particular dietary regimen is given, the different implications on the parameters described are pointed out. The global population is aging, the disease is younger and the influence of modern lifestyle, the clinic promotes personalized anti-aging programs, natural nutritional prescriptions, and preventive medical health management to awaken the body's original anti-aging self-healing power, allowing everyone to reverse the sub-healthy and healthy life, but it does also face the impact of modern diseases. It may be necessary to face the torture of the disease in advance, so the concept of health and advocating naturalness has gradually increased [40].

The ketogenic diet is good for your health. This results in the production of ketones, acetoacetic acid, and β-hydroxybutyric acid. The body uses for acetoacetic acid or β-hydroxybutyric acid to burns body fats, they can lead to weight loss. The possible mechanisms are a decrease in lipogenesis, an increase in lipolysis, and an increase in the metabolic cost of gluconeogenesis. Sarcopenia, obesity and their coexistence, obese sarcopenia, as well as sarcopenic obesity, are among the greatest health concerns in the aging population. A clear age-dependent increased prevalence of sarcopenia and sarcopenic obesity has been registered in the ketogenic diet therapy patients, suggesting mechanistic relationships.

3. Conclusion and future direction

Inflammation aging is a common ground for age-related sarcopenic obesity. Ketogenic diet therapy is observed greater weight loss compared with other balanced diets. The short-term ketogenic diet is by an almost carbohydrate-free oral diet might have weight loss effectively. Therefore, we suggest the benefits of the ketogenic diet and its risks including supports weight loss, reduce risk of cancers, improve heart health, protect brain function, aging-related sarcopenic obesity, and potentially reduces seizures. In this Chapter, we discuss the aging-related sarcopenic obesity. Nutrition, β-hydroxybutyric acid, in the early development of sarcopenic obesity, cardiomyopathy, dysbiosis and age-associated diseases is our future project. We want to know about sarcopenic obesity during COVID-19 lockdown restrictions. Like many difficult global health problems, the COVID-19 solutions maybe apparent but the logistics of implementing them may be lacking.

Author details

Sergey Suchkov[2], Tahereh Seifi Salmi[3], Chyi-Huey Bai[4], Javad Alizargar[1] and Jia-Ping Wu[1]*

1 Research Center for Healthcare Industry Innovation, National Taipei University of Nursing and Health Sciences, Taipei City, Taiwan, R.O.C

2 Immunology and Medicine, Research Center, Department of Pathology, I.M. Sechenov PMGMU, POB, Moscow, Russia

3 Sport Sciences Research Institute of Iran, Tehran, Iran

4 Department of Public Health, College of Medicine, Taipei Medical University, Taipei, Taiwan, R.O.C

*Address all correspondence to: affymax0823@yahoo.com.tw

References

[1] Kayode OT, Owolabi AV, Kayode AAA. Biochemical and histomorphological changes in testosterone propionate-induced benign prostatic hyperplasia in male Wistar rats treated with ketogenic diet. Biomed Pharmacother. 2020;132:110863.

[2] Cunha GM, Guzman G, Correa De Mello LL, Trein B, Spina L, Bussade I, et al. Efficacy of a 2-Month Very Low-Calorie Ketogenic Diet (VLCKD) Compared to a Standard Low-Calorie Diet in Reducing Visceral and Liver Fat Accumulation in Patients With Obesity. Front Endocrinol (Lausanne). 2020;11:607.

[3] Chen CY, Huang WS, Chen HC, Chang CH, Lee LT, Chen HS, et al. Effect of a 90 g/day low-carbohydrate diet on glycaemic control, small, dense low-density lipoprotein and carotid intima-media thickness in type 2 diabetic patients: An 18-month randomised controlled trial. PLoS One. 2020;15:e0240158.

[4] Carroll J, Koenigsberger D. The ketogenic diet: a practical guide for caregivers. J Am Diet Assoc. 1998;98:316-321.

[5] Stafstrom CE. Animal models of the ketogenic diet: what have we learned, what can we learn? Epilepsy Res. 1999;37:241-259.

[6] Taylor R, Agius L. The biochemistry of diabetes. Biochem J. 1988;250:625-640.

[7] Patel MS, Naik S, Wexler ID, Kerr DS. Gene regulation and genetic defects in the pyruvate dehydrogenase complex. J Nutr.1995;125:1753S–1757S.

[8] Ham DJ, Börsch A, Lin S, Thürkauf M, Weihrauch M, Reinhard JR, et al. The neuromuscular junction is a focal point of mTORC1 signaling in sarcopenia. Nat Commun. 2020;11:4510.

[9] Kusakabe T, Yokota S, Shimizu M, Inoue T, Tanaka M, Ohue-Kitano R, et al. Differential effects of sodium-glucose cotransporter 2 inhibitor and low-carbohydrate diet on body composition and metabolic profile in obese diabetic db/db mice. BMJ Open Diabetes Res Care. 2020;8.

[10] Nakao R, Shimba S, Oishi K. Ketogenic diet induces expression of the muscle circadian gene Slc25a25 via neural pathway that might be involved in muscle thermogenesis. Sci. Rep. 2017;7:2885.

[11] Goss AM, Gower B, Soleymani T, Stewart M, Pendergrass M, Lockhart M, et al. Effects of weight loss during a very low carbohydrate diet on specific adipose tissue depots and insulin sensitivity in older adults with obesity: a randomized clinical trial. Nutr Metab. 2020;17:64.

[12] Leite Góes Gitai D, de Andrade TG, Dos Santos YDR, Attaluri S, Shetty AK. Chronobiology of limbic seizures: Potential mechanisms and prospects of chronotherapy for mesial temporal lobe epilepsy. Neurosci Biobehav Rev. 2019;98:122-134.

[13] Weber DD, Aminzadeh-Gohari S, Tulipan J, Catalano L, Feichtinger RG, Kofler B. Ketogenic diet in the treatment of cancer - Where do we stand? Mol Metab. 2019;33:102-121.

[14] Stumpf SK, Berghoff SA, Trevisiol A, Spieth L, Düking T, Schneider LV, et al. Ketogenic diet ameliorates axonal defects and promotes myelination in Pelizaeus-Merzbacher disease. Acta Neuropathol. 2019;138:147-161.

[15] Goss AM, Gower B, Soleymani T, Stewart M, Pendergrass M, Lockhart M,

et al. Effects of weight loss during a very low carbohydrate diet on specific adipose tissue depots and insulin sensitivity in older adults with obesity: a randomized clinical trial. Nutr Metab. 2020;17:64.

[16] Paoli A, Rubini A, Volek JS, Grimaldi KA. Beyond weight loss: a review of the therapeutic uses of very-low-carbohydrate (ketogenic) diets. Eur J Clin Nutr. 2013;67:789-796.

[17] Shah P, Isley WL. Ketoacidosis during a low-carbohydrate diet. N Engl J Med. 2006;354:97-98.

[18] Kossoff EH, Zupec-Kania BA, Amark PE, et al. Optimal clinical management of children receiving the ketogenic diet: recommendations of the International Ketogenic Diet Study Group. Epilepsia. 2009;50:304-317.

[19] Paoli A. Review Ketogenic Diet for Obesity: Friend or Foe? Int J Environ Res Public Health. 2014;11:2092-2107.

[20] Magnusdottir OK, Gunnarsdottir I, Birgisdóttir BE. Dietary guidelines in type 2 diabetes: the Nordic diet or the ketogenic diet? Curr Opin Endocrinol Diabetes Obes. 2017;24:315-319.

[21] Newman J.C. Ketogenic diet reduces midlife mortality and improves memory in aging mice. Cell Metab. 2017;26:547-557.

[22] Hallbook T. The effects of the ketogenic diet on behavior and cognition. Epilepsy Res. 2012;100:304-309.

[23] Yang W, Lee JW, Kim Y, Lee JH, Kang HT. Increased Omega-3 Fatty Acid Intake is Inversely Associated with Sarcopenic Obesity in Women but not in Men, Based on the 2014-2018 Korean National Health and Nutrition Examination Survey. J Clin Med. 2020;9.

[24] Bagheri A, Soltani S, Hashemi R, Heshmat R, Motlagh AD, Esmaillzadeh A. Inflammatory potential of the diet and risk of sarcopenia and its components. Nutr J. 2020;19:129.

[25] Son J, Yu Q, Seo JS. Sarcopenic obesity can be negatively associated with active physical activity and adequate intake of some nutrients in Korean elderly: Findings from the Korea National Health and Nutrition Examination Survey (2008-2011). Nutr Res Pract.13:47-57.

[26] Park WJ, Jung DH, Lee JW, Shim JY, Kwon YJ. Association of platelet count with sarcopenic obesity in postmenopausal women: A nationwide population-based study. Clin Chim Acta. 2017;477:113-118.

[27] Ryu M, Jo J, Lee Y, Chung YS, Kim KM, Baek WC. Association of physical activity with sarcopenia and sarcopenic obesity in community-dwelling older adults: the Fourth Korea National Health and Nutrition Examination Survey. Age Ageing. 2013;42:734-740.

[28] Baek SJ, Nam GE, Han KD, Choi SW, Jung SW, Bok AR, et al. Sarcopenia and sarcopenic obesity and their association with dyslipidemia in Korean elderly men: the 2008-2010 Korea National Health and Nutrition Examination Survey. J Endocrinol Invest. 2014; 37:247-260.

[29] Castaño G, Arruzazabala ML, Fernández L, Mas R, Carbajal D, Molina V, et al. Effects of combination treatment with policosanol and omega-3 fatty acids on platelet aggregation: A randomized, double-blind clinical study. Curr Ther Res Clin Exp. 2006;67:174-192.

[30] Welch C, Greig C, Masud T, Wilson D, Jackson TA. COVID-19 and Acute Sarcopenia. Aging Dis. 2020;11:1345-1351.

[31] Mailer RKW, Hänel L, Allende M, Renné T. Polyphosphate as a Target

forInterference With Inflammation and Thrombosis. Front Med.2019;6:76.

[32] Dedkova EN, Blatter LA. Role of β-hydroxybutyrate, its polymer poly-β-hydroxybutyrate and inorganic polyphosphate in mammalian health and disease. Front Physiol. 2014;5:260.

[33] Elustondo PA, Angelova PR, Kawalec M, Michalak M, Kurcok P, Abramov AY, et al. Polyhydroxybutyrate targets mammalian mitochondria and increases permeability of plasmalemmal and mitochondrial membranes. PLoS One. 2013;8: e75812.

[34] Sato S, Namisaki T, Furukawa M, Saikawa S, Kawaratani H, Kaji K, et al. Effect of L-carnitine on health-related quality of life in patients with liver cirrhosis. Biomed Rep. 2020;13:65.

[35] Ogura Y, Kakehashi C, Yoshihara T, Kurosaka M, Kakigi R, Higashida K, et al. Ketogenic diet feeding improves aerobic metabolism property in extensor digitorum longus muscle of sedentary male rats. PLoS One. 2020;15:e0241382.

[36] Qian M, Wu N, Li L, Yu W, Ouyang H, Liu X, et al. Effect of Elevated Ketone Body on Maternal and Infant Outcome of Pregnant Women with Abnormal Glucose Metabolism During Pregnancy. Diabetes Metab Syndr Obes. 2020; 13:4581-4588.

[37] Long J, Yang Z, Wang L, Han Y, Peng C, Yan C, et al. Metabolite biomarkers of type 2 diabetes mellitus and pre-diabetes: a systematic review and meta-analysis. BMC Endocr Disord. 2020;20:174.

[38] Ogura Y, Kakehashi C, Yoshihara T, Kurosaka M, Kakigi R, Higashida K, et al. Ketogenic diet feeding improves aerobic metabolism property in extensor digitorum longus muscle of sedentary male rats. PLoS One. 2020;15:e0241382.

[39] Si J, Wang Y, Xu J, Wang J. Antiepileptic effects of exogenous β-hydroxybutyrate on kainic acid-induced epilepsy. Exp Ther Med. 2020; 20:177.

[40] Bradshaw PC, Seeds WA, Miller AC, Mahajan VR, Curtis WM. COVID-19: Proposing a Ketone-Based Metabolic Therapy as a Treatment to Blunt the Cytokine Storm. Oxid Med Cell Longev. 2020;2020:6401341.

Section 2

Causes of Obesity

Chapter 6

Lifestyle Factors and Obesity

Anca Mihaela Hâncu

Abstract

Obesity, with growing prevalence around the world, is a disease and a major risk factor for noncommunicable diseases and death. Lifestyle medicine integrates modern lifestyle practices with scientific evidence-based medicine in order to lower risk factors for chronic diseases and to support therapy if the disease is already present. Considering adiposity-based chronic disease conceptual model and new abdominal obesity classification, this article intends to describe healthy lifestyle pillars that must be considered in obesity prevention and treatment. Right nutrition, regular physical activity, optimal sleep, moderation in alcohol consumption, absence of smoking, and mindfulness should be considered in the effort to prevent and treat obesity. Doctor-patient partnership, patient empowerment, and doctor as a role model will complete the basic principle of lifestyle medicine.

Keywords: lifestyle medicine, obesity, overweight, physical activity, sedentarism, nutrition

1. Introduction

Obesity prevalence is growing around the world, since 1975 it has increased by 300%. According to WHO, in 2016, overweight people were 2 billion and obese 650 million, meaning 39% overweight and 13% obesity around the world [1]. In 2020, worldwide, 39 million children under the age of 5 were overweight and obese and for the group between 5 and 19 years, more than 340 million children were overweight or obese [1]. In the USA, there are more recent data, from The National Health and Nutrition Examination Survey, evidenced by the US Department of Health and Human Services, Centers for Disease Control and Prevention, National Center for Health Statistics [2]. According to CDC, in the USA, in 2017–2018, the age-adjusted prevalence of obesity was 42% for adults, without significant differences between men and women. For severe obesity, age-adjusted prevalence is 9.2%, but higher in women vs. men. The age group 40–59 includes the highest prevalence of severe obesity.

1.1 Health concerns associated with obesity

Overweight and obesity represent major risks for noncommunicable diseases (NCDs), linearly correlated with BMI.

- cardiovascular diseases (CVDs) are the leading cause of death, ischemic heart disease representing 16% of total mortality globally in 2019, according to WHO [1].

- diabetes, the ninth position in mortality causes in 2019 [1]
- musculoskeletal disorders
- some cancers—breast, endometrial, ovarian, livers, prostate, gall-bladder, colon, and kidney.

Children's obesity is facing breathing difficulties, hypertension, insulin resistance, higher fractures risk, and psychological effects. Moreover, childhood obesity is correlated with a higher risk of obesity, premature death, and disability in adulthood.

The double burden of malnutrition and obesity is characterizing low- and middle-income countries. Infectious diseases, together with undernutrition, are common; meanwhile, an increase in risk factors such as obesity and overweight can be seen in urban settings. Co-existing undernutrition with obesity is common in the same community, where inadequate dietary patterns combined with lower levels of physical activity have increased childhood obesity in conjunction with an unsolved undernutrition issue.

2. Lifestyle medicine (LM) definition

Described for the first time by the famous Professor James Rippe, cardiologist, in 1989, lifestyle medicine is defined as:

"The integration of lifestyle practices into the modern practice of medicine both to lower the risk factors for chronic disease and/or, if disease is already present, serve as an adjunct in its therapy. Lifestyle medicine brings together sound, scientific evidence in diverse health-related fields to assist the clinician in the process of not only treating disease, but also promoting good health" [3].

3. Obesity new conceptual model

Prof Mechanick introduced, some years ago, a conceptual model that is adiposity-based chronic disease (ABCD), with four stages. The first stage means the risk—genetics, environment, and behavior. The second is when can be noticed an increased amount of adipose tissue with abnormal distribution or function. The disease is named in the third stage, diagnosed by biochemical, anthropometrical tests, measured by body mass index. The fourth stage associates cardiometabolic and biomechanical complications. ABCD is a part of cardiometabolic chronic disease stages that develop through dysglycemia-based chronic disease (DBCD) and cardiometabolic-based chronic disease (CMBCD). This is the new frame describing all metabolic interrelations and evolution through obesity [4]. This is a more comprehensive model to define obesity and explain its treatment.

4. Bioimpedance

The use of bioimpedance to measure tissue's resistance during the passage of low-intensity electric current, based on the principle of variation of the rate of passage of electric current through the body in relation to body composition is widely used, is a good tool in clinical practice. This analysis is offering almost good data about body composition and may be a good tracker of treatment performances [5].

BMI kg/m^2	WC—women (cm)	WC—men (cm)
18,5–24,9	≥80	≥90
25–29,9	≥90	≥100
30–34,9	≥105	≥110
≥35	≥115	≥125

Table 1.
Abdominal obesity classification, adapted after [6].

5. Abdominal obesity classification

A new classification is proposed since February 2020 (**Table 1**) [6].

For each BMI category, another level of waist circumference WC is recommended to identify abdominal fat (adapted after reference [6]) in order to have a more reliable picture of the abdominal distribution of fat.

6. Eating behaviors General indications for people with obesity

This is emphasized by guidelines: European Association for the Study of Obesity EASO 2019 guidelines are emphasizing the importance of eating behaviors [7]. The energetic density of the food should be decreased by eating a lot of vegetables and fruits, within the limit of five portions. Eating less refined carbohydrates and less fatty foods, especially saturated fats and small portions, may support these indications EASO guidelines recommend:

1. To avoid skipping meals but also snacking continuously between meals,

2. Eat slowly, in order to facilitate the satiation sensation that will appear after 20 min,

3. Eat in response to your hungry sensation and stop eating when you feel full,

4. Keep a diary in order to increase awareness of eating habits, and

5. Eating mindfully—slowly, responsible, taking a relaxing moment, sitting down at the table, observing emotions, paying attention to taste, texture, flavor, and temperature of the food.

7. Eating disorders

It describes a group of mental illnesses characterized by disturbed feeding behavior and body weight regulation, compromising key physiological systems, including cardiovascular and gastrointestinal functions [8]. They are as follows:

- anorexia nervosa (AN)

- bulimia nervosa (BN)

- binge eating disorder (BED)

- other unspecified or specified eating disorders that do not fit within these diagnoses.

The shared symptoms for eating disorders are caloric restriction, binging, purging, over-evaluation of body weight.

Detailed anamnesis should reveal these symptoms and a multidisciplinary approach with a psychologist/psychiatrist should be performed in such situations.

8. Nutrition for a healthy lifestyle in treating and managing obesity

Modern nutrition emphasizes that not only singular food or nutrient is important, but also the combination of nutrients in different foods and dishes. That means healthy models will be used instead of pointing out single nutrients.

9. A healthy model

A healthy model, the latest 4-year winner, as the best nutritional model (US News and World Report 2021) is a Mediterranean model (Med Diet).

Mediterranean model: Like was firstly described by Ancel Keys on the occasion of Seven Countries Study, Med Diet is a plant-based diet, with abundant seasonal vegetables, fresh fruits as deserts, olive oil as the main source of fats, fish for 2–3 times/week, regularly nuts and seeds, daily whole cereals, dairies many times per week, red meat only rare, spices and herbs for tasty recipes. The important feature is unprocessed food cooked at home or in small restaurants, in antagonism with the Western diet, characterized mainly by highly processed food [9]. The uniqueness of this model derives from the combination of biologically active foods, with the right proportion between sources of fat, proteins, starches, fibers, minerals, vitamins, and bioactive compounds.

9.1 What are the mechanisms supporting these benefits? Several clinical pathways and molecular mechanisms have been studied, suggesting beneficial changes induced by this dietary pattern

Oxidative stress reduction and anti-inflammatory properties are attributed to bioactive components of food. The high content of polyphenols and low diet inflammatory index (DII) are correlated with all benefits. For example,

- DNA methylation and tumor suppressors are associated with polyphenolic compounds found in grapes, peanuts, extra virgin olive oil (EVOO) [10].
- Anthocyanins—pigments found in eggplants, berries, pomegranates, cruciferous stimulate DNA repair mechanisms [11].
- Fisetin is a flavonoid contained in strawberries, apples, cucumbers, which prevent cancer growth [12].
- Sulforaphane from cruciferous vegetables exerts epigenetic actions through histone deacetylase enzyme inhibition [13].
- A key mechanism explaining Med Diet benefits is gut microbiota, an important player in the relation health/diet, particularly through short-chain fatty acids (SCFAs) metabolites derived from microbial fermentation. Decreased Firmicutes and increased Bacteroides and fecal SCFAs are in line with high adherence to Med Diet, conversely for a healthy microbiota. High SCFAs lead

to increased production of butyrate, acetate, and propionate [14]. High-fiber content is another hallmark of the Med Diet. It has to be mentioned that 2 h of psychological stress may change completely gut bacteria. Butyrate-producing bacteria are increasing the quality of life.

9.2 Studies supporting med diet

Historically, the first study was done in the years 50, Seven Countries Study, which launched the concept defined by Angel Key, Med Diet. Later, Predimed, SUN, and LION are studies that proved different benefits of this eating model.

9.3 Benefits

Benefits proved already in significant studies mentioned before are increased longevity, cardiovascular protection, diabetes decreased incidence, diabetes management, prevention of cognitive decline, dementia, depression, obesity, metabolic syndrome, chronic respiratory diseases but also impact on sustainability [15].

Important in obesity management and higher Med Diet adherence, realized in participants from EPIC-PANACEA study, showed lower weight gain at 5 years vs. participants with low adherence, but also the risk of becoming obese decreased by 10% [16].

Not only a diet, but a lifestyle model, Med Diet means daily consumption of whole grain products, various fresh vegetables and fruits, nuts, seeds, and legumes several times per week. The main source of fat is olive oil and adding herbs and spices will help to decrease salt at recommended intake of <2, 3 mg sodium per day. Sweets will mostly be replaced by fruits. Dairies' daily consumption was mainly represented by yogurt or kefir, cheese in smaller quantities. Up to three times per week were fish and seafood, eggs were 2–4 times/week, and red meat in small portions was very rare (1–2 times monthly). Hydration will be done mainly through water, drinking may be allowed in small quantities, and the wine will be preferred instead of beer (1 drink per day for women, 2 drinks for men). Med Diet means also

Two servings per day	Vegetables like cabbage, tomatoes, eggplants, broccoli Fresh fruits—apples, oranges, cherries, bananas, occasionally fresh juice 100% Whole grains—bread, oat, cereals for breakfast, biscuits
One serving daily	Low GI cereals rice, barley, whole grain pasta Nuts and seeds—almonds, nuts, sunflower seeds, pumpkin seeds Extra virgin olive oil Unflavored yogurt
Four servings/week	Legumes Fish, fresh, frozen, all types white, but also salmon, cod, mackerel, shellfish, tuna
Maximum three portions/ week	White meat—unprocessed turkey, poultry Eggs Cheese—Parmesan, Roquefort, Emmental Milk
Less than two servings/week	Starchy food with high GI—white bread, potatoes, biscuits, refined rice Red meat—unprocessed pork, beef, lamb Butter
Occasionally	Processed meat

Table 2.
Suggested food model for consumption.

a philosophy of cooking at home or with friends, with a preference for local food, minimally processed, connection with nature, respect for nature, sustainability, moderate portion sizes, moderate physical activity, appropriate rest, eating in other people company.

A recent review published in Cardiovascular Research 2021 [17] points some elements related to cardiovascular/atherosclerosis protection. Moderate quantities of cheese and regular yogurt are linked with a protective effect, to replace high glycemic index food with whole grain and low glycemic index (GI) cereal food. A future target will be to promote appropriate food choices for atherosclerosis prevention in the general population, the authors are suggesting.

9.4 A suggested food model for consumption

It is presented in **Table** 2 adapted after [17].

All these recommendations should be followed, in a frame of negative energetic balance, in order to lose weight.

10. Energy balance

Creating a negative energy balance is the first principle for lifestyle intervention in obesity. A daily caloric deficit of 0.5–1 kg will ensure a healthy weight decrease. A healthy weight decrease means 0.5–1 kg/week weight decrease. The decrease has to be mainly from fat mass and not muscular mass, proportion has to be 80% fat and 20% lean mass.

11. As dietary guidelines for Americans for 2020–2025 is mentioning

11.1 Sodium

This is an essential nutrient consumed primarily as salt—sodium chloride—is indicated in a daily maximum intake of 2–3 mg [18].

11.2 Coffee

After some irrelevant studies, a new meta-analysis found that three cups of coffee per day are related to a 10%, respectively, 16% risk reduction of CHD incidence and mortality. But this benefic effect disappears at doses higher than five cups/day [17]. Coffee consumption is associated with higher insulin sensitivity and lower risk of type 2 diabetes together with a low concentration of inflammatory markers such as C reactive protein and E selectin. These benefits are due to its phenolic compounds and magnesium, potassium, and niacin. It has to be mentioned that unfiltered coffee, which contains cafestol may increase total cholesterol levels, with a detrimental effect. Special conditions, like hypertension and arrhythmias, will require special caution for coffee consumption. In conclusion, a moderate coffee consumption, below three cups/day may be suggested.

11.3 Tea

Tea intake is also associated with coronary heart disease (CHD) risk reduction, mainly green tea, and 20% risk decrease being reported at three cups per day. Atherosclerosis prevention is related to catechin content, with high antioxidative properties, contributing to modulate plasma lipid profile, decreasing inflammation at endothelial level, atherogenesis and thrombogenesis.

12. Chrono-nutrition

It is a concept detailed in lifestyle recommendations for the prevention of metabolic syndrome. Potential health problems may arise for shift workers. Overall night working or rotating working is associated with a higher risk of insulin resistance, metabolic syndrome, and heart disease. The recommendation is to eat the main meal of the day before 3 PM [19].

Actual society, westernized, 24/7 means that eating moments are distributed over day and night without a clear schedule. Many people eat late in the evening or even during the night, this leading to a metabolic risk similar to shift workers. Even short-term misalignment, like jet lag or long flights, may cause bowel problems or fatigue. Not surprisingly, circadian misalignment may contribute to different medical conditions, being incriminated in the etiology of type 2 diabetes. The mechanism is insulin resistance at the tissues level, caused by disrupted tissue clocks. As Oosterman is mentioning, it is maybe the time to include in dietary guidelines, in addition to quantity and quality of food the concept of time of meals, which is a critical determinant of metabolic health. Increasing awareness about the relation between eating time and metabolic implications will be a part of the complex system to fight against obesity [20].

13. Sustainability: Food for planet health

In January 2019, The Lancet published the Summary Report of the EAT-*Lancet* Commission, 2019 named Food, Planet, Health [21]. This report is a manifesto for sustainability, proposing a nutrition model for sustainable eating for 10 billion people. This model assumes that until 2050, substantial dietary shifts are necessary. Globally, the consumption of red meat and sugar has to be reduced by more than 50%, and fruits, vegetables, nuts, and legumes have to be doubled. The rich plant-based diet will confer health but also environmental benefits. This model is aspirational and will be implemented step by step, in accordance with country's educational development.

14. Healthy models

DASH and Nordic models are also healthy models, with similarities with Med Diet, and may be applied successfully, in accordance with cultural traditions and personal preferences in order to maximize adherence.

15. Sedentarism

It is the fourth risk factor for death [22] and large studies are revealing a great mortality risk associated with sedentarism. Ekelund investigated in a large meta-analysis sedentary behavior effects on more than 1 million persons, revealing an association between all-cause mortality and the level of physical activity. There have been compared sitting periods of less than 4 h/day with the highest quartile of moderate or intense physical activity. One metabolic equivalent (MET) is defined as the amount of oxygen consumed while sitting at rest and is equal to 3.5 ml O_2 per kg body weight × min. "The metabolic equivalent of task, or simply metabolic equivalent, is a physiological measure expressing the intensity of physical activities. One MET is the energy equivalent expended by an individual while seated at rest.

There is no risk for people sitting more than 8 h/day, but having more than 35, 5 MET h/week of activity (HR = 1.04, 95% CI–1.1). But those being in the lowest physical activity PA quartile, below 2.5 MET h/week and sitting <4 h/day had an increased risk. *The study conclusion is that 60–75 min/day of physical activity may attenuate or even eliminate the detrimental effect of sedentary style on health outcomes* [23, 24]. **Definition of sitting behavior** (SB): The common behavior that is considered a health threat is sitting. There are two modern definitions of SB [25].

1. The first of these definitions is purely physiological and is synonymous with the lower end of the energy expenditure continuum <1.5 METs [25], which includes also standing quietly.

2. The second definition has three components:

   Postural—in a sitting or reclining posture.

   Contextual—walking time.

   Physiological <1,5 METs.

16. Physical activity (PA)

16.1 Definitions (based on WHO 2020 guidelines)

Light PA (1.6–3.0 METs), moderate (3–6 METs), and intense (>6 METs) [26].

Light-intensity physical activity.

Light-intensity physical activity is between 1.6 and 3 METs, that is, activities with energy cost less than three times the energy expenditure at rest for that person. This can include slow walking, bathing, or other incidental activities that do not result in a substantial increase in heart rate or breathing rate.

Moderate-intensity physical activity.

On an absolute scale, moderate-intensity refers to the physical activity that is performed between three and less than six times the intensity of rest. On a scale relative to an individual's personal capacity, moderate-intensity physical activity is usually a 5 or 6 on a scale of 0–10; intense PA is at a level higher than 6 MET's..

16.2 Physical activity

This is essential for health and is an important component of a healthy lifestyle. Promoting continuously all PA benefits will lead finally to a higher percentage of people adopting healthy behaviors. The latest WHO guidelines [26] include the major developments vs. 2010 guidelines, being realized based on larger scientific evidence. Additional health benefits are supported by studies-cognitive health improvement, mental health, sleep, and health-related quality of life, and are emphasized beyond traditionally known benefits for cancer prevention, metabolic diseases prevention, cardiorespiratory fitness improvement, and musculoskeletal and functional health. All these documents are reflecting a maturity of the research, but also the complexity of WHO's definition of health as "a state of complete physical, mental and social wellbeing" [27].

Mentioning that a relation between cardiovascular cause mortality, all-cause mortality, and PA is well proved, WHO guidelines are reaffirming that any level and all intensities of PA are associated with low mortality risk. The incidence of type 2 diabetes is decreasing proportionally with PA level. Benefits are also proven in hypertension, cardiovascular disease, colon cancer, and breast cancer. Meanwhile, adiposity is inversely related to PA and sleep and quality of life (QOL) may be considerably improved according to the level of PA. Development of depression and anxiety may be slower for active people. Guideline's conclusions are that any level of any intensity of PA is associated with lower mortality from all causes but also with reduced incidence for type 2 diabetes, hypertension, and cardiovascular disease.

16.3 Recommendations for adults 18: 64 years

- Regular physical activity for all adults, a strong recommendation.
- Period: About 150–300 min of moderate PA or at least 75–150-min high-intensity PA or a combination of both, also a strong recommendation.
- Muscle training activities have to be performed >2 days/week, providing supplementary benefits and strong recommendation.
- Period of PA may be extended to more than 300 min/150 min for moderate/ intense PA in order to gain additional benefits for health, and this is just a conditional recommendation.
- In conclusion, any type of PA is better than none, even if not meeting these recommendations, at least some PA will be beneficial.
- The level of PA should be increased gradually in frequency and intensity, adapted to the training stage.

There are specific recommendations for limiting sedentary behavior, which are as follows:

- The time spent sedentary should be limited and replaced with PA of any intensity, even if light PA in order to provide some health benefits.
- For compensating the detrimental effect of sedentarism, levels of PA should be overcome.

16.4 Recommendations for older adults

Older adults (> 64y) usually have a very low level of physical activity. WHO guidelines are emphasizing rules even for this period of life, bringing the same benefits as for the other adults. Additionally, for older adults, PA may prevent falls and injuries, a decline in bone density and functionality also will attenuate the decline of muscular mass.

Recommendations for older adults are (as described by WHO guidelines 2020) as follows:

- PA should be regularly performed by any older adults.

- For moderate level, 150–300 min/week.
- For intense level, 75–150 min/week will be enough, bringing substantial health benefits.
- Additionally, 2 or more days for strengthening major muscle groups will substantiate benefits.
- Weekly training should be performed in multiple activities that support functional balance 3 days/week.
- If possible, the period of moderate activities will be increased, together with additional benefits for health and quality of life.

Important for older adults is that any activity is better than inactivity and PA should be increased gradually, based on personal functional capacities and fitness level.

17. Optimal sleep

Optimal sleep is a condition for a healthy lifestyle. The quality of good sleep will be recognized by three elements:

- Duration, that has to be sufficient for remaining alert and rested for the whole day
- Continuity, sleeping without fragmentation
- Depth, in order to restore functional capabilities

17.1 Sleep disorders

These disorders, like insomnia or sleep apnea, are related to obesity. In the obesity management process, Sleep Hygiene guidelines elaborated by the World Sleep Society may prevent poor quality nocturnal sleep, fragmentation of sleep, short duration of sleep, and even sleep deprivation in adults.

17.2 Ten lessons for a healthy sleep for adults, recommended by world sleep society (2021 world sleep day), will be simple and concrete lifestyle advice in obesity management

1. To fix the bedtime and constant awakening time [28]
2. Siesta's habit should not exceed 45 min/day
3. About 4 h before bedtime avoids alcohol ingestion and smoking
4. Avoid caffeine (tea, coffee, sodas, chocolate) for a period of 6 h before bedtime.
5. Before bedtime only a light snack may be accepted, but not heavy meals with spicy, sugary foods, 4 h before sleep.

6. Regular physical activity may not be prolonged before sleep time.

7. Try to use a comfortable bedroom

8. The bedroom should have a comfortable setting temperature for sleeping and good ventilation.

9. All distracting noise should be avoided in the bedroom and light as much as possible.

10. The bed must be used for sleep and sex. No eating, working, or sitting in bed.

17.3 Sleep deprivation risks

Short sleep duration is associated with hypercaloric food and an elevated intake of fats. Sleep may impact the time of meals, being related to intake behaviors. Specific evidence points out altered eating behavior, with frequent snacks, which are described as highly palatable and energy-dense throughout the whole day but also concentrated during the night for some short sleepers. These are important aspects, contributing to an unhealthy diet, predisposing people to noncommunicable diseases, and obesity. During anamnesis, a question about the duration and quality/depth of sleep is mandatory, as short sleep or sleep disorders are closely related to obesity [29].

18. Smoking

A healthy lifestyle means no smoking. Continuous efforts should be done by the medical community to stop smoking and decrease the number of people starting smoking.

18.1 Smoking cessation and weight gain

Smoking cessation is a real challenge and weight gain associated has to be carefully managed [30].

Particularly important for people with type 2 diabetes, due to their high cardiovascular risk augmented by insulin resistance and smoking. However, if smoking cessation is accompanied by weight gain—usually 4 kg/year of abstinence—this will dilute the health benefits of quitting. Nutritional counseling should be done in parallel with smoking cessation in order to maintain weight.

19. Alcohol

A healthy lifestyle may allow two glasses of wine for men/one glass of wine per day for women, or one can of beer. A level of 24 g of alcohol/day, for example, two glasses of wine is associated with 32% total CVD risk reduction in a meta-analysis with total CVD as the endpoint. How could be explained this risk reduction? Benefits exerted on lipid and glucose/insulin metabolism synergically with systemic subclinical anti-inflammatory and anticoagulation effects are the answer. Certainly, higher quantities are associated with a progressive increase of risk. Meanwhile, this meta-analysis shows a 20% lower risk of CVD for beer drinkers (one can per day) vs. abstainers, in concordance with previous studies. The dose–response analysis suggests a J shape curve, after initial risk decreases, and an immediate growing positive trend is seen when doses are increasing. About 10 g per day of alcohol—a small intake, may be the dose correlated with the highest risk reduction. But, as Prof Riccardi emphasized, this dose should be considered maximal allowed intake and not daily recommended dose [18].

20. Mindfulness

The balance between mind, thoughts, body, and emotions is the concept that may be the base of creating the right, positive mindset for treating obesity. People should be able to build motivation and create positive energy, to have meaning in life. All of these will build the mindset of a winner, with the right approach in front of the disease named obesity. People should understand that obesity is a disease, and treatment is the right mindset, applied in daily life. Mindful eating principles, eating smart, but also intuitively, responsible, as an assumed decision for health are fundamental in the obesity management [31].

21. Healthy lifestyle, not dieting

Increasing populational awareness about lifestyle medicine for obesity prevention and treatment is mandatory in order to further control NCDs expansion. WHO defines obesity as a disease and emphasizes that the treatment is a whole life treatment. Lifestyle education is mandatory in the future. Intervention in obesity should be a lifelong intervention and the doctor should be a partner for the patient, guiding him/her in this process. "Food is medicine" is a concept released some years ago in order to motivate more people to connect each eating decision with health benefits. Intuitive eating is an eating type that could influence an individual's awareness of food choices. It is negatively related to weight cycling and disordered eating and positively associated with weight stability and body satisfaction [32]. There is a way of eating in response to hunger/satiety and to create a positive relationship with food. The key is to prioritize behavioral changes, targeting not only the weight but with a focus on overall well-being. Flexible restraint may reduce binge eating and increase weight loss. Eating for health must balance social, hedonic, and environmental reasons to eat. Intuitive eating could help people to reconnect with signals of hunger and satiety. Eating in the absence of hunger is very frequent, triggered by social, emotional, or advertising factors. Clinicians are in the position to help patients to recognize various factors influencing eating choices and they should support their patients to make healthy choices [31].

22. Doctor-patient partnership

The key to lifestyle changes is negotiation and cooperation. Physicians will be role models for their patients, adopting a "coach" approach, instead of the previous "expert" style. But they will not only educate patients and have to empower them, motivating and planning a healthy lifestyle with sustainable change [33].

23. Conclusion

Health is built every moment by right decisions or, on the contrary, is destroyed. The success of health promotion at the populational level requires a different approach. Lifestyle starts from everyone's small daily decisions to community engagement and populational measures, all with a long-term impact.

By creating a doctor-patient partnership, it will be possible to create an optimal motivational approach that will change behaviors. Firstly, medical doctors should adopt healthy lifestyles and become role models for their patients and the whole community.

Conflict of interest

The authors declare no conflict of interest.

Author details

Anca Mihaela Hâncu
Nutriscience Clinic, Bucharest, Romania

*Address all correspondence to: ancahancu@gmail.com

References

[1] He H, Wang B, Zhou M, Cao L, Qiu W, Mu G, et al. Systemic inflammation mediates the associations between abdominal obesity indices and lung function decline in a Chinese general population. Diabetes, Metabolic Syndrome and Obesity: Targets and Therapy. 2020;**13**:141-150 141

[2] Craig M. Hales, M.D., Margaret D. Carroll, M.S.P.H., Cheryl D. Fryar, M.S.P.H., and Cynthia L. Ogden, Ph.D. Prevalence of Obesity and Severe Obesity Among Adults: United States, 2017-2018. NCHS Data Brief. No. 360 February 2020.

[3] Rippe J. Lifestyle medicine. 3rd ed. CRC Press, Taylor & Francis Group; 2019 May 19

[4] Mechanick JI, Farkouh ME, Newman JD, Garvey WT. Cardiometabolic-based chronic disease, addressing knowledge and clinical practice gaps JACC state-of-the-art review. 2020;**75**(5) This is a more comprehensive model to define obesity and to explain its treatment

[5] Dehghan M, Merchant AT. Is bioelectrical impedance accurate for use in large epidemiological studies? Nutrition Journal. 2008;**7**:26

[6] Waist circumference as a vital sign in clinical practice: A consensus Statement from the IAS and ICCR Working Group on Visceral Obesity, published online, 04.02.2020, Nature Reviews Endocrinology

[7] Schutz D et al. Management of obesity by GP's. Obesity Facts. 2019;**12**:40-66

[8] Lam YY, Maguire S, Palacios T, Caterson ID. Are the gut bacteria telling us to eat or not to eat? Reviewing the role of gut microbiota in the etiology, disease progression and treatment of eating disorders. Nutrients. June 2017

[9] Dominguez LJ, Di Bella G, Veronese N, Barbagallo M. Impact of mediterranean diet on chronic non-communicable diseases and longevity. Nutrients. 2021;**13**:2028

[10] Selvakumar P, Badgeley A, Murphy P, Anwar H, Sharma U, Lawrence K, et al. Flavonoids and other polyphenols act as epigenetic modifiers in breast cancer. Nutrients. 2020;**12**:761

[11] Ratovitski EA. Anticancer natural compounds as epigenetic modulators of gene expression. Current Genomics. 2017;**18**:175-205

[12] Kashyap D, Sharma A, Sak K, Tuli HS, Buttar HS, Bishayee A. Fisetin: A bioactive phytochemical with potential for cancer prevention and pharmacotherapy. Life Sciences. 2018;**194**:75-87

[13] Kaufman-Szymczyk A, Majewski G, Lubecka-Pietruszewska K, Fabianowska-Majewska K. The role of sulforaphane in epigenetic mechanisms, including interdependence between histone modification and DNA methylation. International Journal of Molecular Sciences. 2015;**16**:29732-29743

[14] De Filippis F, Pellegrini N, Vannini L, Jeffery IB, La Storia A, Laghi L, et al. High-level adherence to a Mediterranean diet beneficially impacts the gut microbiota and associated metabolome. Gut. 2016;**65**:1812-1821

[15] Estruch R, Ros E, Salas-Salvado J, Covas MI, Corella D, Aros F, et al. Primary prevention of cardiovascular disease with a mediterranean diet supplemented with extra-virgin olive oil or nuts. The New England Journal of Medicine. 2018;**378**:e34

[16] Romaguera D, Norat T, Vergnaud AC, Mouw T, May AM,

Agudo A, et al. Mediterranean dietary patterns and prospective weight change in participants of the EPIC-PANACEA project. The American Journal of Clinical Nutrition. 2010;**92**:912-921

[17] Riccardi G, Giosue A, Calabrese I, Vaccaro O. Dietary recommendations for prevention of atherosclerosis. Cardiovascular Research. 2021;**00**:1-17

[18] www.dietaryguidelines.gov

[19] Pérez-Martınez P, Mikhailidis DP, Athyros VG, Bullo M, Couture P, Covas MI, et al. Lifestyle recommendations for the prevention and management of metabolic syndrome: an international panel recommendation. Nutrition Reviews. 2017;**75**(5):307-326

[20] Oosterman JE, Wopereis S, Kalsbeek A. The circadian clock, shift work, and tissue specific insulin-resistance. Diabetologia. 2020;**63**:2253-2259

[21] Summary Report of the EAT-*Lancet* Commission, 2019 named Food, Planet, Health

[22] WHO Global Health Risks: Mortality and Burden of Disease Attributable to Selected Major Risks. Geneva, Switzerland: WHO Press; 2009, 2009

[23] Wartderton DE, Nicol CW, Bredin SS. Health benefits of physical activity. CMAJ. 2006;**1**:74801-74809

[24] Ekelund U, Steene-Johannessen J, Brown WJ, Fagerland MW, Owen N, Powell KE, et al. Does physical activity attenuate, or even eliminate, the detrimental association of sitting time with mortality? A harmonised meta-analysis of data from more than 1 million men and women. Lancet. 2016;**388**:1302-1310

[25] Stamatakis E et al. Is the time right for quantitative public health guidelines on sitting? A narrative review of sedentary behaviour research paradigms and findings. British Journal of Sports Medicine. 2019;**53**:377-382

[26] WHO Guidelines on Physical Activity and Sedentary Behavior. Geneva: World Health Organization; 2020

[27] www.who.int

[28] www.worldsleepsociety.org; 2021 World Sleep Day

[29] Dashti H, Scheer FAJL, Jacques PF, Fava SL, Ordovas JM. Short sleep duration and dietary intake: Epidemiologic evidence, mechanisms and health implications. Advances in Nutrition. 2015:6648-6659

[30] Liu G, Zong G, et al. Smoking cessation and weight change in relation to cardiovescular disease incidence and mortality in people with type 2 diabetes: a population based cohort study. The Lancet Diabetes & Endocrinology. 2020 Feb;**8**(2):125-133 Epub 2020 Jan 7

[31] Meredith D. Sorensen, Katherine R. Arlinghaus, Tracey A. Ledoux, Craig A. Johnston, Integrating mindfulness into eating behaviors, Behavioral medicine review, American Journal of Lifestyle Medicine, vol XX, nr X, 2019.

[32] Riccardi G, Giosue A, Calabrese I, Vaccaro O. Dietary recommendations for prevention of atherosclerosis. Cardiovascular Research. 2021;**00**:1-17 January 2021

[33] Hâncu A et al. Lifestylemedicine, lifestyle partnership. Internal Medicine. 2019;**XVI**(1). DOI: 102478/inmed-2019-0054

Chapter 7

The Multiple Causes of Obesity

Indu Saxena, Suwarna Suman, Amar Preet Kaur, Abhilasha, Prasenjit Mitra, Praveen Sharma and Manoj Kumar

Abstract

Obesity is known to cause physical and metabolic diseases. It is often assumed by people (including the healthcare workers) that the person with obesity lacks self-control in matters of diet and physical exercise, and is therefore responsible for his or her weight. Persons with obesity have to face sarcasm, barbs, and discrimination due to their condition. They often have difficulty in getting jobs or have to accept lower than standard pay for their work. Although weight gain requires calorie intake in excess of calorie expenditure, it is sometimes not easy for the person to restrict calories due to the underlying causes of obesity. The body resists losing weight, and attempts to hoard calories by reducing the metabolic rate. In this chapter we have explained and classified the causes of obesity into endogenous and exogenous. The endogenous causes include genetic and epigenetic causes, maternal factors, and hormonal causes, while exogenous causes include obesogenic environment, life-style, and weight-gain promoting medicines. It must be realized that losing weight and keeping it off is not easy for a person with obesity.

Keywords: Obesity, Endocrine causes of obesity, Endogenous causes of obesity, Exogenous causes of obesity, Genetics of obesity

1. Introduction

Calorie intake that exceeds body requirements results in storage of the excess calories in the body. Although proteins are highly versatile in function, they cannot be used to store excess energy. The amount of glycogen that can be stored in adult liver is 100–120 grams, the skeletal muscle can store about 400 gram glycogen in a 70 kg adult. Small amounts are also present in other cells. The triacylglycerols (TAGs) are the best suited for energy storage purpose: they are energy-dense, hydrophobic (therefore do not associate with space-filling calorie empty water molecules), and can be stored in huge amounts. However, excess storage of the TAGs is often associated with ailments and early mortality. The Obesity Medicine Association has defined obesity as a 'chronic, relapsing, multi-factorial, neurobehavioral disease, wherein an increase in body fat promotes adipose tissue dysfunction and abnormal fat mass physical forces, resulting in adverse metabolic, biomechanical, and psychosocial health consequences' [1]. Since measurement of body fat content is tedious and requires sophisticated instruments, it is easier to define overweight and obesity on the basis of the Body Mass Index (BMI). BMI is calculated easily by dividing the weight of the person in kilograms by the square of height in meters. According to the World Health Organization, persons with BMI < 18.5 kg/m^2 are underweight, those with BMI 18.5 to < 25 kg/m^2 fare of normal weight, those with BMI 25 to < 30 kg/m^2 are overweight, and those with BMI > 30 kg/m^2 are obese [2]. Besides affecting the patient on the individual level (posing increased risk of obesity-related diseases), obesity affects families and nations in terms of healthcare requirements, reduced working capacity, and economic burden. Annual healthcare costs for obesity exceed $700 billion [3]. With the global increase in the incidence of obesity and obesity-related diseases, healthcare costs for obesity have exceeded those for smoking [4].

Thermodynamics can explain the excess storage of TAGs in a simple, succinct manner: storage of calories occurs when calorie intake exceeds calorie expenditure. Decreasing the intake and increasing the expenditure should melt away the excess fat. Research conducted in the past 70 years reveals that adipose tissue that has grown out of size wants more of itself and persuades the body to devise ways to hoard calories. Thus, obesity is not merely a case of poor self-control. Also, all persons with obesity do not develop obesity-related diseases, as the type of adipose tissue and the site of deposition influence the risks to health.

2. Identifying obesity and determining the adipose content

The fact that weight is related to longevity of the person was realized by life insurance companies [5]. A higher health risk was predicted for weight more than 20% the ideal weight for that height. This is equivalent to a BMI of 27.8 kg/m^2. BMI cannot differentiate muscle from fat, or inform about the distribution of fat. It cannot detect changes in body composition due to sarcopenia or osteopenia. It has been observed that some races are at a higher risk of type 2 diabetes mellitus and cardiovascular diseases at BMI values lower than what are normal for persons of European descent. Distribution of body fat is different in different races, Asians tend to have more central adiposity compared to the Caucasians [6]. Males have higher lean mass and bone mineral mass compared to females, however, females have more peripheral distribution of fat [7]. Pregnancy, age, and menopause cause redistribution of body fat, promoting central obesity [8]. It is important to determine the fat content of the body as well as the distribution of the body fat. The best method for determining fat content and fat distribution is cadaver analysis, as no in vivo technique can be that accurate [9].

Anthropometric methods are the most convenient and most popular for estimating the extent of fatness. Besides BMI, these include waist and hip circumferences, waist-to-hip ratio (WHR), skin fold thickness, and waist-to stature ratio (WSR). Since shorter individuals usually weigh less, weight alone cannot be used as a criterion to determine the amount of fat stores. WSR and waist circumference are easy and relatively accurate techniques to estimate visceral fat [10]. The body adiposity index (BAI) does not require weight measurement; it is the ratio of hip circumference to height. It is a fairly accurate measure of adiposity and can be easily used in remote areas without accessibility to reliable scales [11].

According to the two compartment (2C) model, the mass of the human body can be categorized into anhydrous Fat Mass (FM) and Fat Free Mass (FFM). The FFM includes water, minerals, and proteins. FM is assumed to have a density of 0.9007 g/cm^3 while the FFM is assumed to have a density of 1.1000 g/cm^3. Water content of the body is assumed to be 73.72% [12]. Techniques based on two-component model are bioelectric impedance analysis, whole body counting of total body potassium, densitometry methods (hydrostatic underwater weighing and air displacement plethysmography), and hydrometry using isotope dilution technique. The water content (hydration fraction), bone mineral content, and density of the FFM vary with age, pubertal status, and pregnancy. These values are altered in patients with deranged hydration and in those who have recently lost weight. Differences related to ethnicities have also been observed.

In the 3 compartment (3C) model of body composition assessment, the FFM is sub-divided into lean tissue mass (LTM) and bone mineral content (BMC). This method requires densitometry as well as hydrometry measurements and includes dual energy X-ray absorptiometry (DEXA), a rapid non-invasive method for regional as well as whole body measurement in which high- and low-energy X-rays are transmitted through the body.

The 4 compartment model further categorizes LTM into total body water (TBW) and protein. It requires a combination of several measurement techniques: hydrodensitometry like under-water weighing or air-displacement plethysmography (to measure fat), DEXA (to measure mineral), isotope dilution (to measure water), and residual techniques (to measure protein) [13, 14]. It is an expensive, elaborate, and time requiring technique.

Multi-component models have also been used that incorporate results from many techniques, and are therefore more accurate. Simple methods can be used in the field, while lab-based methods or CT, MRI, X-ray techniques can be used only in clinical settings.

Anthropometric methods and bioelectric impedance analysis are considered indirect methods of assessment. Direct methods include measurement of total body water by isotope dilution technique, total body counting to measure radioactive potassium, and neutron activation techniques with a body scan to measure different elements. Criterion methods include underwater weighing, air-displacement plethysmography, DEXA, computed tomography (CT) scan, and magnetic resonance imaging (MRI) [15].

Vague in 1947 [16] noted that pear-shaped body with higher fat distribution in hips and thigh regions is associated with protection against metabolic diseases. Deposition of fat in the abdominal region (usually seen in males) is associated with development of metabolic diseases [17, 18]. Most of the adipose tissue in the adult human is white adipose tissue (WAT), the main function of which is to store excess calories as triacylglycerols. The brown adipose tissue (BAT), present in small quantities in the interscapular region, is responsible for non-shivering thermogenesis. WAT present in visceral regions is called visceral adipose tissue (VAT), and that present below the skin for insulation is called subcutaneous adipose tissue (SAT). Excess VAT is associated with the metabolic complications of obesity, like metabolic syndrome, type 2 diabetes mellitus, dyslipidemia, and cardiovascular diseases. TAGs may deposit in tissues other than the adipose; this is called ectopic fat. Ectopic fat in viscera, heart, and vasculature can be seen in lipodystrophy, characterized by little subcutaneous fat and high amounts of ectopic fat. Deposition of thoracic peri-aortic fat and peripheral artery disease is considered local toxic effect of the ectopic fat. The renal sinus fat has been associated with hypertension and chronic kidney disease [19]. Although BMI is the most common method to identify overweight and obesity, it is unable to differentiate VAT and SAT, and central and global obesity. CT and MRI can be used to quantify the amount of visceral fat accurately. DEXA can also be used, however, it tends to underestimate VAT in people with normal BMI, and overestimates VAT in people with severe obesity [20].

It has been noted that some individuals classified as overweight or obese according to their BMI do not show insulin resistance or increased risk of metabolic diseases. Such people are said to have metabolically healthy obesity (MHO), which can be a transient stage of variable duration that progresses towards metabolically unhealthy obesity (MUO) [21]. A person with obesity can be classified as metabolically healthy if blood pressure, blood glucose, TAG, and high density lipoprotein cholesterol levels are normal without medication [22]. Metabolically unhealthy obesity results when adipocytes of SAT are unable to proliferate and differentiate. Such tissue shows hypertrophy instead of hyperplasia, leading to ectopic and visceral deposition of fat.

3. What causes overweight and obesity?

The imbalance between energy intake and expenditure can result from various causes that can be broadly classified into endogenous and exogeneous. In his paper on obesity, Pennington has described how the concept of endogenous obesity originated in 1907 [23].

3.1 Endogenous causes of obesity

Genetic and epigenetic disorders, hormonal imbalances, maternal and birth-related factors, microbiome, and infections are included in the endogenous causes of obesity. In case of children, pathologic cause can be suspected if the patient shows hyperphagia with absence of satiety signals, shows food-seeking behavior, hides or steals food, has neuroendocrine abnormalities, has skin and hair that are lighter than those of siblings, or is gaining weight rapidly before the age of 5 years.

3.1.1 Genetic causes of obesity

Ethnic differences in obesity have been observed; admixture mapping studies show that obesity correlates with percentage of ancestry derived from ethnic groups [24]. Studies on individual families and animal models revealed rare obesity causing genes like leptin and leptin receptor genes, melanocortin 4 receptor gene, and the proopiomelanocortin genes, etc. Studies on obesity concordant monozygotic twins show BMI and other anthropometric measures like WHR are 40–60% heritable in children and adults [25]. The genome-wide association studies (GWAS) using massive study populations identified 119 independent loci associated with BMI [26]. The human obesity gene map discussed by Rankinen et al. [27] lists single-gene mutations in 11 different genes, 50 loci related to Mendelian syndromic obesity, 253 quantitative trace loci (QTL) for obesity-related phenotypes. On the basis of clinical presentations, genetic obesity can be classified into monogenic non-syndromic, monogenic syndromic, and polygenic obesity.

A. **Non-syndromic monogenic obesity.** Rare, early-onset severe obesity that is mainly caused by mutations in genes whose products are involved in the regulation of food intake. Most mutations require two dysfunctional copies of genes as homozygous or compound heterozygous condition in order to affect the phenotype. Around 200 single gene mutations have been associated with human obesity, but all are confined to more than 10 genes.

1. **Leptin.** The name leptin has been derived from the Greek word 'leptos' which means 'thin'. Leptin (product of *ob* or *LEP* gene) is a 167 amino acid protein synthesized mainly in the adipocytes and enterocytes, and also in gastric epithelium and placenta. It is also called the satiety hormone as it regulates fat stores by diminishing hunger. Since its discovery in 1994 [28], leptin has been considered a potential target in the treatment of obesity.

   Mutations in leptin gene are very rare, lead to hyperphagia and obesity, and can be ameliorated by leptin administration [29]. Administration of exogenous leptin reduces hyperphagia that is spontaneous or induced by fasting [30]; chronic administration causes weight loss by reducing food intake [31, 32]. In most persons with obesity, circulating leptin levels are high, indicating that leptin resistance rather than leptin deficiency is the underlying reason for weight gain.

2. **Leptin receptor.** Multiple isoforms of leptin receptor (Ob-R or LEPR) have been identified, which are produced by alternative splicing of the mRNA or by post-translational modifications [33]. Ob-Rb, the long form of leptin receptor expressed widely in the hypothalamus and appetite-modulating pathways of brain stem, has an intracellular domain that binds Janus kinases (JAK) and signal transducers and activators of transcription (STAT)-3 factors [34, 35]. The activated JAK–STAT-3 pathway induces expression of suppressor of cytokine signaling (SOCS)-3. SOCS are a family of eight proteins that negatively regulate the JAK–STAT pathway, i.e., the very pathway that increases their synthesis.

Obesity-related leptin-resistance may be due to overexpression of the SOCS-3. This has been supported by the fact that *SOCS-3* deletion in specific neurons in mice [36] or mice with heterozygous global *SOCS-3* deficiency [37, 38] are more leptin-sensitive and resistant to weight gain. Ob-Rb, the long form of leptin receptor, is expressed in the arcuate nucleus of the hypothalamus in two neuronal groups: orexigenic neurons expressing neuropeptide (NP)Y and agouti-related peptide (AgRP), and by anorexigenic neurons expressing proopiomelanocortin (POMC) and cocaine-amphetamine-regulated transcript (CART) [39]. Leptin inhibits the expression of the orexigenic peptides NPY and AgRP, and activates the neurons producing the anorexigenic peptides POMC and CART [40, 41], thus reducing food intake. Low circulating levels of leptin lead to increased expression of NPY and AgRP, decreased expression of POMC and CART, and increased hunger. High levels of leptin in blood decrease the expression of NPY and AgRP, increase the expression of POMC and CART, and decrease hunger. Viral-mediated gene expression used to produce chronic leptin overexpression in the arcuate and paraventricular nuclei and ventromedial hypothalamus resulted in reduced food intake [42].

The secretory isoform of the leptin receptor binds circulating leptin and modulates its biologic availability, while the short isoform of the leptin receptor is involved in the transport of leptin across the blood–brain barrier [43]. Leptin resistance may be due to defect in leptin receptor, or in the transport of leptin across the blood–brain barrier. Such persons have early-onset obesity and hypogonadism, however, the obesity is not as severe as in the case of persons lacking plasma leptin [42]. In rodents, a high-fat diet produces leptin resistance, prior to the weight gain [43].

Mutations in leptin receptor gene (*LEPR*) produce a phenotype similar to that of leptin deficiency, with normal or high leptin levels [44, 45]. Often, LEPR mutations are accompanied with deficiencies of growth hormone or thyroid hormone [46, 47].

3. **Proopiomelanocortin.** The precursor protein pre-proopiomelanocortin is a 267 amino acid protein synthesized in the corticotrophs and melanotrophs of the anterior and intermediate lobes of the pituitary [48]. A 26 amino acid signal peptide is removed to form proopiomelanocortin (POMC) with 241 amino acids. Cleavage of POMC forms multiple peptide hormones (α-, β-, and

γ-melanocyte stimulating hormones (MSH), adrenocorticotropic hormone (ACTH), and β-endorphin). The cleavage is brought about by pro-hormone convertase (PC)1/3 (encoded by PCSK 1 gene in humans), carboxypeptidase (CP) E, and other enzymes. Mutations in PCSK1 and CPE are known to cause monogenic obesities (discussed later). The peptide products are packaged into vesicles and released by exocytosis. The processed products of POMC bind to different types of melanocortin receptors (MCRs), and to the μ-opioid receptor [49]. Five MCRs (MC1R to MC5R) have been identified on the basis of their binding properties and tissue locations. MC1R is mainly located on the melanocytes of skin and preferentially binds α-MSH. ACTH can also bind to MC1R. When ACTH is present at high concentrations, as in Cushing's disease, it can cause hyperpigmentation. MC2R is mainly expressed in the adrenal cortex, and binds only ACTH to activate glucocorticoid synthesis. MC3R binds α-, β-and γ-MSH with equal affinity, is present on POMC neurons in the arcuate nucleus, and acts as an inhibitory auto-receptor. MC4R has a very high expression in the paraventricular nucleus of the hypothalamus and is involved in energy balance (discussed later). The primary agonist for MC4R is α-MSH released from the anorexigenic POMC neurons in the paraventricular nucleus. The primary antagonist of this receptor is agouti-related protein AgRP), released by the orexigenic AgRP/NPY neurons, also located in the paraventricular nucleus. MC5R is not expressed in the central nervous system. It is expressed in a variety of peripheral tissues during embryogenesis and binds with α-MSH with a slightly higher affinity. The μ-opioid receptor is expressed in the cortex, hippocampus, and brain stem, and in peripheral tissues. It binds β-endorphin mediating analgesic effect, and is also involved in feeding behavior.

Mutations in the *POMC* gene are autosomal recessive and cause early-onset severe obesity accompanied by hyperphagia, adrenal insufficiency, mild hypothyroidism, and red/ginger hair [50]. Very few patients with this condition have been diagnosed worldwide. Heterozygous individuals have intermediate increase in BMI.

4. **Prohormone convertase 1 and carboxypeptidase E.** Prohormone convertase (PC1/3), also called PCSK1 (pro-protein convertase subtilisin/kexin type 1), is present only in neuroendocrine cells and is involved in the conversion of prohormones to active hormones. It is a serine protease, activated by calcium. CPE, also called enkephalin convertase, releases terminal arginine or lysine residues from polypeptides. It is involved in the production of nearly all neuropeptides and peptide hormones.

   Mutations in *PC1/3* gene are extremely rare [51] and cause severe obesity in childhood. Since this enzyme is involved in the maturation of many hormones, its deficiency is also associated with adrenal, gonadotropic, somatotropic, and thyrotropic insufficiency and postprandial insulin deficiency. Proinsulin levels are high. Patients have severe malabsorptive neonatal diarrhea and may show central diabetes insipidus.

   Only a few patients with *CPE* mutations have been identified throughout the world. Such patients have morbid obesity, intellectual disability, type 2 diabetes, and hypogonadotropic hypogonadism [52].

5. **Melanocortin 4 receptor.** This is encoded by the *MC4R*, an intron-less gene with open reading frame of 999 bp located on chromosome 18. The MC4R is

glycosylated and has 332 amino acids. It is mainly expressed by brain cells and by the enteroendocrine cells. Besides the neurons, it is also expressed by the astrocytes in brain [53].

The MC4R plays a key role in weight regulation. It is activated by α-MSH, and cocaine- and amphetamine-regulated transcript (CART) to decrease food intake and increase energy expenditure. The orexigenic peptides neuropeptide Y (NPY) and AgRP are the natural antagonists of MC4R, and increase appetite and reduce energy expenditure by binding to MC4R [54]. Leptin stimulates the secretion of POMC, and inhibits that of AgRP and NPY.

Heterozygous mutations in *MC4R* gene reported in different ethnic groups are associated with dominantly inherited obesity. MC4R deficiency is the commonest monogenic cause of obesity. In a cohort of 500 children with obesity, 5.8% were found to have mutations in the *MC4R* gene [55]. Homozygous mutations and double heterozygous mutations are rare; about 25% mutations are heterozygous frame shift or nonsense with complete loss of function. Around 20% of the missense mutations are non-pathogenic. Heterozygous carriers of *MC4R* mutations have hyperphagia, impaired satiety, hyperinsulinemia, higher bone mineral density, and higher stature (big boned), especially in childhood. Patients homozygous for the condition have severe obesity and hyperinsulinemia which can be blocked by the administration of an α-adrenergic blocker. The hyperinsulinemia shows an age-related decrease and parallels amelioration of hyperphagia. Adults with MC4R deficiency have lower blood pressure and heart rate than age and BMI matched controls suggesting impaired activation of sympathetic nervous system. Diet-induced weight loss is not easy, but can be achieved by bariatric surgery in heterozygous persons. Liraglutide promotes weight loss in patients with MC4R deficiency.

6. **Single-Minded Homolog 1 (SIM1).** The single-minded (sim) is a basic helix–loop–helix-PAS domain transcription factor in *Drosophila melanogaster* that regulates gene expression in midline cells in the embryo [56]. SIM1, the human homolog, may have pleiotropic effects during embryogenesis. The *SIM1* gene is located on chromosome 6; chromosomal abnormalities like deletion of 6q16.2 region, translocation between 6q16.2 and 1p22.1, or point mutations in the 6q16.2 region cause severe childhood obesity or SIM1-related Prader-Willi-like syndrome. Homozygous SIM1 knockout mice do not survive due to absence of hypothalamic neurons [57].

7. **Brain Derived Neurotrophic Factor (BDNF).** BDNF, also called neurotrophin and abrineurin, is encoded by the *BDNF* gene on human chromosome 11 [58]. The BDNF preproprotein with 247 amino acid residues is processed to mature 119 amino acid protein. Pro-BDNF can be stored in dendrites and axons and undergoes cleavage either inside or outside the cell. BDNF and pro-BDNF are associated with opposing functions. High levels of BDNF are present in the hippocampus, amygdala, cerebellum, and cerebral cortex. Lower levels have been detected in the liver, heart, lung, etc. BDNF is a member of the neurotrophin family of growth factors required for the differentiation, maturation, and survival of neurons. In adverse conditions like hypoglycemia, cerebral ischemia, neurotoxicity, and glutamatergic stimulation, BDNF has a neuroprotective effect. It is also involved in plastic changes related to learning and memory [59].

Receptors for BDNF include TrkB, encoded by the *NTRK2* gene, and LNGFR (low affinity nerve growth factor receptor). The TrkB receptor belongs to the family of tyrosine kinase receptors and is coupled to the Ras, Cdc42/Rac/RhoG, MAPK, PI3K, and PLC-γ signaling pathways. Binding of BDNF with TrkB causes autophosphorylation of TrkB and is important for the development of short term memory and growth of neurons. LNGFR is also called p75. Pro-BDNF preferentially binds to LNGFR, leading to NFκB receptor activation, triggering apoptosis pathway.

WAGR syndrome involves disorders of many body systems and is named for its main features: Wilms tumor (a childhood kidney cancer), aniridia, genitourinary anomalies, and intellectual disability (formerly referred to as mental retardation). A subtype of the WAGR syndrome called WAGRO (characterized by childhood onset obesity) has been reported to be strongly associated with haploinsufficiency for BDNF [60]. Nineteen patients with deletions in any portion of the *BDNF* gene were reported to become obese by 10 years of age.

8. **NTRK2.** The *NTRK2* gene encodes TrkB receptor for BDNF. In case of mice, homologous *NTRK2* mutations are lethal. Heterozygous missense mutations in *NTRK2* have been reported in patients with severe hyperphagia, obesity, impaired nociception, and intellectual disability [61].

9. **Kinase Suppressor of Ras 2.** This protein is a molecular scaffold that coordinates Raf/MEK/ERK signaling and regulates activation of AMP-kinase. It is a product of *KSR2* or the *Fat* gene located on chromosome 12q. Both KSR 1 and KSR2 phosphorylate Raf, MEK, and ERF at several serine and threonine residues and cause their activation [62]. On stimulation by growth factor, the KSR proteins translocate to the plasma membrane to regulate the dynamics of Ras–Raf–MEK signaling.

   Targeted deletion of *Ksr2* in mice leads to obesity with hyperinsulinemia and low glucose tolerance.

10. **SH2B Adaptor Protein 1.** The Src homology 2b family members are adaptor proteins for several members of the tyrosine kinase receptor family. They contain SH2 and PH domains and can form homo or hetero dimers via their N-terminal dimerization domains. The SH2 domain present on the C-terminus binds proteins phosphorylated at their tyrosine residues: TrkA, insulin receptors, IGF2-receptors, insulin receptor substrate (IRS)-1 and 2, and JAK2 [63].

    The SH2B1 is a product of the *SH2B1* gene located on chromosome 16p. It stimulates JAK2 activity and assembles JAK2/IRS1/2 complex to enhance leptin signaling. It also enhances catalytic activity of insulin receptor and protects IRS from dephosphorylation, thus increasing insulin signaling. Deletion of SH2B1 in mice leads to leptin resistance, hyperphagia, obesity, insulin resistance, and type 2 diabetes.

    Several *SH2B1* mutations have been associated with obesity in humans and are known to increase the risk of type 2 diabetes mellitus. Partial deletions of about 200 bp are associated with early-onset severe obesity, while larger interspersed deletion extending through a 593 kb region on chromosome 16p11.2-p12.2 has been associated with developmental delay, feeding difficulties, dysmorphic facial features, and obesity [64].

11. **Adiponectin.** This 244 amino acid protein is also called adipocyte complement-related protein (Acrp), GBP-28, apM1, and adipo Q [65]. The *ADIPOQ* gene is present on chromosome 3. This hormone is produced mainly by the adipocytes and also by other tissues like osteoblasts, liver, myocytes, epithelial cells, and placenta. It is secreted as trimer, (67 kDa, also called low molecular weight or LMW), hexamer, and a multimer with at least 18 monomers (300 kDa, high molecular weight or HMW). Globular adiponectin is generated from full length adiponectin by proteolysis. Plasma levels of adiponectin are inversely proportional to the amount of adipose. Adiponectin levels are high after weight loss due to calorie restriction or gastric bypass surgery in patients with obesity [66, 67], and also in patients anorexia nervosa [68].

    Administration of adiponectin to rodents, and transgenic mice with increased adiponectin showed increased energy expenditure and oxygen consumption without affecting food intake [69, 70]. Adiponectin has been shown to suppress obesity [71], insulin resistance, type 2 diabetes [72, 73], atherosclerosis, and non-alcoholic fatty liver disease [74].

    Adiponectin receptor AdipoR1 is more in the skeletal muscle, and AdipoR2 is more in the liver. Expression of receptors is proportional to insulin levels, and in case of receptors on the muscle cells, the number is increased with exercise [75]. AdipoR1 has a higher affinity for globular adiponectin while AdipoR2 has higher affinity for full length adiponectin. The T-cadherin receptor for adiponectin recognizes hexameric and HMW forms of adiponectin. It is present in the vasculature and is involved in the cardioprotective action of adiponectin. Action of adiponectin on receptor requires adaptor proteins APPL1 or its isoform APPL2.

    Binding of adiponectin to its receptor leads to activation of the AMP-activated protein kinase (AMPK) and the mitogen-activated protein kinase (MAPK). This causes increased NO production, adiponectin-induced glucose uptake, degradation of ceramide by ceramidase, and fatty acid oxidation, ultimately increasing insulin sensitivity.

    Adiponectin deficiency has been associated with increased atherosclerosis while increased expression of adiponectin protects against atherosclerosis in mice [76]. Thiazolidinediones (TZD) used in the treatment of type 2 diabetes mellitus, are known to activate transcription factor peroxisome proliferator-activated receptor (PPAR)-γ, which has been shown to increase adiponectin levels in plasma [77].

    Adiponectin mutations have been associated with type 2 diabetes mellitus [78] and hypoadiponectinemia [79]. Recently, mutation in ADIPOQ has been associated with early-onset obesity and metabolic syndrome [80].

12. **Adenylate Cyclase Type 3.** Adenylate cyclase type 3 belongs to the adenylate cyclase family of enzymes that synthesize cAMP from ATP. The gene for this enzyme *ADCY3* is located on chromosome 2 and codes for a 1144 amino acid protein. The protein shows highest expression in lungs and placenta, intermediate expression in brain, heart, kidney, and skeletal muscle. Lowest expression is seen in liver and pancreas. It is also present in the olfactory cilia. Saeed et al. [81] reported loss-of-function mutations in *ADCY3* gene in 4 severely obese children from 3 consanguineous Pakistani families, and in

an obese boy from a non-consanguineous European American family. Interestingly, a gain-of-function mutation in *ADCY3* gene in a line of N-ethyl-N-nitrosourea (ENU)-mutagenized mice, Jll, with dominantly inherited resistance to diet-induced obesity, protects mice from diet-induced obesity [82].

13. **Other Monogenic Causes of Obesity.** Mutations in the *INSIG2* gene [83, 84] and in gene for peroxisome proliferator-activated receptor gamma (PPAR-γ) [85, 86] are associated with obesity. INSIG2 gene present on chromosome 2 encodes for insulin-induced gene 2 protein which is involved in lipid homeostasis. The gene for PPAR-γ (*PPARG*), present on chromosome 3p, can be activated by fatty acids and their metabolites. The protein is produced predominantly in liver and adipose and is crucial for the differentiation of fat cells. Besides obesity, mutations in this gene can cause insulin resistance, hypertension, and certain cancers.

    Insulin-sensitizing drugs thiazolidinediones are potent agonists of PPAR-γ. This can also lead to increased adiponectin levels (see above).

B. Syndromic Obesity. Patients with obesity (children or adults) who also show cognitive delay, dysmorphic features, organ-specific abnormalities, hyperphagia, and/or signs of hypothalamic dysfunction are considered to have syndromic obesity. Syndromic obesity may show autosomal or X-linked inheritance pattern, or may occur due to de novo mutations. Since comorbidities are present that require additional treatment, it is important to correctly diagnose syndromic obesity, which can be of the following types:

1. **Fat Mass and Obesity-Associated Protein (FTO) or Alpha-Ketoglutarate-Dependent Dioxygenase Deficiency.** This enzyme is coded by the *FTO* gene located on chromosome 16 in humans. The FTO proteins participate in adipogenesis and tumorigenesis and FTO inhibitors have been found to have anti-obesity and anti-cancer effects in vivo. *FTO* is one of the genes known to contribute to polygenic obesity. In fact, it was the first one to be identified by genome wide association studies (GWAS) [87]. In humans, complete deficiency of FTO is associated with an autosomal recessive syndrome with growth retardation, malformations, and premature death. A loss-of-function non-synonymous mutation at position 316 in the *FTO* gene in which arginine is replaced by glutamine has been identified in nine members of a Palestinian family. The afflicted members showed post-natal growth retardation, dysmorphism of head and face, psychomotor delay, and in some patients, brain, cardiac, genital, and palate defects. Complete/partial inactivation of *FTO* gene in mice protects from obesity while overexpression leads to increased food intake and obesity. Evidence suggests that certain mutations of *FTO* may increase the risk of obesity in humans.

2. **Prader-Willi syndrome (PWS).** This is caused by loss-of-function mutation of specific genes on chromosome 15 [88]. In most cases, a part of chromosome 15 from the father is deleted. In some cases, the patient lacks father's chromosome 15 and has two copies from the mother. Some parts of the mother's chromosomes are turned off by imprinting. This is usually not an inherited condition and affects 1 in 10,000 to 1 in 25,000 neonates. Polyhydramnios, reduced fetal movements, and abnormal fetal position may be present. New born may have hypogonadism, lethargy, poor muscle tone and difficulty in feeding. Afflicted children show delayed milestones, short stature, poor physical coordination,

crossed eyes. Hyperphagia begins between the ages of two and eight years and continues throughout life. The child gains excess weight. Adults with this condition have central obesity, hypogonadism, infertility, subnormal intelligence, extreme flexibility, and light skin and hair. More than 50% patients have strabismus.

3. **Bardet-Biedl syndrome (BBS).** This is a rare pleiotropic, autosomal recessive ciliopathy, the estimated incidence is 1 in 1,60,000 in north European populations [89]. About 16 genes are associated with this disorder, accounting for 80% cases. Diagnosis is based on clinical features: post-axial polydactyly, renal dysfunction, obesity, retinal dystrophy, hypogonadism, and learning difficulties.

   The BBS phenotype is less apparent in the first decade of life and the condition is usually diagnosed in late childhood or early adulthood.

4. **Alstrom syndrome (ALMS).** This is also called Alstrom-Halgren Syndrome [90]. It is a very rare autosomal recessive disorder due to defect in the *ALMS1* gene located on chromosome 2p13. The encoded protein is implicated in ciliary function, control of cell cycle, and intracellular transport. About 900 people with this syndrome have been reported worldwide. This syndrome is characterized by childhood obesity (but normal birth weight), hyperphagia, hyperinsulinemia, and type 2 diabetes mellitus. Other features include progressive cone-rod dystrophy leading to blindness (occurring usually prior to 15 months of age) and sensorineural hearing loss (usually bilateral, beginning in the first decade of life). Otitis media with glue ear has been reported. About 70% patients develop dilated cardiomyopathy during infancy or adolescence. Renal failure, pulmonary, hepatic, and urologic dysfunction are often observed, and systemic fibrosis develops with age. Unlike the Bardet-Biedl syndrome, there is no mental defect, polydactyly, or hypogonadism. Retinal lesion causes nystagmus and early loss of central vision in contrast to loss of peripheral vision first, as in other pigmentary retinopathies. Height is normal or more than normal in children, but growth slows down so that adults are usually of short stature. The symptoms and rate of progression of disease varies in patients, even amongst members of the same family.

5. **Pseudohypoparathyroidism (PHP).** This is a heterogeneous group of very rare endocrine disorders, primarily due to resistance to the parathyroid hormone (PTH) [91]. It was first described by Fuller Albright in 1942 to describe patients with PTH-resistant hypocalcaemia and hypophosphatemia and a constellation of skeletal defects called Albright hereditary osteodystrophy (AHO). Features of AHO (seen in PHP-1a and -1c) include short stature, stocky built, rounded face, short fourth metacarpal and other bones of the hands and feet, and ectopic ossifications.

   Gene encoding the alpha-subunit of the stimulatory G protein (*GNAS1*) is defective resulting in at least 4 different forms of PHP: PHP-1 a, b, and c, and PPHP (pseudo pseudohypoparathyroidism). Molecular defect in PHP-2 is yet to be identified. The exact prevalence of PHP is not known.

6. **Cohen syndrome or Pepper syndrome or Cervenka syndrome.** This was first described by M Michael Cohen Jr. in 1973 in two siblings and one isolated case [92]. More than a hundred cases have been identified over the world, with 35 from Finland [93]

The phenotype in Finnish patients is homogeneous: non-progressive psychomotor retardation, microcephaly, characteristic facial features, myopia, progressive retinochoroidal dystrophy, neutropenia, and cheerful disposition. Non-Finnish patients have a confusing phenotype. Affected persons have low birth weight but develop abnormal truncal fat distribution in teenage. This is an autosomal recessive condition, with mutation in the vacuolar protein sorting 13 homolog B (VPS13B, also called COH1 gene) located on chromosome 8q. This transmembrane protein is involved in vesicle-mediated intracellular protein transport.

7. **Other syndromes associated with obesity.** Down syndrome (trisomy 21) and Turner syndrome (45, X) have been reported to be associated with adult obesity [94, 95].

C. Polygenic obesity. More than an hundred polygenic loci harboring genetic variants associated with overweight and obesity have been identified [96–98]. Polygenic obesity is caused by the cumulative effect of obesogenic environment and weight-gain promoting genes. The contribution of a single gene is very small, of only a few hundred grams, but the combined effect of many such genes in a person can have a significant effect on weight gain. Khera et al. [98] have derived and validated a polygenic predictor of weight gain.

3.1.2 Epigenetic causes of obesity

Although the DNA in every cell of the multicellular organism is the same (exception: mosaicism [99]), the expression of genes is different in different cell types. The mechanisms that regulate the expression of genes can be heritable. Epigenetic modifications are mitotically and meiotically heritable modulation of gene function without changes in the sequence of the DNA [100]. Such modifications allow or silence the expression of specific genes. Epigenetic programming can be influenced by environmental and dietary factors as well as by the gut microbiota.

The epigenetic modifications are brought about by DNA methylation (by DNA methyltransferases, DNMTs, at distinct CpG sites), histone modification (methylation, acetylation, ubiquitination, or phosphorylation), and by short non-coding RNA species called micro-RNAs or miRNAs.

a. **DNA methylation.** The CpG sites where methylation occurs are usually present in the promoter regions of genes. Addition of methyl group hinders the attachment of transcription factors and represses transcription of the gene. Some of these genes are involved in appetite control, obesity, metabolism, insulin signaling, inflammation, and growth. Examples of genes associated with obesity having CpG in the promoter regions are the HIF3A, LEP, ADIPOQ, NPY, IGF-2, IRS-1, and POMC, etc. Increased methylation of LEP gene was found in maternal blood samples with pre-pregnancy obesity and in cord blood samples in neonates small for gestational age and whose mothers continued to smoke during pregnancy [101]. Tobi et al. [102] reported higher LEP methylation in men born after prenatal exposure to wartime (Dutch hunger winter) famine in 1944–1945 compared to their unexposed same-sex siblings.

b. **Histone modification.** Histone modifications control the accessibility of the DNA to transcription factors. The five key regulatory genes of adipogenesis: pre-adipocyte factor-1 (Pref-1), CCAAT-enhancer-binding protein β (C/EBP β), C/EBPα,

PPARγ, and adipocyte protein 2 (aP2), are modulated via histone modification during adipocyte differentiation [103].

c. **Micro RNA.** miRNA are short (18–25 nt) non-coding RNA sequences that regulate gene expression [104]. Certain miRNA species have been identified that are associated with insulin resistance and low-grade inflammation seen in obesity [105]. Childhood obesity is associated with specific miRNAs while some miRNAs are associated with weight changes [106–108].

Epigenetic changes influence embryo formation and development, inactivation of X chromosome in female, genomic imprinting, cell differentiation, stable inheritance of gene expression, and immune cell function. In case of mice it was observed that pregnant animals exposed to polycyclic hydrocarbons during pregnancy gave birth to offspring with higher weight and fat mass. These offspring showed higher expression of PPAR-γ, C/EBP α, Cox2, FAS and adiponectin and lower DNA methylation of PPAR γ. This epigenetic change was heritable, as it was also observed in the subsequent generation [109]. Female mice born following perinatal exposure to bisphenol A showed significantly different DNA methylated regions compared to controls [110].

3.1.3 Maternal factors influencing obesity

Certain factors related to the mother cannot be altered but are known to influence body weight or metabolic processes of the offspring. A U-shaped association between maternal age and fasting glucose concentration in adult offspring has been reported [111]. Adult offspring of younger or older mothers had blood glucose levels higher by about 0.05 mmol/L higher than the reference group. Early maternal menarche [112], maternal diabetes [113], and maternal smoking during pregnancy [114] are associated with a higher BMI in offspring. Low maternal education influences obesity, however, the relationship is different in different ethnicities [115, 116]. Maternal employment has also been found to influence children's weight [117].

3.1.4 Hormonal causes of obesity

Secondary obesity (consequence of some other illness) due to endocrine causes is relatively less common.

1. **Hypothyroidism.** Triiodothyronine (T3) and thyroxine (T4) are tyrosine-derived iodine-containing hormones produced by the thyroid gland that act on almost all cells of the body to regulate a variety of metabolic functions. T4 is converted to the 4-times more potent T3 by deiodinases in cells, however, since T4 has a longer half-life, it is the major form in circulation (ratio of T4/T3 in blood is approximately 14).

   Weight gain has been reported in thyroid insufficiency. About 54% patients with overt hypothyroidism report gain of weight compared to 13.8% control subjects [118]. Hypothyroidism is also associated with dyslipidemia with increased cholesterol levels. The thyroid gland secretes prohormone thyroxine or T4 (3,5,3′,5′-tetraiodothyronine) along with small quantities of active T3 (3,5,3′-triiodothyronine), on receiving the signal from the pituitary gland in the form of thyroid stimulating hormone (TSH) or thyrotropin. TSH is released from the pituitary under the influence of thyrotropin releasing hormone (TRH), the master regulator of thyroid function, produced in the paraventricular nucleus of the hypothalamus. Depending on the underlying cause, hypothyroidism can be primary (decreased production of thyroxine by thyroid due to various reasons), secondary (due to decreased TSH), tertiary (due to deficiency of TRH), and peripheral or consumptive hypothyroidism (due to increased activity of deiodinase 3 which degrades thyroid hormone). Secondary and tertiary hypothyroidism are together called central hypothyroidism [119].

Every organ system and cell in the body is influenced directly or indirectly by the thyroid hormones. Gut motility, heart rate, body temperature, perfusion of lungs, and muscle contraction modulate the effect of catecholamines. In females, thyroid hormones influence menstruation, ovulation, and fertility. Bone growth and brain maturation in children are also influenced by these hormones, while in adults they affect the mood [120]. Thyroid hormones regulate the basal metabolic rate (BMR) and therefore are responsible for increase/decrease/maintenance of body weight.

Decreased thyroxine levels cause accumulation of hyaluronic acid in the dermis which causes water retention and non-pitting edema [121]. Decreased blood flow to kidneys resulting in lowered glomerular filtration rate in hypothyroidism causes water retention and increase in body weight [122]. This is aided by decreased tubular resorption and secretion in thyroxine deficiency. Thyroid hormones also regulate the number of adrenergic receptors and dopaminergic activation of the tubular cells, thus affecting the renin-angiotensin-aldosterone (RAA) axis [123].

Hypothyroidism has been shown to cause decreased mitochondrial biogenesis and decreased levels of uncoupler proteins [124, 125].

Thyroid dysfunction has been associated with decreased insulin sensitivity [126]. This may be a consequence of increased adipose deposition from decreased BMR. Increased adipose tissue is known to cause insulin resistance in obese subjects.

2. **Polycystic Ovarian Syndrome (PCOS).** This is a heterogeneous disorder with ovarian dysfunction, hirsutism, hyperandrogenism, obesity, and insulin resistance. PCOS has multifactorial etiology with both genetic and environmental components [127]. More than 50% of adult women with PCOS are overweight or obese and weight reduction alleviates menstrual irregularity [128]. Weight deposition is more around the waist (android pattern of fat distribution), and is both the cause as well as effect of hyperandrogenaemia [129]. Increased adipose tissue leads to higher production of adipokines. Abnormally high leptin levels have been noted in PCOS [130], although some authors report that the serum levels of leptin correlate with obesity rather than with PCOS [131]. Houjeghani et al. have reported higher levels of insulin, testosterone, luteinizing hormone (LH), and higher LH to FSH (follicle stimulating hormone) ratio in women with PCOS compared to normal age and BMI matched controls [132]. Lower concentrations of sex hormone binding globulins were reported in PCOS.

3. **Cushing Syndrome.** The corticosteroid hormones produced by the adrenal cortex are of two types: glucocorticoids and mineralocorticoids. The glucocorticoids e.g., cortisol affect metabolism of carbohydrates, fats, and proteins, and are involved in anti-inflammation, immunosuppressive, anti-proliferative, and vasoconstrictive processes. The mineralocorticoids like aldosterone are involved in regulation of water and electrolyte balance.

All conditions in which cortisol level is higher than normal are classified under Cushing syndrome, while Cushing disease is pituitary dependent [133]. Cushing syndrome can be classified into ACTH-dependent, ACTH-independent, and pseudo-Cushing syndrome. Cushing disease, ectopic ACTH syndrome, ectopic CRH syndrome, macronodular adrenal hyperplasia, and iatrogenic treatment with ACTH are included in the ACTH-dependent variety of Cushing syndrome. The ACTH-independent Cushing syndrome includes adrenal adenoma and carcinoma, primary pigmented adrenal nodular hyperplasia and Carney's syndrome, McCune-Albright syndrome, aberrant receptor expression, and iatrogenic Cushing caused by pharmacotherapy by steroids. Chronic alcoholism and depression can cause pseudo-Cushing syndrome. A rare condition with repeated episodes of cortisol excess interspersed by regular or irregular periods of normal cortisol secretion is called the cyclic Cushing syndrome.

Chronically elevated levels of cortisol in Cushing's syndrome cause redistribution of fat and central obesity [133]. Glucocorticoids (GCs) increase hypothalamic endocannabinoids, hypothalamic AMPK activity, and gene expression of orexigenic NPY and agouti-related peptide, resulting in increased appetite. GCs promote adipocyte differentiation and sensitize preadipocytes to insulin. Visceral adipose tissue (VAT) shows differential response to GCs: increased deposition and insulin resistance occurs in VAT compared to subcutaneous adipose tissue (SAT). Excess glucocorticoids also produce hyperglycemia, dyslipidemia, and increased protein degradation.

4. **Growth Hormone Deficiency.** Growth hormone (GH) or somatotropin exists as several isoforms; the major isoform is a 191 amino acid protein. Secretion of growth hormone by the somatotropic cells of anterior pituitary is under control of the cells of neurosecretory nuclei of hypothalamus, which release GH releasing hormone (GHRH) or somatocrinin and GH inhibiting hormone (GHIH) or somatostatin. Release of GHRH and GHIH is influenced by physiologic stimulators: sleep, exercise, and nutrition, and by the level of free fatty acids in blood. GH is released in a pulsatile manner, the peak occurs an hour after the onset of sleep. During the day, secretion of GH occurs at 3–5 h intervals [134]. Age, sex, diet, exercise, and stress influence GH secretion, which is also influenced by the other hormones.

   Congenital, acquired, or idiopathic deficiency of GH may be associated with increased adipose deposition, especially in the waist region, and insulin resistance. However, reduced GH levels have been reported in some patients with obesity [135, 136]. Usually, deficiency of GH in children is due to insufficient production of growth hormone releasing hormone in the hypothalamus. Damage to the pituitary or hypothalamus (due to tumor or tumor-related surgery, stroke, bleeding, infection, etc) in adulthood may lead to decreased GH production. GH increases lipolysis in the adipose tissue, and reduces storage of TG in a non-uniform manner. Thus it promotes loss of intra-abdominal fat. Scacchi et al. [137] reported that a primary growth hormone deficiency causes centripetal adiposity, while obesity with increase in visceral adipose tissue produces secondary growth hormone deficiency.

5. **Laron syndrome or primary growth hormone insensitivity (GHI).** GHI [138] is a group of rare disorders caused by mutations either in the GH receptor gene, or in genes of signaling proteins within the cell that are activated on binding of GH to its receptor. Various mutations and their effects have been summarized by Boro et al. [139]. Synthesis of insulin-like growth factor (IGF)-

1 is prevented although GH levels in blood are normal or high. Such children show improved growth when IGF-1 is administered before puberty, but no improvement if only GH treatment is given. Children with GHI show delayed onset of puberty, short limbs, reduced muscle strength and endurance, prominent forehead, low blood sugar, and obesity in adulthood.

6. **Ghrelin (Lenomorelin).** Ghrelin is a 28 amino acid peptide hormone discovered in 1999 by Kojima et al. [140]. It is a fast-acting orexigenic hormone produced by the endocrine cells (ghrelin cells) in gastric fundus and to a lesser extent in the body of the stomach, intestinal mucosa, lungs, urogenital organs, and brain. It has a role in meal initiation. Pre-prandial ghrelin surges occur at fixed feeding schedules, or at food-related cues. The post-prandial decrease in ghrelin levels is due to increased intestinal osmolarity and increased insulin. Ghrelin regulates the input and output of calories, and therefore influences the body weight, via the G-protein-coupled growth hormone secretagogue receptor (GHSR)1a. Besides regulating appetite, ghrelin stimulates secretion of GH and ACTH, increases gut motility and gastric acid secretion, modulates sleep, stress, and anxiety, influences taste sensation and reward-seeking behavior, regulates glucose metabolism, reduces lipid degradation, and suppresses thermogenesis in brown adipose tissue. It has been shown to protect muscle from atrophy and improve cardiovascular function [141].

Two distinct forms of ghrelin are present in blood: acylated ghrelin (AG) and unacylated ghrelin (UAG). About 90% of the circulating ghrelin in unacylated (UAG). The AG acts on GHSR 1a mediating growth hormone release, while UAG acts on GHSR 1a on pancreatic cells stimulating the release of insulin and glucose utilization. AG opposes the action of UAG, inhibiting the release of insulin. In obesity, UAG levels decrease while the AG levels remain unchanged.

Highest levels of ghrelin in blood are immediately before a meal, and drop to lowest levels immediately after the meal. Ghrelin administration increases appetite in both humans and rats. Ghrelin and synthetic ghrelin mimetics bind to the GHSR1a in hypothalamus, brain stem, and in the mesolimbic pathway, cause secretion of orexigenic neuropeptide Y (NPY) and agouti-related protein (AgRP). GHSR 1a is also expressed in vagal efferent neurons. Under influence of ghrelin, the gastric vagal efferents become less sensitive to gastric distension, increasing food intake.

Plasma level of ghrelin is lower in persons with obesity, except in patients with Prader-Willi syndrome, where ghrelin levels are proportional to the food intake. AG and UAG levels were compared in insulin-resistant and insulin-sensitive subjects with obesity. It was found that UAG and total ghrelin was lowered in insulin-resistant subjects, while only AG levels were lowered in the insulin-sensitive subjects [142]. In patients with anorexia nervosa and with cancer-induced cachexia, ghrelin levels are high [143, 144]. Obese rodents with low levels of ghrelin in plasma have reduced levels of ghrelin-receptor mRNA as compared to the normal lean controls. Experiments on rodents showed that central ghrelin signaling activates reward centres in response to alcohol, food, high-fat diet, and psychosomatic drugs like cocaine [145, 146].

Besides being the hunger signal, the ghrelin-GHSR 1a system is related to the rewarding aspects of food intake. It is activated in anticipation of food intake, negative energy balance, and psychological stress. In times of food scarcity, the effect of the ghrelin/GHSR 1a system on the mesolimbic pathway is advantageous for the animal's survival.

In developed countries, as well as in the rapidly developing countries, the changes in environment are favoring sedentary lifestyle, easy availability of calorie-dense tasty affordable foods, and increased stress levels are promoting increased appetite. The action of ghrelin on the mesolimbic system increases the appetite, acting as a spice to further increase food intake. In the current scenario of easy availability of food, the ghrelin/GHSR 1a system is no longer an evolutionary advantage but is in part responsible for the obesity epidemic and the associated diseases [147].

Weight gain may also be influenced by insulin, estrogen, progesterone, prolactin, and melatonin.

3.2 Exogenous causes of obesity

Certain factors that are preventable and influence the person from outside the body are classified as exogenous causes.

3.2.1 Depression, sleep deprivation, gut microbiota, and infections

1. **Depression.** Previously it was believed that depression was associated with a loss of appetite and sleep, with an inability to persuade oneself to cheer up and get going. Later, atypical depression was noted for increased eating, hypersomnia, frequent, relatively short episodes, and a proclivity to obesity [148]. Murphy et al. [149] reported that many patients with depression felt like eating when they felt bad. From their study on 1396 subjects, they concluded that patients with obesity tended to experience more severe depression, compared to the non-obese. It is possible that the stigma of obesity contributed to the depression.

2. **Sleep deprivation.** Lack of sufficient sleep has been reported to be associated with high fat intake, night-time snacking, binge-eating, and gain of weight [150]. Altered sleep patterns due to shift work, trans-continental travel, sleep apnoea, or due to new parenthood can lead to sleep insufficiency. Sleep restriction causes increased fat and carbohydrate intake and increased intake of total calories, with no corresponding increase in energy expenditure. Ding et al. [151] note that sleep dysregulation perturbs appetite-regulating hormones like leptin and ghrelin, affecting eating behavior and metabolism.

3. **Gut microbiota (GM).** Ninety-nine percent of the gut microbiota are bacteria, of which 90% are of the phyla Firmicutes and Bacteroidetes [152]. Some fungal, protozoan, and archaeal species have also been isolated. Some bacteria belong to the phyla Proteobacteria, Actinobacteria, Verrucomicrobia, and Fusobacteria. Most GM share a commensal relationship with the host, enhancing the overall fitness. A 20% increase in Firmicutes and a corresponding decrease in Bacteroidetes is associated with the increase in energy intake, thus inducing obesity. GM composition is involved in diseases like obesity, diabetes, inflammatory and immune disorders, and cancer.

   Type of food taken influences the population of gut biota. High fat Western diet reduces Bacteroidetes and increases in Firmicutes population, similar to what is seen in obesity. Increased ratio of Bacteroidetes to Firmicutes is linked with diminished body mass. *L. rhamnosus* and *Lactobacillus plantarum* are probacteria that convert dietary linoleic acid to conjugated linoleic acid (CLA). In mice, these bacteria prevent weight gain on a high fat diet. Various probiotic strategies are being developed to tailor the GM in such a way that they can help reduce weight of the host. GM are also associated with low-grade inflammation and metabolic syndrome via endotoxemia [153].

4. **Viral infections.** Four animal (canine distemper virus, Rous-associated virus type 7, Borna disease virus, and SMAM-1) and three human viruses (adenovirus (Ad) 36, Ad-37, and Ad-5) are known to cause obesity [154]. Scrapie agent has been shown to produce obesity in mice [155]. The infection affects fat cell differentiation, modulates appetite, or cause inflammation that dysregulates the feeding centre of the brain [156]. SMAM-1 is an avian adenovirus that is associated with human obesity. The human viruses stimulate enzymes and transcription factors that cause differentiation of preadipocytes into mature adipocytes and accumulation of TAGs.

3.2.2 Obesogenic environment

1. **Sedentary lifestyle and neighborhood safety.** Rapid urbanization has brought about various energy-saving techniques that promote sedentary lifestyle: convenient and cheap motorized transport, elevators, household appliances, etc. Entertainment is available 24 x 7, on the television or the mobile phone. Instead of playing games in the fields, children and adults prefer to play video games on a comfortable couch. Built environment, especially in areas inhabited by people with low socioeconomic status, is devoid of safe parks and walkways. Often in unsafe neighborhoods parents prefer their children to stay at home rather than venture out in the parks. Physical inactivity results in reduced energy expenditure, and if calorie intake is not reduced, it will ultimately lead to weight gain [157, 158].

2. **Diet.** With the abundance of calorie-dense food in attractive flavors and affordable prices, calorie-intake has increased for many persons. Fast-food is available at nearby stalls and it has become easier to purchase ready-to-eat food rather than cook at home. With increase in the number of nuclear families and double-incomes, home-cooked meals have been replaced by take-aways, home deliveries, and restaurant dinners. Calorie, carbohydrate, fat, and salt intake has increased, while intake of fruits and vegetables has decreased. Sweetened beverages and alcohol add empty calories [159, 160].

3. **Socioeconomic status (SES).** In case of developed countries, the incidence of obesity decreases with increased income and education [161], as people enjoy food security, are aware of healthy choices, and can afford healthy lifestyles in socially secure neighborhoods. In developing countries, the situation is complex. Low SES is associated with lack of food and medicines, ignorance regarding health, hygiene, and family size, and unwillingness to change [162]. An increase in family income brings about weight gain that can exceed the healthy limit. This is promoted by food insecurity. High SES shows slight decrease in obesity, however, this may not hold true for obesity in children, as high purchasing power and lack of self-control may lead to splurging on unhealthy foods.

4. **Unhealthy food advertisements.** Many people, especially children, are susceptible to food advertisements [163]. Aggressive marketing of calorie-dense food, sweetened beverages, cereals, snacks, etc. on the television, in print, on hoardings, and in shops affects vulnerable people. The message is clear: eat to

feel good. Many adults, especially those prone to depression, are affected in the same manner as children. Children who are overweight or obese usually grow into adults with weight issues.

5. **Culture and Ethnicity.** Certain cultures prefer chubbiness in children and adults and consider it a sign of health [164]. In Asian cultures, hospitality and affection are demonstrated through food. Asian men and women are more prone to develop central obesity [165]. Reward eating also promotes intake of unrequired calories in the form of high fat/high sucrose foods.

6. **Endocrine Disrupting Chemicals (EDCs).** The endocrine disrupting chemicals are man-made chemicals that block connections between hormones and their receptors [166]. The number of EDCs in the environment is increasing rapidly, even though their use has been banned. Their role in obesity has been highlighted by Brown et al. [167], who have used the U.S. National Health and Nutrition Examination Survey data, collected over nearly 4 decades, showing increase in calorie intake and BMI over time. For a given amount of calorie and macronutrient intake and leisure-time physical activity, the predicted BMI was significantly higher in 2006 than in 1998, indicating that factors other than diet and physical activity are contributing to the weight gain.

   More than 800 EDCs have been identified [168]. Persistent organic pollutants (POPs) and certain heavy metals have been classified into EDCs, metabolism disrupting chemicals (MDCs), and mitochondrial function disrupting chemicals (MtDCs). They can interact with nuclear and mitochondrial genes and bring about epigenetic changes, decrease insulin sensitivity, promote inflammation and obesity, decrease basal metabolic rate (BMR), and narrow down the vasculature.

   EDCs may be classified into obesogens and diabetogens. The obesogens (e.g. tributyltin, bisphenol A, phthalates, and metals like arsenic) can increase adipocyte differentiation and adipose tissue depots, disrupt normal lipid metabolism leading to obesity. The compound atrazine inhibits the electron transport chain in the mitochondrion. It has been shown to decrease BMR. Diabetogens either destroy beta cells of pancreas or disrupt their function leading to diabetes [169]. Bisphenol A blocks insulin receptor site causing insulin resistance.

7. **Weight-gain caused by pharmacotherapy.** Certain drugs can lead to weight gain or redistribution of fat. Large increase in weight may be accompanied by dyslipidemia, insulin resistance, metabolic syndrome, and increased risk of type 2 diabetes, non-alcoholic fatty liver disease (NAFLD), CVD, and cancer. Drugs associated with weight gain are described below.

a. **Antidepressants**. Drugs causing up to 5 kilogram per year weight gain include the following:

Tricyclic agents like amitriptyline and doxepine.

Selective serotonin reuptake inhibitors (SSRIs) like paroxetine and citalopram.

Serotonin and norepinephrine uptake inhibitors (SNRIs) like venlafaxine and duloxetine.

Monoamine oxidase inhibitors (MAOIs) like moclobemide, phenelzine.

Others like mirtazapine, mianserine, and maprotiline.

Bupropion is a norepinephrine and dopamine reuptake inhibitor that reduces food cravings. In US bupropion and naltrexone combination has been approved as an anti-obesity drug.

b. **Mood Stabilizer.** Lithium used in the treatment of bipolar disorders causes a weight gain of more than 5% of the initial body weight.

c. **Antipsychotics.** Typical antipsychotics like haloperidol and perphenazine cause weight gain of up to 5 kg/year. Some atypical antipsychotics like clozapine and olanzapine can cause more than 5 kilogram weight gain in a year (4.5–16.2 kg/year). Atypical antipsychotics like amisulpiride, quietapine, and sertindole cause weight gain of up to 5 kg/year.

d. **Anticonvulsants.** Topiramate and zonisamide produce weight loss. Gabapentine and pregabalin cause weight gain of up to 5 kg/year. Valproate and carbamazepine cause weight gain of more than 5 kg/year [170].

e. **Antihyperglycemics.** Type2 diabetes is strongly associated with diabetes. Many of the drugs used in the treatment can cause weight gain. Insulin, meglitinides, and sulfonylureas are known to cause weigh gain. Sulfonylureas like glimepiride, glyburide, glibenclamide, and gliclazide) and meglitinides (e.g. repaglinide) stimulate insulin secretion from the pancreas. Thiazolidinediones (TZD) or glitazones (e.g. pioglitazone) improve insulin sensitivity by acting on transcription factor PPAR-γ, which is involved in glucose and fat oxidation. Insulin increases lipogenesis and fat storage resulting in weight gain [171].

f. **Antihypertensives.** Weight gain is often associated with hypertension, and certain medicines used in the treatment of hypertension can cause weight gain. These include beta-blockers (atenolol, propranolol), angiotensin receptor blocker valsartan, and calcium channel blocker diltiazem [172].

g. **Corticosteroids.** Although short-term use of corticosteroids is not associated with significant change of weight, long-term use (> 3 months) is associated with significant gain of weight. Some patients showed a weight gain of >10 kg/year with prednisone [173].

Since many of the patients are already struggling with the problem of overweight or obesity, it is important to prescribe drugs that are weight neutral or promote weight loss.

4. Direction of future research

The obesity pandemic has spread across the globe and a lot of research is being done regarding its control. If the cause of obesity is known, it is easier to cure or limit the disease. Most of the current research is related to diagnosis of the underlying causes of the condition, as removal of the cause can ameliorate the condition. Suitable lifestyle changes and pharmacotherapies are being designed to reduce weight. Different types of surgical interventions have been improvised to stop weight gain/promote weight loss in patients with severe obesity.

5. Conclusion

Obesity prevalence is increasing worldwide to assume pandemic proportions. Since many diseases are associated with obesity, it is important to identify the presence and causes behind overweight and obesity. We have attempted to list the various causes behind obesity, but we may have missed out some inadvertently or due to lack of space. The purpose behind this work is to generate awareness about how overweight and obesity are sometimes beyond the patient's control. People with obesity of all ages have to face discrimination in the society, teaching institutes, and at the workplace. Often this discrimination leads to depression, stress, and overeating and aggravates the problem. It is important to remove this stigma and to consider people who are having to deal with this stigma as victims, rather than justifying the discrimination.

The World Health Organization has recognized obesity as a disease. It is important for physicians and healthcare workers to treat patients with obesity with compassion and empathy, to be open to endogenous and exogenous causes of obesity, and to suggest weight loss remedies if the patient is unable to achieve it himself/herself.

Conflict of interest

The authors declare no conflict of interest.

Author details

Indu Saxena[1]*, Suwarna Suman[2], Amar Preet Kaur[1], Abhilasha[2], Prasenjit Mitra[3], Praveen Sharma[2] and Manoj Kumar[4]

1 All India Institute of Medical Sciences, Gorakhpur, India

2 All India Institute of Medical Sciences, Jodhpur, India

3 Post-Graduate Institute of Medical Education and Research, Chandigarh, India

4 Maharishi Vashishtha Autonomous State Medical College, Basti, India

*Address all correspondence to: indu.saxena@rediffmail.com

References

[1] Bays HE, McCarthy W, Christensen S, Tondt J, Karjoo S, Davisson L, Ng J, Golden A, Burridge K, Conroy R, Wells S, Umashanker D, Afreen S, DeJesus R, Salter D, Shah N, Richardson L. Obesity algorithm slides, presented by the Obesity Medicine Association. www.obesityalgorithm.org. 2020. https://obesitymedicine.org/obesity-algorithmpowerpoint (Accessed = May 19, 2021)

[2] https://www.who.int/news-room/fact-sheets/detail/obesity-and-overweight. Accessed on May 20, 2021

[3] Panuganti KK, Nguyen M, Kshirsagar RK. Obesity. [Updated 2020 Dec 8]. In: StatPearls [Internet]. Treasure Island (FL): StatPearls Publishing; 2021 Jan. Available from: https://www.ncbi.nlm.nih.gov/books/NBK459357/

[4] Sturm R. The effects of obesity, smoking, and drinking on medical problems and costs. Obesity outranks both smoking and drinking in its deleterious effects on health and health costs. Health Aff (Millwood). 2002;21:245-253. DOI: 10.1377/hlthaff.21.2.245

[5] Metropolitan Life Insurance Company. New weight standards for men and women. Stat Bull Metrop Insur Co 1959;40:1

[6] Sikaris KA. The clinical biochemistry of obesity. Clin Biochem Rev. 2004; 25:165-181

[7] Wells JC. Sexual dimorphism of body composition. Best Practice & Research Clinical Endocrinology & Metabolism. 2007; 21(3):415-430

[8] Toth MJ, Tchernof A, Sites CK, Poehlman ET. Effect of menopausal status on body composition and abdominal fat distribution. Int J Obes Rel Metab Disorders. 2000; 24(2):226-231

[9] Wells JCK, Fewtrell MS. Measuring body composition. Arch Dis Child. 2006;91:612-617. DOI: 10.1136/adc.2005.085522

[10] Parente, EB, Mutter, S, Harjutsalo, V, Ahola AJ, Forsblom C, Groop PH. Waist-height ratio and waist are the best estimators of visceral fat in type 1 diabetes. Sci Rep 10. 2020; 18575. https://doi.org/10.1038/s41598-020-75667-5

[11] Bergman RN, Stefanovski D, Buchanan TA, Sumner AE, Reynolds JC, Sebring NG, Xiang AH, Watanabe RM. A better index of body adiposity. Obesity (Silver Spring). 2011;19(5):1083-1089. DOI: 10.1038/oby.2011.38

[12] Brozek J, Grande F, Anderson JT, Keys A. Densitometric analysis of body composition: Revision of some quantitative assumptions. Ann N Y Acad Sci. 1963;110:113-140. DOI: 10.1111/j.1749-6632.1963.tb17079.x

[13] Lee SY, Gallagher D. Assessment methods in human body composition. Curr Opin Clin Nutr Metab Care. 2008;11(5):566-572. DOI: 10.1097/MCO.0b013e32830b5f23

[14] Toomey CM, Cremona A, Hughes K, Norton C. A review of body composition measurement in the assessment of health. Top Clin Nutrn. 2015;30(1): 16-32

[15] Duren DL, Sherwood RJ, Czerwinski SA, Lee M, Choh AC, Siervogel RM, Cameron Chumlea W. Body composition methods: Comparisons and interpretation. J Diabetes Sci Technol. 2008;2(6): 1139-1146. DOI: 10.1177/193229680800200623.

[16] Vague J. [Sexual differentiation; Factor determining forms of obesity]. Presse Med. 1947;55(30):339. French. PMID: 18918084.

[17] Lapidus L, Bengtsson C, Larsson B, Pennert K, Rybo E, Sjöström L. Distribution of adipose tissue and risk of cardiovascular disease and death: a 12 year follow up of participants in the population study of women in Gothenburg, Sweden. Br Med J (Clin Res Ed). 1984;289(6454):1257-61. DOI: 10.1136/bmj.289.6454.1257. PMID: 6437507; PMCID: PMC1443498.

[18] Donahue RP, Abbott RD, Bloom E, Reed DM, Yano K. Central obesity and coronary heart disease in men. Lancet. 1987;1(8537):821-824. DOI: 10.1016/s0140-6736(87)91605-9.

[19] Britton KA, Fox CS. Ectopic fat depots and cardiovascular disease. Circulation. 2011;124(24): e837-e841. DOI: 10.1161/CIRCULATIONAHA.111.077602

[20] Neeland IJ, Grundy SM, Li X, Adams-Huet B, Vega GL. Comparison of visceral fat mass measurement by dual-X-ray absorptiometry and magnetic resonance imaging in a multiethnic cohort: The Dallas heart study. Nutr Diabetes. 2016; 6: e221.

[21] Sims EAH. Characterization of the syndromes of obesity, in Brodoff BN, Bleicher SJ (eds): Diabetes Mellitus and Obesity. Baltimore, MD, Williams & Wilkins, 1982, pp. 219-226

[22] Lavie CJ, Laddu D, Arena R, Ortega FB, Alpert MA, Kushner RF. Healthy weight and obesity prevention. JACC Health Promotion Series, JACC. 2018; 72(13):1506-1531. https://doi.org/10.1016/j.jacc.2018.08.1037

[23] Pennington AW. A reorientation on obesity. N Engl J Med. 1953 Jun 4;248(23):959-964. doi: 10.1056/NEJM195306042482301. PMID: 13046654.

[24] Redden DT, Divers J, Vaughan LK. Regional admixture mapping and structured association testing: Conceptual unification and an extensible general linear model. PLoS Genet. 2006;2:e137

[25] Wardle J, Carnell S, Haworth CM, Plomin R. Evidence for a strong genetic influence on childhood adiposity despite the force of the obesogenic environment. Am J Clin Nutr. 2008;87:398-404.

[26] Yazdi FT, Clee SM, Meyre D. Obesity genetics in mouse and human: Back and forth, and back again. Peer J. 2015; 3:e856

[27] Rankinen T, Zuberi A, Chagnon YC. The human obesity gene map: The 2005 update. Obesity (SilverSpring) 2006;14(4):529-644.

[28] Zhang Y, Proenca R, Maffei M, Barone M, Leopold L, Friedman JM. Positional cloning of the mouse obese gene and its human homologue. Nature. 1994; 372(6505):425-432.

[29] Funcke JB, von Schnurbein J, Lennerz B, Lahr G, Debatin KM, Fischer-Posovszky P, Wabitsch M. Monogenic forms of childhood obesity due to mutations in the leptin gene. Mol Cell Pediatr. 2014;1(1):3. DOI: 10.1186/s40348-014-0003-1.

[30] Farooqi IS, Jebb SA, Langmack G, Lawrence E, Cheetham CH, Prentice AM, Hughes IA, McCamish MA, O'Rahilly S. Effects of recombinant leptin therapy in a child with congenital leptin deficiency. N Engl J Med. 1999; 341: 879-884

[31] Licinio J, Caglayan S, Ozata M, Yildiz BO, de Miranda PB, O'Kirwan F, Whitby R, Liang L, Cohen P, Bhasin S, Krauss RM, Veldhuis JD, Wagner AJ,

DePaoli AM, McCann SM, Wong ML. Phenotypic effects of leptin replacement on morbid obesity, diabetes mellitus, hypogonadism, and behavior in leptin deficient adults. Proc Natl Acad Sci USA. 2004; 101: 4531-4536

[32] Ahima RS, Prabakaran D, Mantzoros C, Qu D, Lowell B, Maratos-Flier E, Flier JS. Role of leptin in the neuroendocrine response to fasting. Nature. 1996; 382: 250-252

[33] Chua SC Jr, Koutras IK, Han L, Liu SM, Kay J, Young SJ, Chung WK, Leibel RL. Fine structure of the murine leptin receptor gene: Splice site suppression is required to form two alternatively spliced transcripts. Genomics. 1997;45: 264-270

[34] Tartaglia LA. The leptin receptor. J Biol Chem. 1997;272: 6093-6096

[35] Lee GH, Proenca R, Montez JM, Carroll KM, Darvishzadeh JG, Lee JI, Friedman JM. Abnormal splicing of the leptin receptor in diabetic mice. Nature. 1996;379: 632-635

[36] Kievit P, Howard JK, Badman MK, Balthasar N, Coppari R, Mori H, Lee CE, Elmquist JK, Yoshimura A, Flier JS. Enhanced leptin sensitivity and improved glucose homeostasis in mice lacking suppressor of cytokine signaling-3 in POMC-expressing cells. Cell Metab. 2006; 4(2):123-32. DOI: 10.1016/j.cmet.2006.06.010. PMID: 16890540.

[37] Vaisse C, Halaas JL, Horvath CM, Darnell JE Jr, Stoffel M, Friedman JM. Leptin activation of Stat3 in the hypothalamus of wild-type and Ob/Ob mice but not db/db mice. Nat Genet. 1996;14: 95-97

[38] Mori H, Hanada R, Hanada T, Aki D, Mashima R, Nishinakamura H, Torisu T, Chien KR, Yasukawa H, Yoshimura A. Socs3 deficiency in the brain elevates leptin sensitivity and confers resistance to diet-induced obesity. Nat Med. 2004;10: 739-743

[39] Howard JK, Cave BJ, Oksanen LJ, Tzameli I, Bjorbaek C, Flier JS. Enhanced leptin sensitivity and attenuation of diet-induced obesity in mice with haploinsufficiency of Socs3. Nat Med. 2004; 10: 734-738

[40] Cheung CC, Clifton DK, Steiner RA. Proopiomelanocortin neurons are direct targets for leptin in the hypothalamus. Endocrinology. 1997;138: 4489-4492

[41] Elias CF, Aschkenasi C, Lee C, Kelly J, Ahima RS, Bjorbaek C, Flier JS, Saper CB, Elmquist JK. Leptin differentially regulates NPY and POMC neurons projecting to the lateral hypothalamic area. Neuron. 1999; 23:775-786

[42] Bagnasco M, Dube MG, Kalra PS, Kalra SP. Evidence for the existence of distinct central appetite, energy expenditure, and ghrelin stimulation pathways as revealed by hypothalamic site-specific leptin gene therapy. Endocrinology. 2002;143: 4409-4421

[43] El Haschimi K, Pierroz DD, Hileman SM, Bjorbaek C, Flier JS. Two defects contribute to hypothalamic leptin resistance in mice with diet-induced obesity. J Clin Invest. 2000;105: 1827-1832

[44] Clement K, Vaisse C, Lahlou N, Cabrol S, Pelloux V, Cassuto D, Gourmelen M, Dina C, Chambaz J, Lacorte JM, Basdevant A, Bougneres P, Lebouc Y, Froguel P, Guy-Grand B. A mutation in the human leptin receptor gene causes obesity and pituitary dysfunction. Nature. 1998;392: 398-401

[45] Farooqi IS, Wangensteen T, Collins S, et al. Clinical and molecular genetic spectrum of congenital deficiency of the leptin receptor. N Engl

J Med. 2007; 356(3):237-47. [PubMed: 17229951]

[46] Nunziata A, Funcke JB, Borck G, von Schnurbein J, Brandt S, Lennerz B, Moepps B, Gierschik P, Fischer-Posovszky P, Wabitsch M. Functional and Phenotypic Characteristics of Human Leptin Receptor Mutations. J Endocr Soc. 2018 Sep 17;3(1):27-41. doi: 10.1210/js.2018-00123. PMID: 30560226; PMCID: PMC6293235.

[47] Clément K, Vaisse C, Lahlou N, et al. A mutation in the human leptin receptor gene causes obesity and pituitary dysfunction. Nature. 1998; 392(6674):398-401. [PubMed: 9537324]

[48] Cawley NX, Li Z, Loh YP. 60 YEARS OF POMC: Biosynthesis, trafficking, and secretion of pro-opiomelanocortin-derived peptides. J Mol Endocrinol. 2016;56(4):T77-97. DOI: 10.1530/JME-15-0323. PMID: 26880796; PMCID: PMC4899099.

[49] Harno E, Gali Ramamoorthy T, Coll AP, White A. POMC: The Physiological Power of Hormone Processing. Physiol Rev. 2018;98(4):2381-2430. doi: 10.1152/physrev.00024.2017. PMID: 30156493; PMCID: PMC6170974.

[50] Krude H, Biebermann H, Luck W, Horn R, Brabant G, Grüters A. Severe early-onset obesity, adrenal insufficiency and red hair pigmentation caused by POMC mutations in humans. Nat Genet. 1998;19(2):155-157. DOI: 10.1038/509. PMID: 9620771.

[51] Ramos-Molina B, Martin MG, Lindberg I. PCSK1 Variants and human obesity. Prog Mol Biol Transl Sci. 2016;140:47-74. DOI: 10.1016/bs.pmbts.2015.12.001. PMID: 27288825; PMCID: PMC6082390

[52] Alsters SIM, Goldstone AP, Buxton JL, Zekavati A, Sosinsky A, Yiorkas AM, et al. Truncating homozygous mutation of carboxypeptidase E (CPE) in a morbidly obese female with type 2 diabetes mellitus, intellectual disability and hypogonadotrophic hypogonadism. PLoS ONE. 2015;10(6):e0131417. DOI: 10.1371/journal.pone.0131417

[53] Tao YX. The melanocortin-4 receptor: physiology, pharmacology, and pathophysiology. Endocr Rev. 2010;31(4):506-43. DOI: 10.1210/er.2009-0037. PMID: 20190196; PMCID: PMC3365848.

[54] Fani L, Bak S, Delhanty P, van Rossum EFC, van den Akker ELT. The melanocortin-4 receptor as target for obesity treatment: A systematic review of emerging pharmacological therapeutic options. Int J Obesity. 2014; 38:163-169. DOI: 10.1038/ijo.2013.80

[55] Farooqi IS, Keogh JM, Yeo GSH, Lank EJ, Cheetham K, O'Rahilly S. Clinical spectrum of obesity and mutations in the melanocortin 4 receptor gene. N Engl J Med. 2003;348:1085-1095. DOI: 10.1056/NEJMoa022050

[56] https://www.genecards.org/cgi-bin

[57] Bonnefond A, Raimondo A, Stutzmann F, Ghoussaini M, Ramachandrappa S, Bersten DC, Durand E, Vatin V, Balkau B, Lantieri O, Raverdy V, Pattou F, Van Hul W, Van Gaal L, Peet DJ, Weill J, Miller JL, Horber F, Goldstone AP, Driscoll DJ, Bruning JB, Meyre D, Whitelaw ML, Froguel P. Loss-of-function mutations in SIM1 contribute to obesity and Prader-Willi-like features. J Clin Invest. 2013;123(7):3037-41. DOI: 10.1172/JCI68035. PMID: 23778136; PMCID: PMC3696559

[58] Pandit M, Behl T, SachdevaM, Arora S. Role of brain derived neurotropic factor in obesity. Obes Med.

2020; 17:100189. DOI: 10.1016/j.obmed.2020.100189

[59] Miranda M, Morici JF, Zanoni MB, Bekinschtein P. Brain-derived neurotrophic factor: A key molecule for memory in the healthy and the pathological brain. Front Cell Neurosci. 2019; 13:363. DOI: 10.3389/fncel.2019.00363

[60] Han JC, Liu Q-R, Jones M, Levinn RL, Menzie CM, Jefferson-George KS, Adler-Wailes DC, Sanford EL, Lacbawan FL, Uhl GR, Rennert OM, Yanovski JA. Brain-derived neurotrophic factor and obesity in the WAGR syndrome. New Eng J Med. 2008;359: 918-927. DOI: 10.1056/NEJMoa0801119

[61] Gray J, Yeo G, Hung C, Keogh J, Clayton P, Banerjee K, McAulay A, O'Rahilly S, Farooqi IS. Functional characterization of human NTRK2 mutations identified in patients with severe early-onset obesity. Int J Obes. 2007; 31, 359-364. DOI: 10.1038/sj.ijo.0803390

[62] Pearce LR, Atanassova N, Banton MC, Bottomley B, van der Klaauw AA, Revelli JP, Hendricks A, Keogh JM, Henning E, Doree D, Jeter-Jones S, Garg S, Bochukova EG, Bounds R, Ashford S, Gayton E, Hindmarsh PC, Shield JP, Crowne E, Barford D, Wareham NJ; UK10K consortium, O'Rahilly S, Murphy MP, Powell DR, Barroso I, Farooqi IS. KSR2 mutations are associated with obesity, insulin resistance, and impaired cellular fuel oxidation. Cell. 2013;155(4):765-77. DOI:10.1016/j.cell.2013.09.058. PMID: 24209692; PMCID: PMC3898740.

[63] Rui L. SH2B1 regulation of energy balance, body weight, and glucose metabolism. World J Diabetes. 2014; 5(4): 511-526. DOI: 10.4239/wjd.v5.i4.511

[64] Walters RG, Jacquemont S, Valsesia A, de Smith AJ, Martinet D, Andersson J, Falchi M, Chen F, Andrieux J, Lobbens S, Delobel B, Stutzmann F, El-Sayed Moustafa JS, Chèvre JC, Lecoeur C, Vatin V, Bouquillon S, Buxton JL, Boute O, Holder-Espinasse M, Cuisset JM, Lemaitre MP, Ambresin AE, Brioschi A, Gaillard M, Giusti V, Fellmann F, Ferrarini A, Hadjikhani N, Campion D, et al. A new highly penetrant form of obesity due to deletions on chromosome 16p11.2. Nature. 2010; 463: 671-675. DOI: 10.1038/nature08727.

[65] Achari AE, Jain SK. Adiponectin, a Therapeutic Target for Obesity, Diabetes, and Endothelial Dysfunction. Int J Mol Sci. 2017;18(6):1321. doi: 10.3390/ijms18061321. PMID: 28635626; PMCID: PMC5486142.

[66] Hotta K, Funahashi T, Arita Y, Takahashi M, Matsuda M, Okamoto Y, Iwahashi H, Kuriyama H, Ouchi N, Maeda K, Nishida M, Kihara S, Sakai N, Nakajima T, Hasegawa K, Muraguchi M, Ohmoto Y, Nakamura T, Yamashita S, Hanafusa T, Matsuzawa Y. Plasma concentrations of a novel, adiposespecific protein, adiponectin, in type 2 diabetic patients. Arterioscler Thromb Vasc Biol. 2000;20: 1595-1599

[67] Yang WS, Lee WJ, Funahashi T, Tanaka S, Matsuzawa Y, Chao CL, Chen CL, Tai TY, Chuang LM. Weight reduction increases plasma levels of an adipose-derived anti-inflammatory protein, adiponectin. J Clin Endocrinol Metab. 86:3815-3819

[68] Cawthorn WP, Scheller EL, Learman BS, Parlee SD, Simon BR, Mori H, Ning X, Bree AJ, Schell B, Broome DT, Soliman SS, DelProposto JL, Lumeng CN, Mitra A, Pandit SV, Gallagher KA, Miller JD, Krishnan V, Hui SK, Bredella MA, Fazeli PK, Klibanski A, Horowitz MC, Rosen CJ, MacDougald OA. Bone marrow adipose tissue is an endocrine organ that contributes to increased circulating adiponectin during caloric

restriction. Cell Metabolism. 2014; 20 (2): 368-375. doi:10.1016/j.cmet.2014.06.003

[69] Bauche IB, El Mkadem SA, Pottier AM, Senou M, Many MC, Rezsohazy R, Penicaud L, Maeda N, Funahashi T, Brichard SM. Overexpression of adiponectin targeted to adipose tissue in transgenic mice: Impaired adipocyte differentiation. Endocrinology. 2007 148 (4): 1539-1549. doi:10.1210/en.2006-0838. PMID 17204560.

[70] Fruebis J, Tsao TS, Javorschi S, Ebbets-Reed D, Erickson MR, Yen FT, Bihain BE, Lodish HF. Proteolytic cleavage product of 30-kDa adipocyte complement-related protein increases fatty acid oxidation in muscle and causes weight loss in mice. Proc Natl Acad Sci USA. 2001;98:2005-2010

[71] Berg AH, Combs TP, Du X, Brownlee M, Scherer PE. The adipocyte-secreted protein Acrp30 enhances hepatic insulin action. Nat Med 7: 947-953, 2001.

[72] Yamauchi T, Kamon J, Waki H, Terauchi Y, Kubota N, Hara K, Mori Y, Ide T, Murakami K, Tsuboyama-Kasaoka N, Ezaki O, Akanuma Y, Gavrilova O, Vinson C, Reitman ML, Kagechika H, Shudo K, Yoda M, Nakano Y, Tobe K, Nagai R, Kimura S, Tomita M, Froguel P, Kadowaki T. The fat-derived hormone adiponectin reverses insulin resistance associated with both lipoatrophy and obesity. Nat Med. 2001;7: 941-946

[73] Díez JJ, Iglesias P. The role of the novel adipocyte-derived hormone adiponectin in human disease. European Journal of Endocrinology. 2003 148 (3): 293-300. DOI:10.1530/eje.0.1480293.

[74] Fang X, Sweeney G. Mechanisms regulating energy metabolism by adiponectin in obesity and diabetes. Biochemical Society Transactions. 2006; 34 (Pt 5): 798-801. DOI:10.1042/BST0340798.

[75] Okamoto Y, Folco EJ, Minami M, Wara AK, Feinberg MW, Sukhova GK, Colvin RA, Kihara S, Funahashi T, Luster AD, Libby P. Adiponectin inhibits the production of CXC receptor 3 chemokine ligands in macrophages and reduces T-lymphocyte recruitment in atherogenesis. Circ Res. 2008; 102(2):218-225

[76] Ouchi N, Walsh K. Adiponectin as an anti-inflammatory factor. Clin Chim Acta. 2007; 380(1-2):24-30. DOI: 10.1016/j.cca.2007.01.026. Epub 2007 Feb 2. PMID: 17343838; PMCID: PMC2755046.

[77] Eggleton JS, Jialal I. Thiazolidinediones. [Updated 2021 Apr 6]. In: StatPearls [Internet]. Treasure Island (FL): StatPearls Publishing; 2021 Jan-. Available from: https://www.ncbi.nlm.nih.gov/books/NBK551656/

[78] Waki H, Yamauchi T, Kamon J, et al. Impaired multimerization of human adiponectin mutants associated with diabetes. Molecular structure and multimer formation of adiponectin. J Biol Chem. 2003;278: 40352-40363.

[79] Vendramini MF, Kasamatsu TS, Crispim F, Ferreira SR, Matioli SR, Moisés RS. Novel mutation in the adiponectin (ADIPOQ) gene is associated with hypoadiponectinaemia in Japanese-Brazilians. Clin Endocrinol. 2009;71:50-55

[80] Bueno AC, Sun K, Martins CS, Elias Junior J, Miranda W, Tao C, Foss-Freitas MC, Barbieri MA, Bettiol H, de Castro M, Scherer PE, Antonini SR, A novel ADIPOQ mutation (p.M40K) impairs assembly of high-molecular-weight adiponectin and is associated with early-onset obesity and metabolic syndrome. J Clin Endocrinol Metab. 2014; 99(4):E683–E693. DOI: 10.1210/jc.2013-3009

[81] Saeed S, Bonnefond A, Tamanini F, Mirza MU, Manzoor J, Janjua QM,

Din SM, Gaitan J, Milochau A, Durand E, Vaillant E, Haseeb A, De Graeve F, Rabearivelo I, Sand O, Queniat G, Boutry R, Schott DA, Ayesha H, Ali M, Khan WI, Butt TA, Rinne T, Stumpel C, Abderrahmani A, Lang J, Arslan M, Froguel P. Loss-of-function mutations in ADCY3 cause monogenic severe obesity. Nat Genet. 2018 Feb;50(2):175-179. doi: 10.1038/s41588-017-0023-6. Epub 2018 Jan 8. PMID: 29311637.

[82] Pitman JL, Wheeler MC, Lloyd DJ, Walker JR, Glynne RJ, Gekakis N. A gain-of-function mutation in adenylate cyclase 3 protects mice from diet-induced obesity. PLoS One. 2014 Oct 16;9(10):e110226. doi: 10.1371/journal.pone.0110226. PMID: 25329148; PMCID: PMC4199629.

[83] Talbert ME, Langefeld CD, Ziegler JT, Haffner SM, Norris JM, Bowden DW. INSIG2 SNPs associated with obesity and glucose homeostasis traits in Hispanics: the IRAS Family Study. Obesity (Silver Spring). 2009;17(8):1554-62. DOI: 10.1038/oby.2009.94. PMID: 19360016; PMCID: PMC2916685

[84] Prakash J, Mittal B, Apurva S, Shally A, Pranjal S, Neena S. Common genetic variant of insig2 gene rs7566605 polymorphism is associated with severe obesity in North India. Iran Biomed J. 2017;21(4):261-9. DOI: 10.18869/acadpub.ibj.21.4.261. PMID: 28160769; PMCID: PMC5459941

[85] Freake HC. A genetic mutation in PPAR gamma is associated with enhanced fat cell differentiation: Implications for human obesity. Nutr Rev. 1999;57(5 Pt 1):154-156. DOI: 10.1111/j.1753-4887.1999.tb01796.x. PMID: 10391018

[86] Celi FS, Shuldiner AR. The role of peroxisome proliferator-activated receptor gamma in diabetes and obesity. Curr Diab Rep. 2002;2(2):179-185. DOI: 10.1007/s11892-002-0078-2. PMID: 12643137

[87] Tung YCL, Yeo GSH, O'Rahilly S, Coll AP. Obesity and FTO: Changing focus at a complex locus. Cell Metabolism, 20 (5) (2014), pp. 710-718. DOI: 10.1016/j.cmet.2014.09.010

[88] Driscoll DJ, Miller JL, Schwartz S, et al. Prader-Willi Syndrome. 1998 Oct 6 [Updated 2017 Dec 14]. In: Adam MP, Ardinger HH, Pagon RA, et al., editors. GeneReviews® [Internet]. Seattle (WA): University of Washington, Seattle; 1993-2021. Available from: https://www.ncbi.nlm.nih.gov/books/NBK1330/

[89] Forsythe E, Beales P. Bardet–Biedl syndrome. Eur J Hum Genet. 2013; 21:8-13. DOI:10.1038/ejhg.2012.115

[90] Tahani N, Maffei P, Dollfus H, Paisey R, Valverde D, Milan G, Han JC, Favaretto F, Madathil SC, Dawson C, Armstrong MJ, Warfield AT, Duzenli S, Francomano CA, Gunay-Aygun M, Dassie F, Marion V, Valenti M, Leeson-Beevers K, Chivers A, Steeds R, Barrett T, Geberhiwot T. Consensus clinical management guidelines for Alström syndrome. Orphanet J Rare Dis. 2020; 15, 253. DOI: 10.1186/s13023-020-01468-8

[91] Mantovani G, Bastepe M, Monk D, de Sanctis L, Thiele S, Usardi A, Ahmed SF, Bufo R, Choplin T, De Filippo G, Devernois G, Eggermann T, Elli FM, Freson K, Ramirez AG, Germain-Lee EL, Groussin L, Hamdy N, Hanna P, Hiort O, Juppner H, Kamenicky P, Knight N, Kottler M-L, Le Norcy E, Lecumberri B, Levine MA, Makitie O, Martin R, Martos-Moreno GA, Minagawa M, Murray P, Pereda A, Pignolo R, Reinmark L, Rodado R, Rothenbuhler A, Saraff V, Shoemaker AH, Shore EM, Silve C, Turan S, Woods P, Zillikens MC, de Nanclares GP, Linglart A. Diagnosis and management of

pseudohypoparathyroidism and related disorders: First international consensus statement. Nat Rev Endocrinol. 2018; 14, 476-500. DOI: 10.1038/ s41574-018-0042-0

[92] Cohen MM Jr, Hall BD, Smith DW, Graham CB, Lampert KJ. A new syndrome with hypotonia, obesity, mental deficiency, and facial, oral, ocular, and limb anomalies. J Pediatr. 1973; 83(2):280-284

[93] Rodrigues JM, Fernandes HD, Caruthers C, Braddock SR, Knutsen AP. Cohen syndrome: Review of the literature. Cureus. 2018;10(9):e3330. DOI: 10.7759/cureus.3330. PMID: 30473963; PMCID: PMC6248805.

[94] Bertapelli F, Pitetti K, Agiovlasitis S, Guerra-Junior G. Overweight and obesity in children and adolescents with down syndrome-prevalence, determinants, consequences, and interventions: A literature review. Res Dev Disabil. 2016;57:181-192. DOI: 10.1016/j. ridd.2016.06.018. PMID: 27448331.

[95] Lebenthal Y, Levy S, Sofrin-Drucker E, Nagelberg N, Weintrob N, Shalitin S, de Vries L, Tenenbaum A, Phillip M, Lazar L. The Natural History of Metabolic Comorbidities in Turner Syndrome from childhood to early adulthood: Comparison between 45,X monosomy and other karyotypes. Front Endocrinol (Lausanne). 2018;9:27. DOI: 10.3389/fendo.2018.00027. PMID: 29479339; PMCID: PMC5811462.

[96] Hinney A, Giuranna J. (2018) Polygenic obesity. In: Freemark M. (eds) Pediatric Obesity. Contemporary Endocrinology. Humana Press, Cham. https://doi.org/10.1007/ 978-3-319-68192-4_10

[97] Pigeyre M, Yazdi FT, Kaur Y, Meyre D. Recent progress in genetics, epigenetics and metagenomics unveils the pathophysiology of human obesity. Clin. Sci. 2016;130: 943-986

[98] Khera AV, Chaffin M, Wade KH, Zahid S, Brancale J, Xia R, Distefano M, Senol-Cosar O, Haas ME, Bick A, Aragam KG, Lander ES, Smith GD, Mason-Suares H, Fornage M, Lebo M, Timpson NJ, Kaplan LM, Kathiresan S. Polygenic prediction of weight and obesity trajectories from birth to adulthood. Cell. 2019;177(3):587-596.e9. DOI: 10.1016/j.cell.2019.03.028. PMID: 31002795; PMCID: PMC6661115.

[99] https://www.yalemedicine.org/ conditions/mosaicism

[100] Ouni M, Schürmann A. Epigenetic contribution to obesity. Mamm Genome. 2020; 31, 134-145. DOI:10.1007/s00335-020-09835-3

[101] Lesseur C, Armstrong DA, Paquette AG, Koestler DC, Padbury JF, Marsit CJ. Tissue-specific leptin promoter DNA methylation is associated with maternal and infant perinatal factors. Mol Cell Endocrinol. 2013; 381(1-2):160-167

[102] Tobi EW, Lumey LH, Talens RP, Kremer D, Putter H, Stein AD, Slagboom PE, Heijmans BT. DNA methylation differences after exposure to prenatal famine are common and timing- and sex-specific. Hum Mol Genet. 2009; 18(21):4046-4053

[103] Zhang Q, Ramlee MK, Brunmeir R, Villanueva CJ, Halperin D, Xu F. Dynamic and distinct histone modifications modulate the expression of key adipogenesis regulatory genes. Cell Cycle. 2012; 11(23):4310-4322

[104] Pasquinelli AE. MicroRNAs and their targets: Recognition, regulation and an emerging reciprocal relationship. Nat Rev Genet. 2012; 13(4):271-282

[105] Cruz KJC, de Oliveira ARS, Morais JBS, Severo JS, Marreiro DDN. Role of microRNAs on adipogenesis, chronic low-grade inflammation, and insulin resistance in obesity. Nutrition. 2017; 35():28-35.

[106] Prats-Puig A, Ortega FJ, Mercader JM, Moreno-Navarrete JM, Moreno M, Bonet N, Ricart W, López-Bermejo A, Fernández-Real JM. Changes in circulating microRNAs are associated with childhood obesity. J Clin Endocrinol Metab. 2013; 98(10):E1655-E1660.

[107] Zhao H, Shen J, Daniel-MacDougall C, Wu X, Chow WH. Plasma MicroRNA signature predicting weight gain among Mexican-American women. Obesity (Silver Spring). 2017; 25(5):958-964.

[108] Hubal MJ, Nadler EP, Ferrante SC, Barberio MD, Suh JH, Wang J, Dohm GL, Pories WJ, Mietus-Snyder M, Freishtat RJ. Circulating adipocyte-derived exosomal MicroRNAs associated with decreased insulin resistance after gastric bypass. Obesity (Silver Spring). 2017; 25(1):102-110.

[109] Yan Z, Zhang H, Maher C, Arteaga-Solis E, Champagne FA, Wu L, McDonald JD, Yan B, Schwartz GJ, Miller RL. Prenatal polycyclic aromatic hydrocarbon, adiposity, peroxisome proliferator-activated receptor (PPAR) γ methylation in offspring, grand-offspring mice. PLoS One. 2014; 9(10):e110706.

[110] Anderson OS, Kim JH, Peterson KE, Sanchez BN, Sant KE, Sartor MA, Weinhouse C, Dolinoy DC. Novel epigenetic biomarkers mediating bisphenol a exposure and metabolic phenotypes in female mice. Endocrinology. 2017; 158(1):31-40.

[111] Fall CHD, Sachdev HS, Osmond C, et al. For the COHORTS investigators. Association between maternal age at childbirth and child and adult outcomes in the offspring: A prospective study in five low-income and middle-income countries (COHORTS collaboration). Lancet Glob Health. 2015; DOI: 10.1016/S2214-109X(15)00038-8

[112] Wang H, Zhang Y, Tian Y, Li F, Yan C, Wang H, Luo Z, Jiang F, Zhang J. Maternal age at menarche and offspring body mass index in childhood. BMC Pediatr. 2019; 19, 312. DOI: 10.1186/s12887-019-1659-4

[113] Dabelea D. The predisposition to obesity and diabetes in offspring of diabetic mothers. Diabetes Care 2007 Jul; 30(Supplement 2): S169-S174. DOI: 10.2337/dc07-s211

[114] Magalhães EIDS, Lima NP, Menezes AMB, Goncalves H, Wehmeister FC, Assuncao MCF, Horta BL. Maternal smoking during pregnancy and offspring body composition in adulthood: Results from two birth cohort studies. BMJ Open. 2019; 9: e023852. DOI: 10.1136/bmjopen-2018-023852

[115] Ruiz M, Goldblatt P, Morrison J, Porta D, Forastiere F, Hryhorczuk D, Antipkin Y, Saurel-Cubizolles MJ, Lioret S, Vrijheid M, Torrent M, Iñiguez C, Larrañaga I, Bakoula C, Veltsista A, van Eijsden M, Vrijkotte TG, Andrýsková L, Dušek L, Barros H, Correia S, Järvelin MR, Taanila A, Ludvigsson J, Faresjö T, Marmot M, Pikhart H. Impact of low maternal education on early childhood overweight and obesity in Europe. Paediatr Perinat Epidemiol. 2016;30(3):274-284. DOI: 10.1111/ppe.12285. PMID: 26945670.

[116] Muthuri SK, Onywera VO, Tremblay MS, Broyles ST, Chaput J-P, Fogelholm M, et al. (2016) Relationships between parental education and overweight with childhood overweight and physical activity in 9-11 year old children: Results from a 12-country study. PLoS ONE 11(8): e0147746. https://doi.org/10.1371/journal.pone.0147746

[117] Fitzsimons E, Pongiglione B. The impact of maternal employment on children's weight: Evidence from the UK. SSM-Population Health. 2019: 100333. DOI: 10.1016/j.ssmph.2018.100333

[118] Zulewski H, Muller B, Exer P, Miserez AR, Staub JJ. Estimation of tissue hypothyroidism by a new clinical score: Evaluation of patients with various grades of hypothyroidism and controls. J Clin Endocrinol Metab. 1997;82:771-776

[119] Chaker L, Bianco AC, Jonklaas J, Peeters RP. Hypothyroidism. Lancet. 2017;390(10101):1550-1562. DOI: 10.1016/S0140-6736(17)30703-1. PMID: 28336049; PMCID: PMC6619426.

[120] Shahid MA, Ashraf MA, Sharma S. Physiology, Thyroid Hormone. [Updated 2020 May 18]. In: StatPearls [Internet]. Treasure Island (FL): StatPearls Publishing; 2021 Jan-. Available from: https://www.ncbi.nlm.nih.gov/books/NBK500006/ Accessed on May 24, 2021

[121] Smith TJ, Bahn RS, Gorman CA. Connective tissue, glycosaminoglycans, and diseases of the thyroid. Endocr Rev. 1989;10:366-391

[122] Basu G, Mohapatra A. Interactions between thyroid disorders and kidney diseases. Indian J Endocrinol Metab. 2012; 16(2):201-213. DOI: 10.4103/2230-8210.93737. PMID:22470856; PMCID: PMC33133737

[123] Pracyk JB, Slotkin TA. Thyroid hormone differentially regulates development of beta-adrenergic receptors, adenylate cyclase and ornithine decarboxylase in rat heart and kidney. J Dev Physiol. 1991; 16(4):251-261

[124] Joachim M. Weitzel, K. Alexander Iwen. Coordination of mitochondrial biogenesis by thyroid hormone. Molecular and Cellular Endocrinology, Elsevier, 2011, 342 (1-2), pp.1. ff10.1016/j.mce.2011.05.009ff. ffhal-00721652f

[125] Lanni A, Moreno M, Lombardi A, Goglia F. Thyroid hormone and uncoupling proteins. FEBS Lett. 2003; 543(1-3):5-10

[126] B. Havekes and H. P. Sauerwein, Adipocyte-myocyte crosstalk in skeletal muscle insulin resistance; is there a role for thyroid hormone? Curr Opin Clin Nutr Metab Care. 2010; 13(6): 641-646

[127] Rotterdam, consensus, 2003: Revised 2003 consensus on diagnostic criteria and long-term health risks related to polycystic ovary syndrome (PCOS). Hum Reprod 2004;19:41-47

[128] Kiddy DS, Hamilton-Fairley D, Bush A, et al. Improvement in endocrine and ovarian function during dietary treatment of obese women with polycystic ovary syndrome. Clin Endocrinol (Oxf). 1992;36:105-111

[129] Barber TM, McCarthy MI, Wass JA, Franks S. Obesity and polycystic ovary syndrome. Clin Endocrinol (Oxf). 2006;65:137-145

[130] Brzechffa PR, Jakimiuk AJ, Agarwal SK, Weitsman SR, Buyalos RP, Magoffin DA. Serum immunoreactive leptin concentrations in women with polycystic ovary syndrome. J Clin Endocrinol Metab 1996;81:4166-4169

[131] Pirwany IR, Fleming R, Sattar N, Greer IA, Wallace AM. Circulating leptin concentrations and ovarian function in polycystic ovary syndrome. Eur J Endocrinol. 2001;145:289-294

[132] Houjeghani S, Pourghassem Gargari B, Farzadi L. Serum leptin and ghrelin levels in women with polycystic ovary syndrome: Correlation with anthropometric, metabolic, and endocrine parameters. Int J Fertil Steril. 2012;6(2):117-126. PMID: 25493169; PMCID: PMC4258240

[133] Ferraù F, Korbonits M. Metabolic comorbidities in Cushing's syndrome. Europ J Endocrinol. 2015;173: M133-M157. Retrieved May 25, 2021,

from https://eje.bioscientifica.com/view/journals/eje/173/4/M133.xml

[134] Vance ML. Growth-hormone-releasing hormone. Clin Chem. 1990 Mar;36(3):415-420. PMID: 2107038.

[135] Veldhuis JD, Iranmanesh A, Ho KK, Waters MJ, Johnson ML, Lizarralde G. Dual defects in pulsatile growth hormone secretion and clearance subserve the hyposomatotropism of obesity in man. J Clin Endocrinol Metab. 1991;72:51-59.

[136] Heptulla R, Smitten A, Teague B, Tamborlane WV, Ma YZ, Caprio S. Temporal patterns of circulating leptin levels in lean and obese adolescents: Relationships to insulin, growth hormone, and free fatty acids rhythmicity. J Clin Endocrinol Metab. 2001;86:90-96

[137] Scacchi M, Pincelli AI, Cavagnini F. Growth hormone in obesity. Int J Obes Relat Metab Disord. 1999; 23: 260-271

[138] Laron Z. Growth hormone insensitivity (Laron syndrome). Rev Endocr Metab Disord. 2002; 3(4):347-355

[139] Boro H, Rahman SKH, Khatiwada S, Alam S, Khadgawat R. Laron syndrome: An experience of treatment of two cases. J Clin Translational Endocrinology: Case Reports. 2021;19:100076. DOI:10.1016/j.jecr.2020.100076

[140] Kojima M, Hosoda H, Date Y, Nakazato M, Matsuo H, Kangawa K. Ghrelin is a growth-hormone-releasing acylated peptide from stomach. Nature. 1999; 402:656e660.

[141] Müller TD, Nogueiras R, Andermann ML, Andrews ZB, Anker SD, Argente J, et al. Ghrelin. Molecular Metabolism, 4 (6) (2015), pp. 437-460, 10.1016/j.molmet.2015.03.005

[142] St-Pierre DH, Karelis AD, Coderre L, Malita F, Fontaine J, Mignault D, Brochu M, Bastard JP, Cianflone K, Doucet E, Imbeault P, Rabasa-Lhoret R. Association of acylated and nonacylated ghrelin with insulin sensitivity in overweight and obese postmenopausal women. J Clin Endocrinol Metab. 2007;92:264-269.

[143] Tolle V, Kadem M, Bluet-Pajot M-T, Frere D, Foulon C, Bossu C, Dardennes R, Mounier C, Zizzari P, Lang F, Epelbaum J, Estour B. Balance in ghrelin and leptin plasma levels in anorexia nervosa patients and constitutionally thin women. J Clin Endocrinol Metab. 2003; 88 (1):109-116. https://doi.org/10.1210/jc.2002-020645

[144] Garcia JM, Garcia-Touza M, Hijazi RA, Taffet G, Epner D, Mann D, Smith RG, Cunningham GR, Marcelli M. Active ghrelin levels and active to Total ghrelin ratio in cancer-induced Cachexia. The Journal of Clinical Endocrinology & Metabolism. 2005;90(5):2920-2926. https://doi.org/10.1210/jc.2004-1788

[145] Perello M, Sakata I, Birnbaum S, Chuang JC, Osborne-Lawrence S, Rovinsky SA, Woloszyn J, Yanagisawa M, Lutter M, Zigman JM. Ghrelin increases the rewarding value of high-fat diet in an orexin-dependent manner. Biol Psychiatry. 2010; 67: 880-886

[146] Wellman PJ, Davis KW, Nation JR. Augmentation of cocaine hyperactivity in rats by systemic ghrelin. Regul Pept. 2005; 125: 151-154

[147] Perello M, Dickson SL. Ghrelin Signalling on food reward: A salient link between the gut and the mesolimbic system. J Neuroendocrinol. 2015; 27(6): 424-434. DOI: 10.1111/jne.12236

[148] Kendler KS, Eaves LJ, Walters EE, Neale MC, Heath AC, Kessler RC. The identification and validation of distinct depressive syndromes in a population-based sample of female twins. Arch Gen Psychiatry. 1996; 53(5):391-399.

[149] Murphy JM, Horton NJ, Burke JD Jr, Monson RR, Laird NM, Lesage A, Sobol AM. Obesity and weight gain in relation to depression: findings from the Stirling County Study. Int J Obes (Lond). 2009;33(3):335-41. doi: 10.1038/ijo.2008.273. PMID: 19139752; PMCID: PMC2656591.

[150] Colles SL, Dixon JB, O'Brien PE. Night eating syndrome and nocturnal snacking: Association with obesity, binge eating and psychological distress. Int J Obes (Lond). 2007; 31(11):1722-1730.

[151] Ding C, Lim LL, Xu L, Kong APS. Sleep and obesity. J Obes Metab Syndr. 2018; 27(1):4-24. doi: 10.7570/jomes.2018.27.1.4. PMID: 31089536; PMCID: PMC6489488.

[152] Harakeh SM, Khan I, Kumosani T, Barbour E, Almasaudi SB, Bahijri SM, Alfadul SM, Ajabnoor GM, Azhar EI. Gut microbiota: A contributing factor to obesity. Front Cell Infect Microbiol. 2016;6:95. DOI: 10.3389/fcimb.2016.00095. PMID: 27625997.

[153] Everand A, Cani PD. Diabetes, obesity and gut microbiota. Best Practice and Research Clinical Gastroenterology. 2013; 27:73-83. DOI: 10.1016/j.bpg.2013.03.007

[154] Vasilakopoulou, A., le Roux, C. Could a virus contribute to weight gain? Int J Obes. 2007; 31: 1350-1356. DOI:10.1038/sj.ijo.0803623

[155] Kim YS, Carp RI, Callahan SM, Wisniewski HM. Scrapie-induced obesity in mice. JID. 1987; 156 (2):402-405. DOI: 10.1093/infdis/156.2.402

[156] Wierucka-Rybak M, Bojanowska E. Bacteria, viruses, and hypothalamic inflammation: Potential new players in obesity. Postepy Hig Med Dosw (Online). 2014;68:271-279. DOI: 10.5604/17322693.1093928. PMID: 24662795.

[157] Haas GM, Liepold E, Schwandt P. Metabolic risk factors, leisure time physical activity, and nutrition in german children and adolescents. Cholesterol. 2012; 2012():370850.

[158] Ekelund U, Brage S, Froberg K, Harro M, Anderssen SA, Sardinha LB, Riddoch C, Andersen LB. TV viewing and physical activity are independently associated with metabolic risk in children: The European youth heart study. PLoS Med. 2006; 3(12):e488.

[159] Mozaffarian D, Hao T, Rimm EB, Willett WC, Hu FB. Changes in diet and lifestyle and long-term weight gain in women and men. N Engl J Med. 2011; 364(25):2392-2404.

[160] Schulze MB, Manson JE, Ludwig DS, Colditz GA, Stampfer MJ, Willett WC, Hu FB. Sugar-sweetened beverages, weight gain, and incidence of type 2 diabetes in young and middle-aged women. JAMA. 2004; 292(8):927-934.

[161] Wang Y, Beydoun MA. The obesity epidemic in the United States--gender, age, socioeconomic, racial/ethnic, and geographic characteristics: A systematic review and meta-regression analysis. Epidemiol Rev. 2007; 29():6-28.

[162] Sobal J, Stunkard AJ. Socioeconomic status and obesity: A review of the literature. Psychol Bull. 1989;105(2):260-275. DOI: 10.1037/0033-2909.105.2.260. PMID: 2648443.

[163] McClure AC, Tanski SE, Gilbert-Diamond D, Adachi-Mejia AM, Li Z, Li Z, Sargent JD. Receptivity to television fast-food restaurant marketing and obesity among U.S. youth. Am J Prev Med. 2013;45(5):560-8. DOI: 10.1016/j.amepre.2013.06.011. PMID: 24139768; PMCID: PMC3934414.

[164] Crawford PB, Gosliner W, Anderson C, Strode P, Becerra-Jones Y,

Samuels S, Carroll AM, Ritchie LD. Counselling Latina mothers of preschool children about weight issues: Suggestions for a new framework. J Am Diet Assoc. 2004; 104(3):387-394.

[165] Higgins V, Nazroo J, Brown M. Pathways to ethnic differences in obesity: The role of migration, culture and socio-economic position in the UK.SSM-Population Health. 2019; 100394. Doi: 10.1016/j.ssmph.2019.100394

[166] Diamanti-Kandarakis E, Bourguignon JP, Giudice LC, Hauser R, Prins GS, Soto AM, Zoeller RT, Gore AC. Endocrine-disrupting chemicals: An Endocrine Society scientific statement. Endocr Rev. 2009; 30(4):293-342.

[167] Brown RE, Sharma AM, Ardern CI, Mirdamadi P, Mirdamadi P, Kuk JL. Secular differences in the association between caloric intake, macronutrient intake, and physical activity with obesity. Obes Res Clin Pract. 2016; 10(3):243-255.

[168] Kim JT, Lee HK. Childhood obesity and endocrine disrupting chemicals. Ann Pediatr Endocrinol Metab. 2017; 22(4):219-225. DOI: 10.6065/apem.2017.22.4.219. PMID: 29301181; PMCID: PMC5769835.

[169] Pizzorno J. Is the diabetes epidemic primarily due to toxins? Integr Med (Encinitas). 2016;15(4):8-17. PMID: 27574488; PMCID: PMC4991654.

[170] Wharton S, Raiber L, Serodio KJ, Lee J, Christensen RA. Medications that cause weight gain and alternatives in Canada: a narrative review. Diabetes Metab Syndr Obes. 2018;11:427-438. DOI: 10.2147/DMSO.S171365. PMID: 30174450; PMCID: PMC6109660.

[171] Domecq JP, Prutsky G, Leppin A, Sonbol MB, Altayar O, Undavalli C, Wang Z, Elraiyah T, Brito JP, Mauck KF, Lababidi MH, Prokop LJ, Asi N, Wei J, Fidahussein S, Montori VM, Murad MH. Clinical review: Drugs commonly associated with weight change: A systematic review and meta-analysis. J Clin Endocrinol Metab. 2015; 100(2):363-370.

[172] Sharma AM, Pischon T, Hardt S, Kunz I, Luft FC. Hypothesis: Beta-adrenergic receptor blockers and weight gain: A systematic analysis. Hypertension. 2001; 37(2):250-254.

[173] Wung PK, Anderson T, Fontaine KR, Hoffman GS, Specks U, Merkel PA, Spiera R, Davis JC, St Clair EW, McCune WJ, Stone JH, Wegener's granulomatosis Etanercept research group. Effects of glucocorticoids on weight change during the treatment of Wegener's granulomatosis. Arthritis Rheum. 2008; 59(5):746-753.

Section 3

Mechanisms by Which Obesity Influences Health Risks

Chapter 8

Influence of the Basal Metabolic Profile on the Evolution of the Pediatric Patient with Obesity

Belén Fernández, Ainhoa Sarasua Miranda, Isabel Lorente Blázquez and Ignacio Diez López

Abstract

Childhood obesity is a problem of growing importance globally. It is associated with significant health problems. Knowing how to treat it effectively would improve the quality of life of these children. The aim of this chapter is to study how basal metabolism influences the somatometric evolution of the child and adolescent population with obesity in a pediatric endocrinology clinic. Study childhood obesity in a tertiary hospital by means of a multichannel impedanceometry study. All the patients had a basal metabolism lower than the calculated theoretical ideal. In overall terms, weight reduction is not achieved in this pediatric population. However, it is observed a decrease in fat content in the medium term (1-3 years). Bioelectrical impedanceometry measurement is a simple method in clinical practice to evaluate the energy consumption and the body composition. Knowing the body composition of these children would help to intervene more effectively to help control obesity and its health consequences.

Keywords: obesity, childhood obesity, basal metabolism, bioelectrical impedance analysis, body mass analysis, body fat mass, body weight, body composition

1. Introduction

Obesity, in adults and in childhood, is one of the most serious public health problems of the 21st century. The World Health Organization (WHO) describes it as an epidemic since it generally affects all countries.

In 2016, more than 41 million children under the age of five were overweight or obese [1]. That same year, according to UNICEF, the prevalence in children and adolescents between the ages of 5 and 19 was approximately 124 million with obesity and 216 million with overweight [2].

In pediatric age, obesity is already the chronic non-communicable disease and the most frequent nutritional and metabolic disorder [3].

The importance resides in the association of obesity with important health problems and the development of serious non-communicable diseases, such as cardiovascular diseases, high blood pressure, type 2 diabetes mellitus and some types of cancer, which increases social and health costs considerably.

It is suspected that the presence of common causal factors could explain the global nature of this problem. Among other theories arises that of the Thrifty

Genotype [4, 5], whose hypothesis maintains that, due to the way of life of primitive man, the human genome developed a tendency to create energy reserve tissues for periods of famine based on fats since they provide more calories in less volume. This type of genes in a current way of life, characterized by food in abundance, cheap and with high fat contents, and the tendency to sedentary lifestyle of the population, would be responsible for the aforementioned global epidemic of the 21st century: obesity [6–8].

In developing countries, the prevalence of obesity and overweight in preschool children exceeds 30%, which represents a significant risk for them to become adults with metabolic syndrome and obesity [9].

Obesity is defined as an excess of body fat, the result of a positive energy balance persisting over a long period of time [9].

This situation in childhood develops different types of complications [10]. At first, problems such as flat feet, insulin resistance, increase in androgens, increase in cholesterol, LDL (low-density lipoproteins) and triglycerides, as well as pulmonary, menstrual, type 2 diabetes and psychological disorders, such as deteriorated self-image.

After the first two or four years of the onset of obesity, obese children increase the risk of high blood pressure, hypercholesterolemia, increase in LDL, and decrease in HDL (high-density lipoprotein).

If this situation persists, the presence of an increase in coronary diseases, vascular hypertension, vascular kidney disease, atherosclerosis, arthritis and certain neoplasias is added in adulthood, which are those that increase morbidity and explain mortality in adult life.

Furthermore, obesity in pediatric age is related to other comorbidities such as: sleep apnea, nonalcoholic steatohepatitis, cholelithiasis, pseudotumor cerebri, gastrointestinal reflux and polycystic ovary syndrome [10].

A simple tool to assess this problem is the body mass index (BMI), which represents both fat mass and fat-free mass, so it is an indicator of weight and not of adiposity as such. It is independent of height, allowing the comparison of the body weights of individuals of different heights [10].

Body composition is made up of two major components: body fat mass (BFM) and lean body mass (LBM). Fat mass refers to the fat tissue, lipids that the human body has, while lean mass in turn is divided into three main components: total body water (TBW), mineral content, mainly bones, and protein content like muscles.

In the first year of life there is a significant increase in body fat content, followed by a period of decline that ends between the 4 to 6 years of age, increasing later until the end of adolescence, known as adipose rebound. The earlier the rebound begins, the greater the risk of later obesity [11].

Childhood overweight is established above the 85th percentile of BMI, and obesity above the 95th percentile of BMI [12].

Due to the physiological differences between boys and girls, graphics and percentiles are created for each sex [10, 13, 14].

In Spain, the ALADINO study has evaluated the prevalence of childhood overweight and obesity every 4 years since 2011. In 2019, a downward trend is observed since 2011 and stable compared to 2015 [15].

Currently in Spain overweight in the child population is 23.3% and obesity 17.3% [15].

Poor eating habits, low physical activity and low socioeconomic status of the family influence these results. A significant percentage of parents mistakenly perceive their children's overweight or obesity as normal.

The child population with overweight oro bese has, in general, greater weight at birth than thin or normal weight children.

By sex, overweight is more prevalent in girls and obesity in boys.

In children, the frequency of overweight is higher in those of 9 years and regarding obesity in those of 7, 8 and 9, compared to younger age groups. In girls, there are no age differences in overweight, while obesity increases from 6 to 8 years old [15].

Being thin does not necessarily mean having a lower percentage of body fat than people who are thinner, since the latter can be more muscular. A high percentage of fat tissue increases the risk of developing cardiovascular diseases, diabetes, hypertension and certain types of cancer [16, 17].

Accurately assessing the weight of a person is to know the body composition, that is, the amount of lean body mass and fat body mass in their organism. There are different measurement methods, each of them with advantages and disadvantages: [16].

- Octopolar multi-frequency impedance measurement: An electrical current of very low intensity runs through the body, interacts with body water, which has a constant proportion of muscle mass. This data, together with the sex, age and height of the patient, calculates the body muscle mass. Fat mass does not conduct electricity, so it is not directly measured.

- Dual X-ray Absorption (DXA): "Gold standard". It determines the corresponding weights and percentages of fat, bone and muscle tissue. It allows assessing the specific location of an excess of fat or muscle tissue. It evaluates the distribution of android and gynoid fat and these two data are two of the best predictors of health risks.

- Anthropometry: It consists of measuring skin folds using a "caliper", different perimeters and diameters. It needs to be measured by an expert. Applying a series of formulas subsequently, the body composition and the somatotype are determined. It reports the magnitude and distribution of subcutaneous fat. However, it only provides regional body fat data, not the deep fat. Also, it is not useful for measuring folds in obese people.

- Image morphological study: it observes subtle changes in body silhouette, volumes and postural habits.

Metabolism represents energy expenditure at a baseline situation without stress. And it is primarily determined by age, sex, size, and body composition.

The most used technique for its determination is indirect open-circuit calorimetry; its value can also be estimated using predictive equations. The most used in the pediatric population are those of Schofield and those of the WHO [18].

In 2017, a study led by the Imperial College London and the WHO concluded that the number of children and adolescents (between the ages of 5 and 19) with obesity has multiplied by 10 in the world in the last four decades. It is also indicated that in 2022 there will be more children and adolescents with obesity than children with low weight.

Two articles on body composition in the adolescent and adult [19, 20] population have been found in the literature, but not in the child population. Both highlight the fact that the female population has a higher percentage of body fat mass; and that in overall; the obese population has a lower basal metabolism than estimated, higher in men than in women. In general, in terms of intake, this population falls within the normal limits of the FAO/WHO recommendations; at the same time that they present insufficient total energy expenditure.

Detecting excess weight early and preventing it during childhood is essential to achieve a greater impact on health.

With the aim of finding another explanation for excess weight in childhood, apart from those already mentioned, this work will focus on finding a causal relationship between basal metabolism and excess weight in the child population.

2. Hypothesis

Given the importance of the knowledge and management of obesity due to its relationship with certain comorbidities in the child population, it seems necessary to know if children who attend hospital consultation for childhood obesity referred from primary care have a basal metabolism or caloric intake below what is expected for their age and sex. Assuming that this fact is an associated risk factor for obesity or, on the other hand, its usual treatment is more difficult than usual.

3. Aim

To study how basal metabolism influences the somatometric evolution of the child and adolescent population with obesity in a pediatric endocrinology consultation.

4. Material and methods

An anonymized and coded database of a pediatric endocrine clinic in a tertiary hospital was used, which records the body composition of patients by means of impedance measurement at different consultations, up to 3 years of follow-up.

Finally, a sample of 100 people was selected from the database that had 1,400 patients.

Inclusion criteria:

- Patients referred from primary care, less than 14 years of age at the time of referral, who present a lack of weight control.
- Minimum age 6 years, due to impedance measurement limitation.
- Minimum longitudinal follow-up 12 months (at least 2 visits).

Deferral criteria:

- Patients with syndromic or similar diseases that could justify their overweight or obesity.

Children with obesity who meet the criteria are weighed with a bioelectrical impedance scale. Thanks to this type of measurement, we have access to the following measurements for each patient: weight (kg), height (cm), body mass index, basal metabolism (kcal), percentage of body fat mass, percentage of lean body mass and percentage of total body water. Before they step on the scale, they are asked to urinate so that the amount of body water is not overestimated and the calculation is as accurate as possible. Once the child is on the scale, the scale emits an imperceptible electrical signal that interacts with all water-containing body structures. In this way, the fat-free body mass, the lean body mass and indirectly, because there is no water, the body fat of the patient is calculated. In addition, the scale provides the child's height, total weight and basal metabolism. All these data are stored in a database and can be compared at subsequent check-ups. The method is completely painless for the patient and very fast, taking only a few seconds.

5. Results

As shown in **Figures 1** and **2**, the type of patient who mainly attends these consultations are 11-year-old girls. In girls, it is observed that most of them start the follow-up at two different ages or at 8 years of age or, mostly, at 11 years.

On the other hand, as shown in **Figure 3**, males constitute less than half of the sample and, in general, they start their follow-up at the age of 9 years, following a homogeneous trend between 8 and 11 years of age.

The entire sample studied presented a basal metabolism lower than that corresponding to their age and sex, on average the difference was −209 kcal in both boys and girls.

In light of this analysis, **Figure 4** shows that the mean basal metabolic rate at the first visit for boys was 1664 ± 262.54 kcal, and 1408 ± 125.54 kcal for girls. Whereas, according to their theoretical water needs calculated with the TBW prediction equations (18), the ideal basal metabolic rate for boys would be 1740 kcal and for girls an average of 1700 kcal.

All patients who come for obesity control are instructed in standardized child nutrition educational programs.

After the first 12 months of follow-up, basal metabolism in both sexes increased. Boys reached 1738 ± 276.84 kcal and girls reached 1449 ± 123.20 kcal.

The calculated theoretical basal metabolism increases steadily with age. This trend is also observed in **Table 1**, although with lower values than the desired values, it is maintained in the sample analyzed in all age ranges except at 9 years of age; at this age the basal metabolism has values more similar to the calculated theoretical metabolism with a difference of −85 kcal.

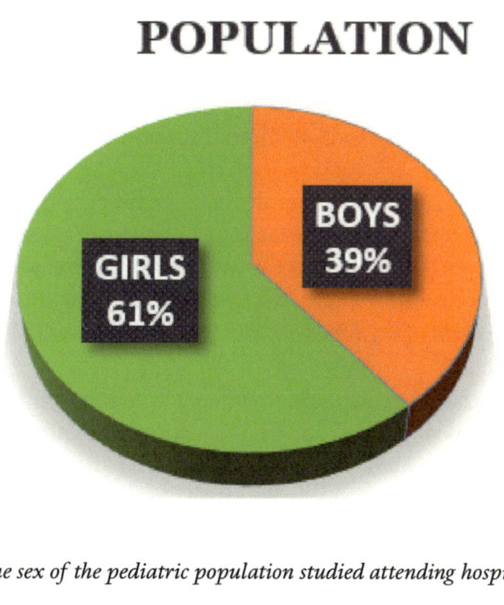

Figure 1.
Percentage distribution of the sex of the pediatric population studied attending hospital consultations for weight control.

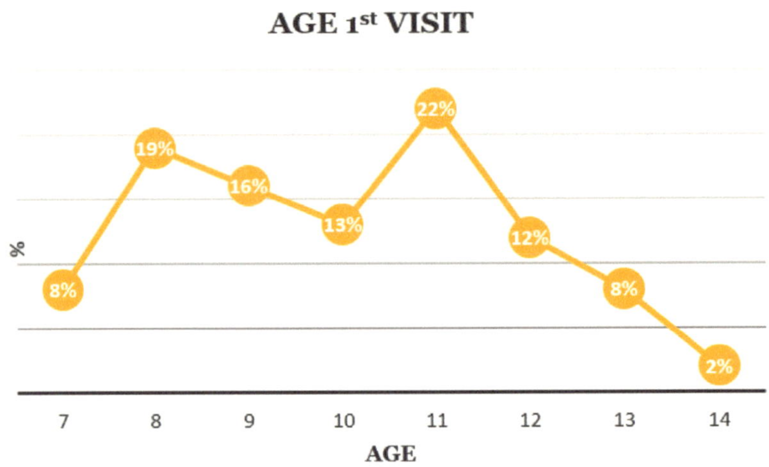

Figure 2.
Percentage age distribution of the pediatric population studied attending hospital consultations for weight control.

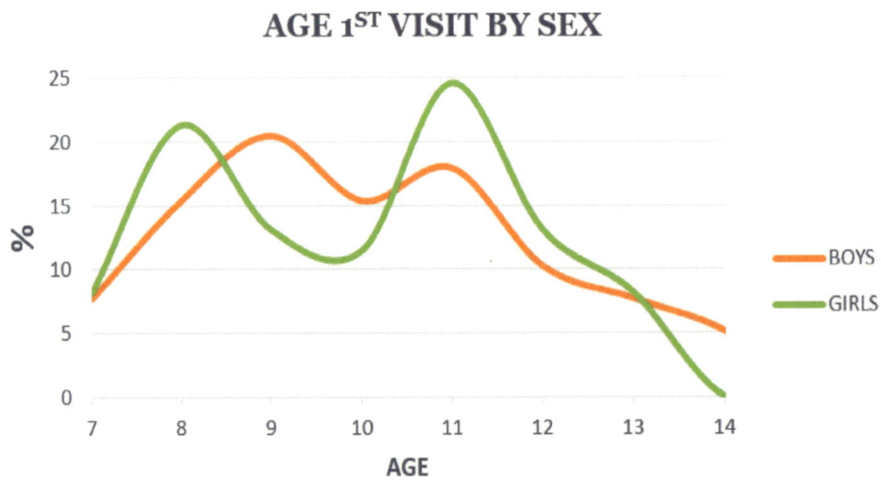

Figure 3.
Percentage distribution of age of onset for hospital weight control, by sex.

After one year of follow-up, all age groups achieved a decrease in body fat mass content. The higher success rate was at 11 years, achieving a reduction of almost 2% in fat mass.

At 9 years of age, despite a basal metabolism more similar to the theoretical one, the lowest rate of reduction in fat content is achieved per year, that is −0.4%.

After three years, there continues to be an overall decrease in the percentage of fat mass. The 7 and 9-year-old groups, after three years of follow-up, show a slight increase in their fat content (+ 1.6% and + 0.9%, respectively), corresponding to the start of adolescence.

Whereas the 10-year-old group, after three years achieved a reduction of 4.5%.

A greater difference is observed in the 14-year-old group, but due to such extreme data and the low prevalence of the sample at this age, they are considered non-representative values.

Regarding the study of body composition by sex:

At the beginning of the control, the boys had an average of 36.4 ± 6% of fat mass and the girls an average of 37.1 ± 3% of fat mass.

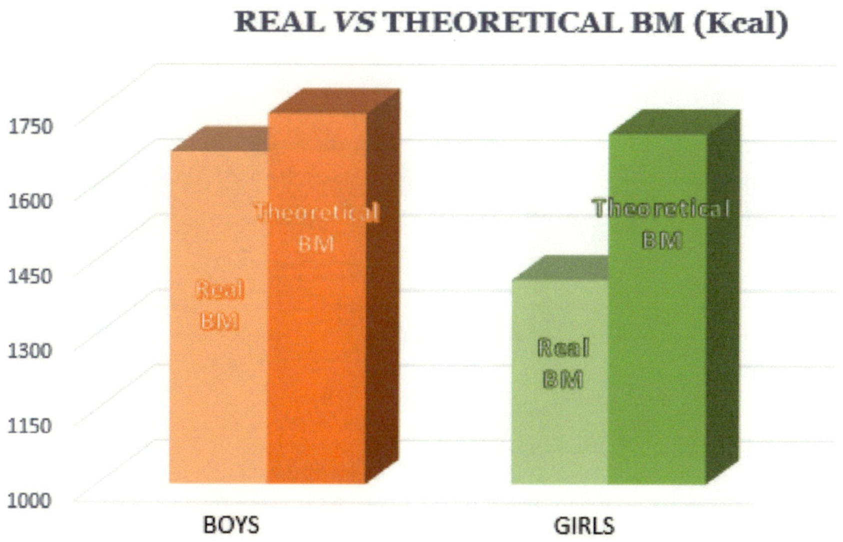

Figure 4.
Real basal metabolism and theoretical basal metabolism calculated by sex of the pediatric population attending hospital for weight control.

AGE at the start of follow-up	BM medium	BM theoretical medium	Mean difference BM	EvoBFM After 12 m	EvoBFM After 36 m
7	1.315 kcal	1.422 kcal	−107	−0,5	1,6
8	1.409 kcal	1.517 kcal	−108	−1,7	−1,5
9	1.534 kcal	1.619 kcal	−85	−0,4	0,3
10	1.481 kcal	1.691 kcal	−210	−1,7	−4,5
11	1.505 kcal	1.817 kcal	−311	−1,9	−2,2
12	1.560 kcal	1.878 kcal	−318	−0,7	−1,0
13	1.717 kcal	2.077 kcal	−360	−2,3	−2,7
14	2.077 kcal	2.237 kcal	−161	−16,2	−11,5

Table 1.
Evolution of actual and theoretical basal metabolic rate and body fat mass in the pediatric population by age group at the beginning of the hospital weight control intervention.

After the first year, as shown in **Figure 5**, there is a decrease in fat content in both sexes. Boys had around 34.2 ± 6% of fat mass (−2.2%) and girls 35.9 ± 4% (−1.2%).

After one year, the boys in the study show an increase of 2.2% (65.8 vs. 63.6%) in lean body mass content. Of this, 72% of this increase corresponds to mineral-protein components. So these boys have increased height and their muscle development.

The girls in the study, after the first check-up per year, increased their lean body mass content by 1.2% (62.9 vs. 64.1%), of which 75% corresponds to mineral-protein component and the remaining 25% to body water.

Looking at **Figure 6** 68% of the patients, regardless of their age or sex, achieved a reduction in fat content after one year of control, so it can be said that they actually managed to lose weight. After three years, 61% of the sample persists in a decrease in their body fat content, the remaining 7% gain fat, that is, they gain weight.

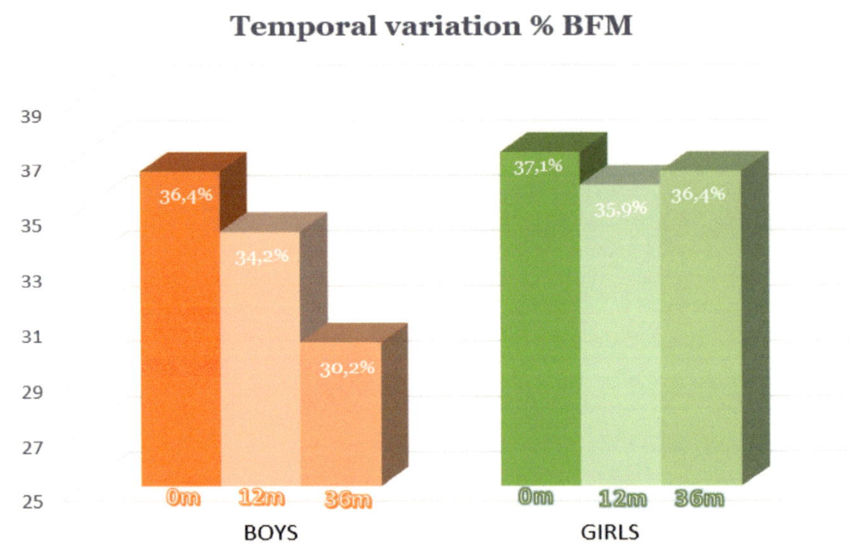

Figure 5.
Evolution over time at the beginning, at 12 months and at 36 months of the percentage of body fat mass in the patients studied for weight control in the hospital. Differentiation between boys and girls.

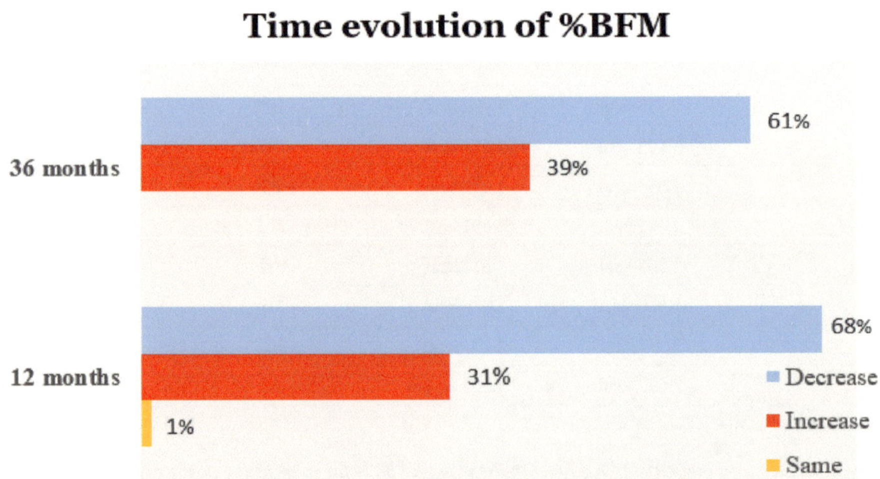

Figure 6.
Evolution of the proportion of patients reducing or increasing body fat mass over time.

After three years, looking again at **Figure 5**, the fat content in boys was reduced to 30 ± 7.5%. Girls, on the other hand, increased the fat content compared to the previous control, (+ 0.5% GM) although they do not reach initial figures.

Despite finding numerical differences, this result of body composition after three years for BFM, LBM and TBW are not statistically significant, since Levene's test for equality of variances show a $p > 0.05$.

54% of boys after three years achieved a reduction in fat mass compared to 36% of girls.

Most of the patients who achieved a reduction in fat mass after three years of follow-up are those who started the control at 11 years.

Regarding the relationship between the kg of weight and the weight situation of the pediatric population: (**Figures 6-10**).

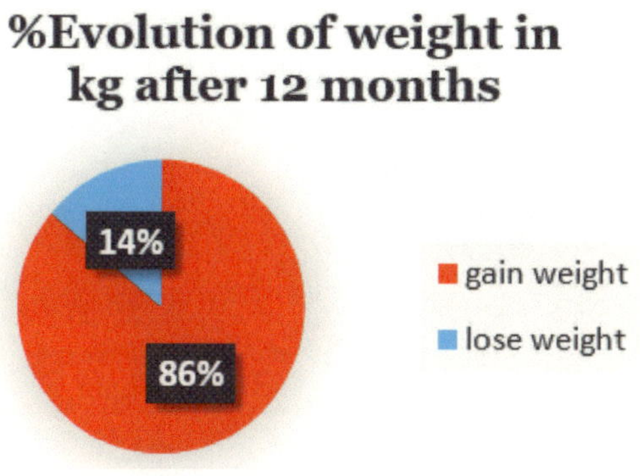

Figure 7.
Percentage evolution of weight in kilograms after 12 months of follow-up in hospital consultations.

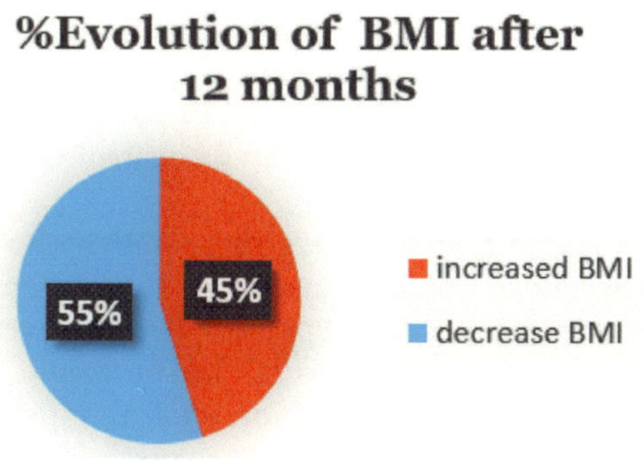

Figure 8.
Percentage evolution of BMI, after 12 months of control in hospital consultations for weight loss.

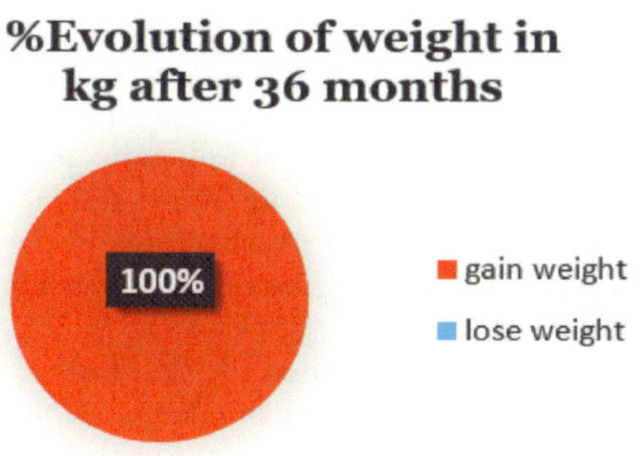

Figure 9.
Percentage evolution of weight in kilograms after 36 months of follow-up in hospital consultations.

In the first year, 86% of the studied sample increased their initial weight and 45% their BMI value. Whereas, in the same time, only 31% increased their body fat content.

The same occurs after three years, 100% increased their initial weight and 86% increased their BMI, but 61% decreased their fat content.

The lack of relationship between weight and body fat content is observed, which is really harmful to health.

Finally, it was studied which of all the available variables had the most influence on these results, and it was the value of the basal metabolism that the patient presents at the beginning of the follow-up was different between girls and boys, better at first one than second one.

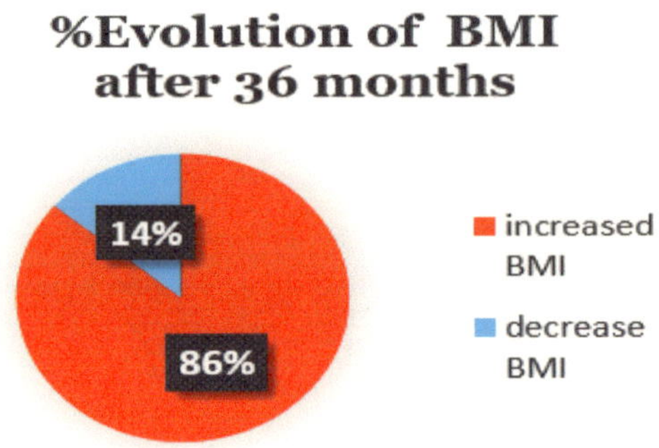

Figure 10.
Percentage evolution of BMI, after 36 months of control in hospital consultations for weight loss.

6. Discussion

Childhood obesity is a problem of increasing importance in our society. Knowing its characteristics would allow different strategies to be taken for a better treatment and diagnosis of these cases.

One of the strategies is to know if those girls and boys who have a worse evolution are those who either move less, consume more food or, on the contrary, their body could have a lower metabolism. The present essay focuses on this possible third cause in which it was called the Thrifty Gene syndrome. Among the main methods of the study of consumption, the bioelectrical impedance measurement was chosen as it is a simple, cheap and easy-to-use method in clinical practice. It has been shown that the basal metabolism of these patients is globally lower than the theoretical one, more noticeable in girls as well as the presence of a higher percentage of fat mass in girls compared to boys, as it has been published in previous studies; In a novel way, it has been concluded that the patients who fare worse over a follow-up time of between 1 and 3 years are girls, who on average had a basal metabolism markedly lower than the theoretical one for their age and sex.

In turn, it is observed that after one year of follow-up and all of them employing standardized educational programs in child nutrition, the boys achieve a greater reduction in the percentage of fat mass. From this it can be deduced that a basal metabolism more similar to the needs intervenes positively when it comes to burning the excess of body fat.

It was observed how 86% of the individuals in the study after one year of follow-up gained weight, while only 31% presented an increase in their fat content. From this it can be deduced that the changes in nutritional habits of these patients, added to their growth, influence weight gain at the expense of increasing other parameters, without the need for an increase in fat content. There is a risk of committing a bias when assessing the total weight by not perceiving that there has been a decrease in fat content at the cost of an increase in muscle mass. In the pediatric population, the gross data of total weight and BMI are not faithful to the seriousness of this disease and its evolution, what makes more interesting to know their body composition. One of the most reliable methods to determine this composition is bioimpedance measurement, such as the one used in this study.

It has previously been shown how after 12 months of follow-up, the boys reduced their LBM by 2.2%, therefore an increase in BFM and that, of this, 72% corresponded to the mineral-protein component. The girls in the same period, reduced the BFM more discreetly, a 1.2%, and the increase of the mineral-protein component was of 75%.

A growth in height and an increase in muscle content can be seen, greater in girls, this can be a result of the fact that they start puberty two years earlier. This growth period would be key to achieving a reduction in fat mass and for overweight or obese patients to be normal weight.

Regarding the fat content by sex, both presented on average very similar percentages, although the girls presented slightly higher numbers. Interestingly, it was observed that the boys after re-evaluating them after 12 months achieved a greater reduction, twice that of the girls. It can be deduced that, given the same adherence to nutritional programs, since both achieve a reduction, boys perform on average more physical activity than girls, which influences basal metabolism and a subsequent decrease in fat content.

One of the purposes was to find out which of the variables, of all available, had the most global influence on the results of the population. Characteristically, the value of the basal metabolism of the boy and girl at the time of the start of follow-up, turned out to be the variable that most influences the evolution of these patients, regardless of other variables such as sex, age, BFM at the beginning, etc.

It can be observed how basal metabolism can influence a person's tendency to gain weight. For example, a person with a low basal metabolic rate (who therefore burns fewer calories while resting or sleeping) will tend to gain more pounds of body fat over time than a similarly tall person with an average basal metabolic rate who eats the same amount of food and practices the same amount of physical exercise.

7. Conclusion

It is observed in our sample that the fat content of the patients in this practice and their body weight do not follow a direct relationship with each other. Our sample describes different types of patients: those who lose weight and those who gain weight, but this is not always related to a change in fat mass, as the study shows that there are patients who gain weight, but on the basis of lean mass. This is important because if we only look at the weight variable we could be biased by continuing to classify a child as overweight when what has actually increased is lean mass and may have increased muscle power.

In our sample of patients, we observed that boys have a higher basal metabolism than girls, which could be due to differences due to sexual dimorphism or, as has been published in several previous studies, to the fact that they are more physically active.

In view of these results and the importance of the situation of obesity in the child population, we propose to carry out a new study that includes variables that were not included in this study to analyze in more detail the child population affected by obesity, such as ethnicity, the type of family to which they belong, the economic resources they have and customs.

On the other hand, it would also be interesting to evaluate body composition, not only by age and sex, but also taking into account pubertal development, that is, the Tanner stage at the time of data collection.

Due to the current mobility restrictions and economic crisis derived from the COVID-19 pandemic worldwide, it would be interesting to study its impact on the weight control and prevalence of this disease in the population, especially in the pediatric population.

We emphasize the importance of the impedance measurement study and to focus efforts on the population with the worst basal metabolism and to contribute to improving the efficiency and effectiveness of the scarce health resources that we have. Achieving an effective action in childhood obesity will improve life expectancy and its quality in adulthood.

Acronyms

BFM	Body fat mass
BM	Basal metabolism
BMI	Body mass index
HDL	High-density lipoprotein
LBM	Lean body mass
LDL	Low-density lipoproteins
TBW	Total body water
WHO	World Health Organization

Author details

Belén Fernández[1], Ainhoa Sarasua Miranda[2], Isabel Lorente Blázquez[2] and Ignacio Diez López[1,2]*

1 Medicine Faculty, Vitoria-Gasteiz University of the Basque Country UPV/EHU, Spain

2 Paediatrics Department, Álava's University Hospital, Vitoria-Gasteiz, Spain

*Address all correspondence to: ignacio.diezlopez@osakidetza.eus

References

[1] World Health Organization. Datos y cifras sobre obesidad infantil [Internet]. World Health Organization; 2017 [cited 2021 Jan 19]. Available from: http://www.who.int/end-childhood-obesity/facts/es/

[2] González-Bueno G, F. Gómez S. Malnutrición, obesidad infantil y derechos de la infancia en España [Internet]. UNICEF Comité Español. Madrid; 2019 [cited 2020 Oct 19]. 28 p. Available from: https://www.unicef.es/sites/unicef.es/files/comunicacion/Malnutricion_obesidad_infantil_y_derechos_de_la_infancia_en_Espana.pdf

[3] Rivero Urgell M, Aznar Moreno L, Dalmau Serra J, MorenoVillares J, Aliaga Pérez A, García Perea A, et al. LIBRO blanco de la Nutrición Infantil en España [Internet]. Libro blanco de la nutrición. Zaragoza: Tipolínea, S. A. U.; 2015. 530 p. Available from: http://www.aeped.es/sites/default/files/documentos/libro_blanco_de_la_nutricion_infantil.pdf

[4] Chacin M, Rojas J, Pineda C, Rodriguez D, Nuñez M, Marquez M, et al. Predisposición humana a la Obesidad, Síndrome Metabólico y Diabetes: El genotipo Ahorrador y la incorporación de los diabetogenes al genoma humano desde la Antropología Biológica. Diabetes Int. 2011;I:11-23.

[5] Valenzuela A. ¿Porqué Comemos Lo Que Comemos? Rev Chil Nutr. 2011;38(2):198-209.

[6] Tarbal A. La obesidad Infantil: una epidemia mundial. Faros St joan Déu Obs salud la Infanc y Adolesc. 2010;5:1-13.

[7] Cascales Angosto M. Obesidad: Pandemia Del Siglo XXI. Real Acad Nac Farm. 2015;14-46.

[8] World Health Organization. Controlling the global obesity epidemic [Internet]. Vol. 7. 2015 [cited 2021 Jan 19]. p. 1-2. Available from: https://www.who.int/activities/controlling-the-global-obesity-epidemic

[9] World Health Organization. Obesidad [Internet]. 2016 [cited 2021 Jan 19]. Available from: https://www.who.int/topics/obesity/es/

[10] Kaufer-Horwitz M, Toussaint G. Indicadores antropométricos para evaluar sobrepeso y obesidad en pediatría. Bol méd Hosp Infant Méx. 2008;65(6):502-18.

[11] Fundación para la Formación e Investigación Sanitarias de la Región de Murcia (FFIS). Rebote Adiposo Precoz [Internet]. Vol. 1. 2014 [cited 2021 Feb 9]. p. 1. Available from: https://www.ffis.es/busqueda.php?ie=utf-8&cx=004778800403451640878%3Adpyc5vgjbqq&cof=FORID%3A11&q=rebote+adiposo+precoz

[12] Martinez Sopena M, Redondo del Rio M. Valoracion Nutricional En La Obesidad Infantil. XXIV Jornada de Pediatría de Gipuzkoa [Internet]. 2011;1-32. Available from: http://www.avpap.org/documentos/gipuzkoa2007/obsvalnutri.pdf

[13] Carrascosa A, Fernández JM, Ferrández Á, López-Siguero JP, López D, Sánchez E, et al. Estudios Españoles de Crecimiento 2010. In: Anales de Pediatría. 2011. p. 1-46.

[14] Güemes-Hidalgo M, Muñoz-Calvo MT. Obesidad en la infancia y adolescencia. Pediatr Integr. 2015;19(6):412-27.

[15] García Solano M, Dal Re Saavedra M, Gutiérrez González E, García López A, Villar Villalba C, Yusta Boyo M, et al. Estudio sobre la Alimentación, Actividad Física, Desarollo Infantil y Obesidad en España

2019. Gobierno de España. Ministerio de Consumo. Agencia Española de Seguridad Alimentaria y Nutrición (AESAN); 2020. 184 p.

[16] Mesa T. ¿Cómo se mide la composición corporal? [Internet]. Neolifeclinic. 2016 [cited 2021 Feb 9]. Available from: https://neolifeclinic.com/blog/como-se-mide-la-composicion-corporal/

[17] De la Fuente Hidalgo E. Conceptos para adelgazar: ¿Sabes qué es la masa magra, la masa grasa y la grasa visceral? [Internet]. Sanitas. 2017 [cited 2021 Feb 10]. Available from: https://muysaludable.sanitas.es/nutricion/la-hora-adelgazar-no-solo-importa-peso-otros-factores-cuenta/

[18] Moráis López A, Rivero de la Rosa M, Galera Martínez R, Ros Arnal I, Herrero Álvarez M, Rodríguez Martínez G. Cálculo de los requerimientos energético-proteicos para el soporte nutricional en la práctica clínica. Acta Pediatr Esp. 2011;69(5):211-6.

[19] Marcela Reyes J, Erick Díaz B, Lydia Lera M, Raquel Burrows A. Ingesta y metabolismo energético en una muestra de adolescentes chilenos con sobrepeso y obesidad. Rev Med Chil. 2011;139(4):425-31.

[20] Xiongfei Liang M, Xianhua Chen M, Jing Li M, Mengdan Yan M, Yifeng Yang M. Study on body composition and its correlation with obesity. Medicine (Baltimore). 2018;97(21).

Chapter 9

Leptin and Its Role in Oxidative Stress and Apoptosis: An Overview

Volkan Gelen, Abdulsamed Kükürt, Emin Şengül and Hacı Ahmet Deveci

Abstract

Adipose tissue (AT) in the body plays a very important role in the regulation of energy metabolism. AT regulates energy metabolism by secreting adipokines. Some of the adipokines released are vaspin, resistin, adiponectin, visfatin and omentin, and leptin. In addition to regulating energy metabolism, leptin plays a role in the regulation of many physiological functions of the body such as regulation of blood pressure, inflammation, nutrition, appetite, insulin and glucose metabolism, lipid metabolism, coagulation, and apoptosis. Among all these physiological functions, the relationship between leptin, oxidative stress, and apoptosis has gained great importance recently due to its therapeutic effect in various types of cancer. For this reason, in this study, the release of leptin, its cellular effects and its effect on oxidative stress, and apoptosis are discussed in line with current information.

Keywords: Apoptosis, leptin, obesity, oxidative stress

1. Introduction

Obesity is defined as a chronic disease that results in an increase in adipose tissue (AT) in the body as a result of the energy intake being more than the energy spent. Today, it has become a common and important health problem in both developed and developing countries due to various reasons such as changes in eating habits and inactivity [1, 2]. Obesity directly or indirectly affects national economies. Obesity causes an increase in the rates of noncommunicable diseases, damage to various organs, shortens the life span, and negatively affects the quality of life [3–5]. In the case of obesity, which is so important, the level of leptin increases. Leptin is an adipokine secreted in fat cells [6]. After leptin is released from the fat cell, it reaches the central nervous system via the blood, binds to its receptor, and reduces food intake through this receptor [7, 8]. Leptin is produced by the obese *(ob)* gene in adipose cells by encoding it into mRNA [9, 10]. As the number of fat cells in the body increases, the plasma leptin level also increases. While leptin decreases plasma glucose and insulin levels, it increases metabolic rate and physical activity, resulting in a decrease in body fat [11]. It has been determined that leptin, which has such important effects on fat cells and hunger, is effective on cancer cells. In line with this information, this study aimed to explain leptin synthesis, its receptor, factors affecting its release, and the relationship between leptin, oxidative stress, and apoptosis.

2. Leptin

Leptin (a fat tissue hormone), the *ob* gene product, was the first adipokine discovered. Its discovery is based on work done in the 1950s. It begins with the researchers' discovery of two genes, called diabetic *(db/db)* and obese *(ob/ob)*, in two separate strains of mice [12, 13]. In a study conducted in these mice, which have the same phenotypic characteristics (such as insulin resistance, morbid obesity, lethargy, and infertility), blood leptin level was found to be deficient in the *ob/ob* gene product, while the *db/db* gene product was found to have a deficient leptin receptor. In addition, in the study where *db* and *ob* genes were examined in detail, *db/db* and *ob/ob* mice were both three times heavier than controls, and both groups of animals had five times more fat than the control [14]. About 40 years after the first studies, the *ob* or *Lep* gene encoding leptin was discovered and given this name because of its weak meaning [15]. About a year later, the isolation of the leptin receptor gene was reported [16].

The mouse leptin gene size is 4.5 kilobases long containing 167 amino acids [15]. Regulation of the leptin gene initiator that controls leptin production, is mediated by glucocorticoid response elements, CCAAT/enhancers, cyclic adenosine monophosphate (cAMP), and specificity protein 1 (SP1) binding sites [17]. Studies have shown that human leptin is 84% similar to mouse leptin and 83% to rat leptin [18]. Besides, a positive correlation was found between plasma leptin concentrations and AT leptin mRNA levels. Therefore, as leptin mRNA increases, plasma leptin concentrations also increase [19].

Human leptin is produced from a gene on chromosome 7. The structure of human leptin, a 16 kilodalton protein, is in the form of a 4 α helical bundle coil, like class-I helical cytokines [20]. The most highly conserved amino acid extension is the GLDFIP sequence [21, 22]. Leptin, synthesized by adipocytes, is a hormone that notifies the brain of energy reserves and affects metabolism, reproduction, growth, and development processes [16, 22]. Circulating leptin levels act at the hypothalamic central level to increase energy expenditure and reduce food intake when the body is well nourished [23]. It induces the storage of triglycerides in AT and has an effect on appetite [7]. When plasma leptin levels increase, it sends a signal of satiety to the brain in the short term, while it sends information about the energy status in the long term [24]. It also influences hypothalamic neuropeptide signaling [25]. The main physiological role of leptin during periods of hunger is to regulate the neuroendocrine system. With regard to obesity, leptin levels rise with increasing adiposity [26]. Circulating leptin levels are high in obese, pointing to the importance of leptin resistance in the obese [24]. Leptin-deficient mice have been found to show neuroendocrine abnormalities similar to starving mice. Leptin supplementation causes neuroendocrine normalization and reduced food intake in leptin-deficient obese rodents and humans, thereby reversing obesity [10]. Mutations of the *ob* gene result in leptin resistance and extreme obesity in mice [15]. *Ob/ob* mice have neuroendocrine abnormalities and they are generally classified as hyperphagic, hypothermic, morbidly obese [27].

It has been reported that leptin plays a proinflammatory role by increasing the inflammatory immune response, and this is associated with the pathogenesis of many complications of obesity [28]. It is noted that leptin can affect both adaptive and innate immunity by inducing proinflammatory response and thus playing a key role in regulating the pathogenesis of various autoimmune/inflammatory diseases [29]. It has been shown that as the degree of obesity increases in adults, the levels of plasminogen activator inhibitor-1 (PAI-1) and leptin, which is a proinflammatory marker, increase. It has been reported that it is responsible for the proinflammatory process, which is associated with an increased level of obesity [30]. Leptin regulates the functions of immune cells, such as natural killer cells, dendritic cells, neutrophils, eosinophils, macrophages, and basophils [23].

3. Leptin synthesis

Effector systems that control energy intake and energy expenditure, hypothalamic control centers where leptin signals from different sources are received, and the size of AT mass are the regulatory steps of leptin synthesis [31]. The major sites of leptin mRNA expression are in the stomach, liver, and AT [32]. Leptin mRNA is also expressed at minor levels in the fetal tissue, placenta, heart, brain, and pituitary gland [18]. Leptin synthesized is generally related to the degree of adiposity. Larger adipocytes express more leptin genes than smaller adipocytes [33]. Mechanical stretching of the fat cell, determined by the amount of stored triglycerides, can generate signals to increase leptin synthesis [24]. In addition, in humans, uridine diphosphate N-acetylglucosamine (UDPGlcNAc) and hexosamine act as potential links between cell size and leptin content. Body mass index is positively correlated with the amount of UDPGlcNAc in subcutaneous AT [34].

The composition of the food, not the amount, affects leptin production [35]. The composition of a meal affects leptin levels; for example, low-fat and high-carb food causes increased leptin levels [36]. Compared to high-carbohydrate meals, high-fat meals lower circulating plasma leptin levels 24 hours after a meal [37]. It has been reported that meals rich in ω-6 polyunsaturated fatty acids (PUFA) increase leptin production [35]. It has been reported that the protein composition of a meal does not affect leptin production [38].

Gender differences have an effect on leptin production. Although there is no difference in leptin levels between girls and boys in the prepubertal period, leptin levels increase in girls and decrease in boys with puberty development [39, 40]. This is explained by the fact that with puberty, the amount of body fat in girls increases more than in boys, and testosterone suppresses leptin levels in boys [41]. In addition, the fact that the subcutaneous AT mass is significantly larger than the omental fat mass of women is also among the factors [39]. Reproductive hormones greatly affect leptin production. Androgenic hormones inhibit leptin synthesis, while estrogens stimulate leptin synthesis [42]. In one study, it was thought that increased estrogen concentrations caused an increase in leptin concentration, which may have been caused by leptin stimulating gonadotrophin releasing hormone (GnRH) synthesis and thus increasing estrogen synthesis [43]. In addition, chronic insomnia and an increase in melatonin concentrations have been reported to decrease plasma leptin concentrations [44].

4. Leptin release factors

The immune system has a role in regulating energy expenditure and AT lipolysis [45]. White adipose tissue (WAT) is the primary energy store; brown adipose tissue (BAT) is associated with heat production. Sympathetic activity in WAT is increased in conditions associated with decreased leptin synthesis/secretion, such as cold exposure and starvation. By the way, catecholamine and β-adrenoceptor agonists inhibit leptin production; this suppressive effect is mediated by β3-adrenoceptor agonists, which actively reduce leptin levels [46]. Leptin also causes sympathetic nervous system activation, resulting in regulatory feedback inhibition [47]. Intracerebroventricular injections of leptin have been noted to increase metabolic rates through increased norepinephrine release from sympathetic nerve terminals innervating BAT [48].

After a meal, plasma insulin and amino acid levels initiate the mammalian target of rapamycin (mTOR) pathway, which stimulates leptin biosynthesis via mechanisms involving the 5′/3′ untranslated region (UTR) [49]. Cyclic AMP activates cyclic AMP-activated exchange proteins (EPACs). Deletion of *EPAC1* genes causes an increase in leptin sensitivity in the hypothalamus. *EPAC1* is also involved in leptin secretion and expression in WAT [50].

Leptin antagonizes orexigenic pathways and stimulates anorexigenic pathways. Leptin exerts its general effects on the nervous system through these pathways [7]. Orexigenic neuropeptides that are down-regulated by leptin are orexins, agouti-related peptides, neuropeptide Y, and melanin-concentrating hormone. By the way, the anorexigenic neuropeptides upregulated by leptin are alpha-melanocyte-stimulating hormone, which acts on corticotropin-releasing hormone, cocaine and amphetamine-regulated transcript, and melanocortin-4 receptor (**Figure 1**) [31].

Glucocorticoids are long-term regulators of leptin expression [52, 53]. They increase leptin mRNA levels by acting on adipocytes; *in vitro* incubation of a synthetic glucocorticoid in rats, adipocytes have been found to increase leptin secretion [54]. Oral glucocorticoids doubled serum leptin levels and leptin mRNA 24–48 hours after absorption. Furthermore, cell cultures incubated with a glucocorticoid and insulin combination synergistically increased leptin mRNA levels [55].

Lactates and hexoses also increase leptin secretion [56]. Because leptin secretion requires ATP, suppressing glucose uptake suppresses leptin secretion. When the energy supply is low, food is needed to increase it. Glucose, the cellular sensor of energy stock, stimulates leptin gene expression and secretion in both muscle and AT via hexosamine biosynthetic [57]. Insulin lowers blood sugar when glucose levels rise above normal and also increases leptin promoter activity [58]. No increase in leptin mRNA levels was observed after adipocytes were incubated with insulin for 1–2 hours, but an increase in leptin release was observed [54].

Regulation of tumor necrosis factor-alpha(TNFα) and leptin may be interdependent and similar as they have comparable functions such as suppressing

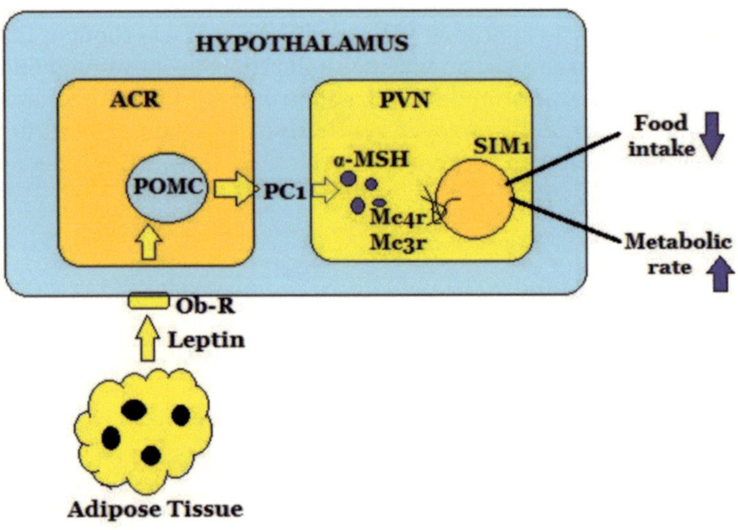

Figure 1.
The leptin/Melanocortin pathway. ARC; the arcuate nucleus of the hypothalamus, POMC; proopiomelanocortin, Ob-R; leptin receptor, PVN; paraventricular nucleus, MSH; melanocyte-stimulating hormone (α-MSH,β-MSH,γ-MSH), MC4R; melanocortin-4 receptor, SIM1; single-minded 1 [51].

lipid synthesis, reducing food intake, and stimulating lipolysis [59]. Leptin limits AT mass. TNFα has the role of stimulating leptin secretion from mature human adipocytes. TNFα therapy has been shown to cause increased leptin levels in humans [60].

5. Leptin receptor and leptin resistance

Leptin receptors are in the family of cytokine receptors. There are six isoforms encoded by the *LepR* gene. The *OB-Rb* receptor is the dominant longest form. Its mutations cause obesity because it cannot bind to the receptor [16]. Obese people have high leptin levels. Circulating leptin levels are correlated with body mass index [61]. On the other hand, in diet-related exogenous obesity, studies in fat mice and humans without leptin deficiency, it has been shown that external leptin treatment does not provide a significant reduction in body weight and food intake [62]. In obese people, leptin levels increase, but hyperglycemia-correcting or appetite-reducing effects are not observed [63]. Despite the increased leptin levels in obese patients, the absence of the functions of leptin, an appetite-reducing hormone, suggests leptin resistance [64]. It has been suggested that leptin resistance plays a role in the pathogenesis of obesity triggered by overeating [65]. However, the molecular mechanisms underlying leptin resistance have not yet been clearly elucidated. The inability of leptin to cross the blood–brain barrier, inhibition of the intracellular leptin signaling pathway in neurons, and/or downregulation of leptin receptors are thought to be the underlying mechanisms of leptin resistance. It has been reported that a high-fat diet causes an increase in fat mass, leading to hyperleptinemia and triggering leptin resistance [66]. In high-fat rats *(fa/fa)*, substitutions in *OB-Rb* result in reduced signaling capacity, leptin binding affinity, and cell surface expression [67]. Obese *fa/fa* rats have leptin resistance and are not sensitive to the effects of leptin. Although obese people may have high plasma leptin concentrations due to leptin resistance, they do not experience the effects of leptin [19].

In gastric chief cells (also known as zymogenic cell or peptic cell), leptin is released upon sensing gastrin and secretin and it is actively inhibited by cholecystokinin [68]. The binding of leptin to its receptor activates the Janus kinase (JAK) signal transducer and activator of the transcription 3 (STAT3) signal transduction pathway, inducing cellular anti-apoptotic events, angiogenesis, and proliferation [69, 70]. The gene product also interacts with IL-1 and Notch cascade, which are involved in promoting tumor growth. Some other pathways activated are mitogen-activated protein kinases/extracellular signal-regulated kinases pathway (MAPK/ERK), phosphatidylinositol 3 kinase (PI3K), 5′AMP activated protein kinase (AMPK), and mTOR [71].

6. Leptin-related cellular pathways

After leptin binds to its receptor on the cell membrane, it acts by stimulating the following signaling pathways in the cell.

6.1 JAK2/ STAT3 signaling pathway

In the activation of this signaling pathway, leptin is activated by phosphorylation of its receptor, binding of STAT3, and phosphorylated by JAK2 [72]. Activated STAT3 enters the nucleus and binds to target sites on DNA; and so cellular activity takes place (**Figure 2**).

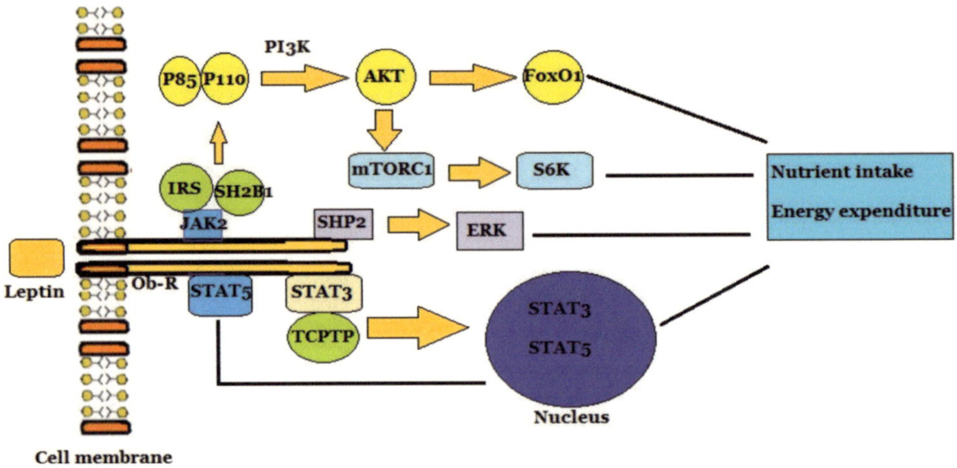

Figure 2.
Leptin signaling pathways. POMC;pro-opiomelanocortin, SOCS3; intracellular suppressor of cytokine signal 3, PTP1B; protein tyrosine phosphatase 1B, SHP2; tyrosine phosphatase 2, IRS; (insulin receptor substrate)/PI3K; (phosphoinositol 3 kinase), FoxO1; (forkhead box O1) and mTOR; (mammalian target of rapamycin), S6K; ribosomal S6 kinase, ERK; extracellular signal-regulated kinase [73].

6.2 SHP2/ERK signaling pathway

Stimulation of the leptin receptor activates the protein tyrosine phosphatase 2 (SHP2), contributing to the activation of the ERK signaling pathway, resulting in a cellular response [72, 74].

6.3 JAK2/STAT5 signaling pathway

As a result of the stimulation of the receptor, it provides activation of STAT5 by JAK2. Activated STAT5 acts by binding to the target region in the nucleus [75].

6.4 IRS/ PI3K Signaling pathway

Leptin also activates the IRS (insulin receptor substrate)/PI3K (phosphoinositol 3 kinase) pathway [76, 77] (**Figure 2**). The SH2B1 adapter protein mediates activation of the PI3K pathway by linking the JAK2 and IRS protein via the SH2 domain [78]. In addition, the IRS/PI3K pathway proceeds in two substeps, FoxO1 (forkhead box O1) and mTOR (the mammalian target of rapamycin) (**Figure 2**).

7. The relationship between leptin and oxidative stress

Oxidative stress results from an imbalance between reactive oxygen species (ROS) and the organism's antioxidant defense. Due to oxidative stress, peroxidative damage to macromolecules and membranes of cells occurs in organisms. Moreover, their metabolic activities in cell components are impaired. Known to tissue and organ pathologies occur in the presence of oxidative stress in the organism [79–86]. It has been reported that high leptin levels can induce the formation of ROS, mainly due to nicotinamide adenine dinucleotide phosphate (NADPH) oxidase activation [87, 88]. However, leptin replacement therapy has also been shown to significantly downregulate NADPH oxidase expression in AT of leptin-deficient *ob/ob* mice [89]. This indicates that leptin has a protective role at normal levels.

Free radical-mediated peroxidation of membrane lipids loses its integrity, increasing membrane fluidity and permeability. The lipid peroxidation process is one of the oxidative conversions of PUFAs to products known as malondialdehyde (MDA). MDA is a highly toxic molecule and its secondary products such as thiobarbituric acid reactive agent are commonly used to assess lipid peroxidation [90–94]. Glutathione (GSH) is an important nonenzymatic component of the cellular antioxidant system and plays an important role in ROS antioxidation [95–97]. It has been suggested that leptin modulates the activity of various antioxidant enzymes such as superoxide dismutase (SOD) and glutathione peroxidase (GPx) in patients with leptin gene mutations [98]. Leptin production is increased by overexpression of the endogenous antioxidant enzyme catalase and correlates with markers of oxidative stress and inflammatory in *ob/ob* mice [99]. In another study, enzymatic antioxidants including catalase and GSH levels were increased by leptin treatment in *ob/ob* mice, and leptin treatment decreased MDA levels in rats exposed to oxidative stress [100, 101]. It is noted that leptin treatment reverses the effect of streptozotocin (STZ)-induced diabetes by lowering glutathione and catalase levels and increasing lipid peroxidation [102, 103] It has been reported that defective antioxidant enzyme activity is recovered after leptin treatment in the plasma of humans with leptin gene mutations and ob/ob mice [97, 104]. They are most likely the result of the modulatory effect of leptin on metabolic and hormonal disorders. Recombinant leptin treatment leads to weight loss by reducing food intake and has a reducing effect on oxidative stress caused by a high-fat diet [105].

Hyperleptinemia is the most prominent feature of obesity and is likely to be involved in the pathogenesis of obesity-related pathologies [19]. Studies in obese individuals have shown a correlation between leptin levels and oxidative stress parameters such as nitric oxide (NO), superoxide anion ($O_2^-.$), peroxynitrite, MDA, hydroperoxides, protein carbonyl (PC) contents, GSH, and SOD [106–108]. Studies in which hyperleptinemia was induced by the administration of exogenous leptin in nonobese animals suggest that leptin increases the level of systemic oxidative stress [109, 110]. In addition, some *in vitro* studies have shown that in the presence of high leptin concentration, ROS production is stimulated by endothelial cells, inflammatory cells, and other cell types [111–113]. In another *in vitro* study, it was noted that leptin significantly decreased pro-oxidant biomarkers such as MDA and NO and increased antioxidant markers such as total antioxidant capacity (TAC), SOD, and GPx against cryopreservation-induced oxidative stress in rabbit embryos. It has been suggested that leptin can be used as an antiapoptotic and antioxidant promoter to support embryonic development *in vitro* under oxidative stress induced by cryopreservation [114]. In one study, treatment with high glucose caused an increase in oxidative stress in pheochromocytoma (PC12) cells with excessive ROS and MDA production and depletion of GSH content, however, leptin treatment caused a decrease in MDA and ROS levels and an increase in GSH content, resulting in hyperglycemic PC12 cells. It has been reported to significantly reduce the oxidative damage mediated by reactive oxygen species caused by the condition. Therefore, it was stated that leptin may have a protective effect against oxidative stress and apoptosis mediated by reactive oxygen species caused by the hyperglycemic state [115]. In addition, hypothalamic oxidative stress induces leptin resistance, which leads to the induction of insulin resistance and obesity. Activation of nuclear factor erythroid 2–related factor 2 (Nrf2) suppresses hypothalamic oxidative stress and improves leptin resistance in the hypothalamus [116].

8. The relationship between leptin and apoptosis

Recently, some studies have shown that there is an important relationship between leptin and apoptosis; such as in a study, it was determined that there is a leptin receptor (Ob-R) on the surface of breast cancer cells. Leptin is thought to stimulate these cancer cells with various effects, such as migration and spread. It has been determined that the expression of Ob-R increases as the tumor grows [117]. Another study reported that leptin may affect the risk of breast cancer by increasing estrogen synthesis [118, 119]. It is believed that leptin, which is associated with breast cancer, exerts this effect by affecting the JAK/STAT and MAPK pathways, as well as increasing the transcriptional expression of vascular endothelial growth factor receptor-2 (VEGFR-2) and VEGF [120]. In another study, it was determined that the ratio between leptin and adiponectin is important in regulating the development of breast cancer [121]. Again, in some studies, it has been determined that leptin triggers cell proliferation by stimulating the MAPK pathway in breast cancer cells [122]. It has been observed that leptin also stimulates estrogen receptors via MAPK in breast cancer cells [123].

It has also been reported that leptin is associated with lung cancer. Ob-Ra and Ob-Rb were expressed on the surface of lung cancer cells. It has been determined that leptin plays a role in the development and progression of lung cancer as well as its migration [124, 125]. It has been reported that leptin also increases cytokine production by stimulating JAK/STAT3, PI3K/AKT, and MEK1/2 signaling pathways [126]. In a study, it was determined that the removal of leptin from the medium in non-small cell lung cancer cell lines inactivates the JAK/STAT3 and Notch signaling pathways, thus stopping cell proliferation and stimulating apoptosis (**Figure 3**) [128].

In some studies, leptin has been shown to stimulate cell proliferation and prevent apoptosis by activation of the PI3K/AKT signaling pathway in thyroid cancer cells [129, 130].

Leptin has been reported to be associated with liver cancer [131]. In one study, they reported elevated leptin levels in patients with hepatocellular carcinoma [132]. It has been determined that leptin increases liver fibrosis by stimulating transforming growth factor-β (TGF-β) synthesis and release. It has also been reported that leptin stimulates the production of a tissue inhibitor of metalloproteinase1 through the JAK/STAT pathway in hepatic stellate cells [133]. Leptin has also been reported to cause the proliferation of hepatocellular cancer cells by altering cyclin D1, *Bcl-2* (B-cell lymphoma-2)-related X protein (Bax), and apoptotic gene activity [134].

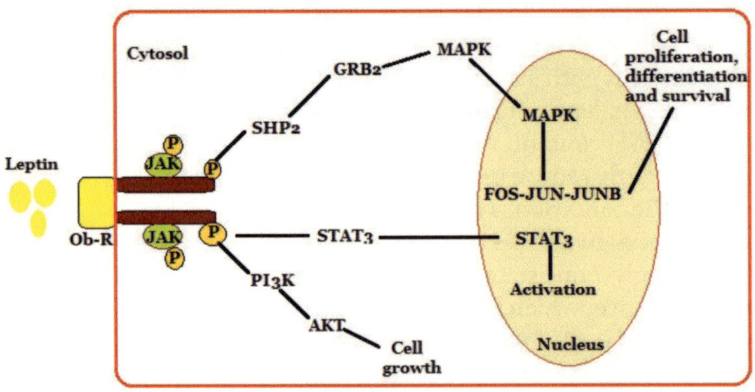

Figure 3.
Leptin signaling. AKT; protein kinase B, GRB2; growth factor receptor-bound protein 2, JAK; Janus kinase, Ob-R; leptin receptor, MAPK; mitogen-activated protein kinase, FOS, JUN, JUNB; GENES PI3K; phosphatidylinositol 3 kinase, SHP2; Src homology 2-containing tyrosine phosphatase, STAT3; signal transducer and activator of transcription 3 [127].

Another study demonstrated the presence of leptin receptors on the surface of human colon tumor cells [135]. In colorectal cancer, leptin acts as a very potent mitogen and antiapoptotic cytokine. It has been determined that leptin plays a role in many stages of this type of cancer [136, 137]. It has been reported that leptin increase is proportional to tumor development and tumor metastasis [138]. It has been determined that leptin exerts this effect via JAK and the extracellular signal-regulating kinase (ERK) pathway [139]. In another study, they found that leptin prevented apoptosis and stimulated cell proliferation via PI3K/AKT/mTOR pathways in colon cancer cells (**Figure 4**) [141].

In a study conducted in ovarian cancer, it was determined that leptin is directly related to PI3K/AKT signaling pathways, antiapoptotic proteins XIAP (X-linked inhibitor of apoptosis), and Bcl-XL. By activating these pathways, leptin has been reported to suppress cell proliferation and apoptosis [142]. In another study, it was determined that leptin administration to epithelial ovarian cancer cells increases cancer cell proliferation in a dose-dependent manner, and this increase is done by suppressing genes that inhibit cell proliferation [143].

An increase in leptin levels has been found to be associated with the development of prostate cancer [144]. It has been determined that leptin suppresses apoptosis in prostate cancer cells. Leptin has been reported to exert this effect via the MAPK and PI3K pathways [145]. It has also been reported that leptin stimulates the increase of (hypoxia-inducible factor 1), which is known to play an important role in carcinogenesis in prostate cancer cell culture and stimulates the spread and adhesion of these cells [146].

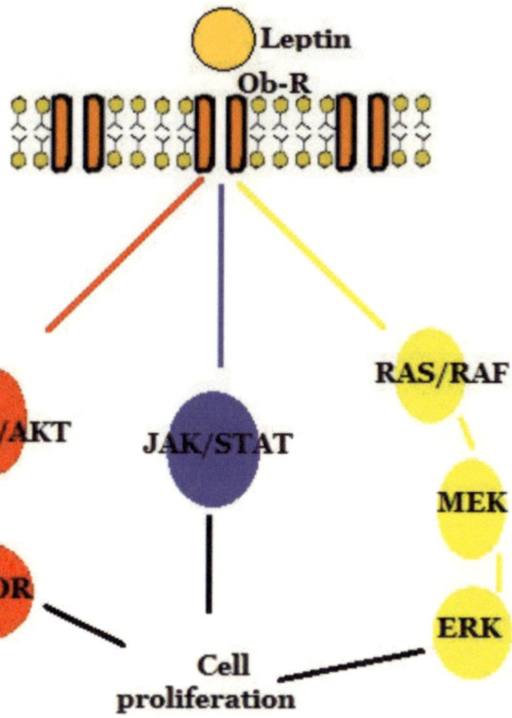

Figure 4.
Intracellular signaling pathways of leptin in connection with cellular proliferation. AKT: Protein kinase B/serine–threonine kinase, ERK: Extracellular signal-regulated kinase, JAK: Janus kinases, MAPK: Mitogen-activated protein kinase, MEK: Mitogen-activated protein kinase, mTOR: Mechanistic/mammalian target of rapamycin, Ob-R: Leptin receptor, PI3K: Phosphatidylinositol3-kinase, STAT: Signal transducer and activator of transcription [140].

9. Conclusion

In conclusion, leptin is adiponectin released from AT. As a result of studies, it has been reported that leptin is associated with oxidative stress and apoptosis, as well as regulating body energy metabolism and food intake. Knowing the release of leptin, its receptor, cellular effects, and especially the relationship between oxidative stress and apoptosis will guide various studies on this subject.

Author details

Volkan Gelen[1*], Abdulsamed Kükürt[2], Emin Şengül[3] and Hacı Ahmet Deveci[4]

1 Faculty of Veterinary Medicine, Department of Physiology, Kafkas University, Kars, Turkey

2 Faculty of Veterinary Medicine, Department of Biochemistry, Kafkas University, Kars, Turkey

3 Faculty of Veterinary Medicine, Department of Physiology, Atatürk University, Erzurum, Turkey

4 Faculty of Health Sciences, Department of Nutrition and Dietetics, Gaziantep University, Gaziantep, Turkey

*Address all correspondence to: gelen_volkan@hotmail.com

References

[1] Wang YC, McPherson K, Marsh T, Gortmaker SL, Brown M. Health and economic burden of the projected obesity trends in the USA and the UK. Lancet. 2011;**378**:815-825. DOI: 10.1016/S0140-6736(11)60814-3

[2] Dhurandhar EJ, Keith SW. The aetiology of obesity beyond eating more and exercising less. Best Practice & Research. Clinical Gastroenterology. 2014;**28**:533-544. DOI: 10.1016/j.bpg.2014.07.001

[3] McAllister EJ, Dhurandhar NV, Keith SW, Aronne LJ, Barger J, Baskin M, et al. Ten putative contributors to the obesity epidemic. Critical Reviews in Food Science and Nutrition. 2009;**49**:868-913. DOI: 10.1080/10408390903372599

[4] Gelen V, Şengül E, Gedikli S, Gür C, Özkanlar S. Therapeutic effect of quercetin on renal function and tissue damage in the obesity induced rats. Biomedicine & Pharmacotherapy. 2017;**89**:524-528. DOI: 10.1016/j.biopha.2017.02.057

[5] Gedikli S, Ozkanlar S, Gur C, Sengul E, Gelen V. Preventive effects of quercetin on liver damages in high-fat diet-induced obesity. Journal of Histology & Histopathology. 2017;**4**:7. DOI: 10.7243/2055-091X-4-7

[6] Koerner A, Kratzsch J, Kiess W. Adipocytokines: leptin—the classical, resistin—the controversical, adiponectin—the promising, and more to come. Best Practice & Research. Clinical Endocrinology & Metabolism. 2005;**19**:525-546. DOI: 10.1016/j.beem.2005.07.008

[7] Friedman JM, Halaas JL. Leptin and the regulation of body weight in mammals. Nature. 1998;**395**:763-770. DOI: 10.1038/27376

[8] Elmquist JK, Elias CF, Saper CB. From lesions to leptin: Hypothalamic control of food intake and body weight. Neuron. 1999;**22**:221-232. DOI: 10.1016/S0896-6273(00)81084-3

[9] Bates SH, Myers MG. The role of leptin receptor signaling in feeding and neuroendocrine function. Trends in Endocrinology and Metabolism. 2003;**14**:447-452. DOI: 10.1016/j.tem.2003.10.003

[10] Zhang F, Chen Y, Heiman M, DiMarchi R. Leptin: Structure, function and biology. Vitamins and Hormones. 2005;**71**:345-372. DOI: 10.1016/S0083-6729(05)71012-8

[11] Montague CT, Farooqi IS, Whitehead JP, Soos MA, Rau H, Wareham NJ, et al. Congenital leptin deficiency is associated with severe early-onset obesity in humans. Nature. 1997;**387**:903-908. DOI: 10.1038/43185

[12] Ingalls AM, Dickie MM, Snell GD. Obese, a new mutation in the house mouse*. Obesity Research. 1996;**4**:101-101. DOI: 10.1002/j.1550-8528.1996.tb00519.x

[13] Hummel KP, Dickie MM, Coleman DL. Diabetes, a New Mutafton in the Mouse. Science (80-). 1966;**153**:1127-1128. DOI: 10.1126/science.153.3740.1127

[14] Coleman DL. Obese and diabetes: Two mutant genes causing diabetes-obesity syndromes in mice. Diabetologia. 1978;**14**:141-148. DOI: 10.1007/BF00429772

[15] Zhang Y, Proenca R, Maffei M, Barone M, Leopold L, Friedman JM. Positional cloning of the mouse obese gene and its human homologue. Nature. 1994;**372**:425-432. DOI: 10.1038/372425a0

[16] Tartaglia LA, Dembski M, Weng X, Deng N, Culpepper J, Devos R, et al.

Identification and expression cloning of a leptin receptor, OB-R. Cell. 1995;**83**: 1263-1271. DOI: 10.1016/0092-8674(95)90151-5

[17] Gong DW, Bi S, Pratley RE, Weintraub BD. Genomic structure and promoter analysis of the human obese gene. The Journal of Biological Chemistry. 1996;**271**:3971-3974. DOI: 10.1074/jbc.271.8.3971

[18] Ahima RS, Flier JS. Leptin. Annual Review of Physiology. 2000;**62**:413-437. DOI: 10.1146/annurev.physiol.62.1.413

[19] Maffei M, Halaas J, Ravussin E, Pratley RE, Lee GH, Zhang Y, et al. Leptin levels in human and rodent: Measurement of plasma leptin and ob RNA in obese and weight-reduced subjects. Nature Medicine. 1995;**1**:1155-1161. DOI: 10.1038/nm1195-1155

[20] Huising MO, Kruiswijk CP, Flik G. Phylogeny and evolution of class-I helical cytokines. The Journal of Endocrinology. 2006;**189**:1-25. DOI: 10.1677/joe.1.06591

[21] Peelman F, Iserentant H, De Smet AS, Vandekerckhove J, Zabeau L, Tavernier J. Mapping of binding site III in the leptin receptor and modeling of a hexameric leptin·leptin receptor complex. The Journal of Biological Chemistry. 2006;**281**:15496-15504. DOI: 10.1074/jbc.M512622200

[22] Denver RJ, Bonett RM, Boorse GC. Evolution of leptin structure and function. Neuroendocrinology. 2011;**94**:21-38. DOI: 10.1159/000328435

[23] Al-Suhaimi EA, Shehzad A. Leptin, resistin and visfatin: The missing link between endocrine metabolic disorders and immunity. European Journal of Medical Research. 2013;**18**:12-18. DOI: 10.1186/2047-783X-18-12

[24] Caro JF, Sinha MK, Kolaczynski JW, Zhang PL, Considine RV. Leptin: The tale of an obesity gene. Diabetes. 1996;**45**:1455-1462. DOI: 10.2337/diab.45.11.1455

[25] Inui A. Feeding and body-weight regulation by hypothalamic neuropeptides - Mediation of the actions of leptin. Trends in Neurosciences. 1999;**22**:62-67. DOI: 10.1016/S0166-2236(98)01292-2

[26] Ahima RS, Prabakaran D, Mantzoros C, Qu D, Lowell B, Maratos-Flier E, et al. Role of leptin in the neuroendocrine response to fasting. Nature. 1996;**382**:250-252. DOI: 10.1038/382250a0

[27] Lutz TA, Woods SC. Overview of animal models of obesity. Current Protocols in Pharmacology. 2012. Chapter 5: Unit 5.61. DOI: 10.1002/0471141755.ph0561s58

[28] Loffreda S, Yang SQ, Lin HZ, Karp CL, Brengman ML, Wang DJ, et al. Leptin regulates proinflammatory immune responses. The FASEB Journal. 1998;**12**:57-65. DOI: 10.1096/fsb2fasebj.12.1.57

[29] Procaccini C, La Rocca C, Carbone F, De Rosa V, Galgani M, Matarese G. Leptin as immune mediator: Interaction between neuroendocrine and immune system. Developmental and Comparative Immunology. 2017;**66**:120-129. DOI: 10.1016/j.dci.2016.06.006

[30] Dos Santos MA, Pisani LP, Corgosinho FC, Testa Carvalho LO, Masquio DCL, Jamar G, et al. The role of leptinemia state as a mediator of inflammation in obese adults. Hormone and Metabolic Research. 2013;**45**:605-610. DOI: 10.1055/s-0033-1343450

[31] Jéquier E. Leptin signaling, adiposity, and energy balance. Annals of the New York Academy of Sciences. 2002;**967**: 379-388. DOI: 10.1111/j.1749-6632.2002.tb04293.x

[32] Friedman JM. Leptin, leptin receptors, and the control of body weight. Scandinavian Journal of Nutrition. 1998;**56**:54-75

[33] Lönnqvist F, Nordfors L, Jansson M, Thörne A, Schalling M, Arner P. Leptin secretion from adipose tissue in women: Relationship to plasma levels and gene expression. The Journal of Clinical Investigation. 1997;**99**:2398-2404. DOI: 10.1172/JCI119422

[34] Considine RV, Cooksey RC, Williams LB, Fawcett RL, Zhang P, Ambrosius WT, et al. Hexosamines regulate leptin production in human subcutaneous adipocytes. The Journal of Clinical Endocrinology and Metabolism. 2000;**85**:3551-3556. DOI: 10.1210/jc.85.10.3551

[35] Takahashi Y, Ide T. Dietary n-3 fatty acids affect mRNA level of brown adipose tissue uncoupling protein 1, and white adipose tissue leptin and glucose transporter 4 in the rat. The British Journal of Nutrition. 2000;**84**:175-184. DOI: 10.1017/s0007114500001409

[36] Havel PJ, Townsend R, Chaump L, Teff K. High-fat meals reduce 24-h circulating leptin concentrations in women. Diabetes. 1999;**48**:334-341. DOI: 10.2337/diabetes.48.2.334

[37] Havel PJ. Role of adipose tissue in body-weight regulation: Mechanisms regulating leptin production and energy balance. The Proceedings of the Nutrition Society. 2000;**59**:256-371. DOI: 10.1017/S0029665100000410

[38] Heini AF, Lara-Castro C, Schneider H, Kirk KA, Considine RV, Weinsier RL. Effect of hydrolyzed guar fiber on fasting and postprandial satiety and satiety hormones: A double-blind, placebo-controlled trial during controlled weight loss. International Journal of Obesity. 1998;**22**:906-909. DOI: 10.1038/sj.ijo.0800680

[39] Rosenbaum M, Leibel RL. Clinical review 107: Role of gonadal steroids in the sexual dimorphisms in body composition and circulating concentrations of leptin. The Journal of Clinical Endocrinology and Metabolism. 1999;**84**:1784-1789. DOI: 10.1210/jcem.84.6.5787

[40] Ahmed ML, Ong KKL, Morrell DJ, Cox L, Drayer N, Perry L, et al. Longitudinal study of leptin concentrations during puberty: Sex differences and relationship to changes in body composition. The Journal of Clinical Endocrinology and Metabolism. 1999;**84**:899-905. DOI: 10.1210/jc.84.3.899

[41] Hims-Hagen J. Physiological roles of the leptin endocrine system: Differences between mice and humans. Critical Reviews in Clinical Laboratory Sciences. 1999;**36**:575-655. DOI: 10.1080/10408369991239259

[42] Jockenhövel F, Blum WF, Vogel E, Englaro P, Müller-Wieland D, Reinwein D, et al. Testosterone substitution normalizes elevated serum leptin levels in hypogonadal men. The Journal of Clinical Endocrinology and Metabolism. 1997;**82**:2510-2513. DOI: 10.1210/jc.82.8.2510

[43] Kuru M, Öğün M, Kulaksiz R, Kükürt A, Oral H. Comparison of oxidative/nitrosative stress, leptin and progesterone concentrations in pregnant and non-pregnant Abaza goats synchronized with controlled internal drug release application. Kafkas Universitesi Veteriner Fakultesi Dergisi. 2018;**24**:887-892. DOI: 10.9775/kvfd.2018.20222

[44] Knutson KL, Spiegel K, Penev P, Van Cauter E. The metabolic consequences of sleep deprivation. Sleep Medicine Reviews. 2007;**11**:163-178. DOI: 10.1016/j.smrv.2007.01.002

[45] Bartness TJ, Bamshad M. Innervation of mammalian white

adipose tissue: Implications for the regulation of total body fat. American Journal of Physiology. Regulatory, Integrative and Comparative Physiology. 1998;**275**:1399-1411. DOI: 10.1152/ajpregu.1998.275.5.r1399

[46] Hardie LJ, Rayner DV, Holmes S, Trayhurn P. Circulating leptin levels are modulated by fasting, cold exposure and insulin administration in lean but not Zucker (fa/fa) rats as measured by ELISA. Biochemical and Biophysical Research Communications. 1996;**223**:660-665. DOI: 10.1006/bbrc.1996.0951

[47] Eikelis N, Schlaich M, Aggarwal A, Kaye D, Esler M. Interactions between leptin and the human sympathetic nervous system. Hypertension. 2003;**41**:1072-1079. DOI: 10.1161/01.HYP.0000066289.17754.49

[48] Mistry AM, Swick AG, Romsos DR. Leptin rapidly lowers food intake and elevates metabolic rates in lean and ob/ob mice. The Journal of Nutrition. 1997;**127**:2065-2072. DOI: 10.1093/jn/127.10.2065

[49] Lee MJ, Fried SK. Integration of hormonal and nutrient signals that regulate leptin synthesis and secretion. American Journal of Physiology. Endocrinology and Metabolism. 2009;**296**:1230-1238. DOI: 10.1152/ajpendo.90927.2008

[50] Hu Y, Robichaux WG, Mei FC, Kim ER, Wang H, Tong Q, et al. Role of exchange protein directly activated by cyclic AMP Isoform 1 in energy homeostasis: regulation of leptin expression and secretion in white adipose tissue. Molecular and Cellular Biology. 2016;**36**:2440-2450. DOI: 10.1128/mcb.01034-15

[51] Foster-Schubert KE, Cummings DE. Emerging therapeutic strategies for obesity. Endocrine Reviews. 2006;**27**:779-793. DOI: 10.1210/er.2006-0041

[52] Russell CD, Petersen RN, Rao SP, Ricci MR, Prasad A, Zhang Y, et al. Leptin expression in adipose tissue from obese humans: Depot-specific regulation by insulin and dexamethasone. American Journal of Physiology. Endocrinology and Metabolism. 1998;**275**:507-515. DOI: 10.1152/ajpendo.1998.275.3.e507

[53] Elimam A, Knutsson U, Brönnegård M, Stierna P, Albertsson-Wikland K, Marcus C. Variations in glucocorticoid levels within the physiological range affect plasma leptin levels. European Journal of Endocrinology. 1998;**139**:615-620. DOI: 10.1530/eje.0.1390615

[54] Bradley RL, Cheatham B. Regulation of ob gene expression and leptin secretion by insulin and dexamethasone in rat adipocytes. Diabetes. 1999;**48**:272-278. DOI: 10.2337/diabetes.48.2.272

[55] Laferrère B, Caixas A, Fried SK, Bashore C, Kim J, Pi-Sunyer FX. A pulse of insulin and dexamethasone stimulates serum leptin in fasting human subjects. European Journal of Endocrinology. 2002;**146**:839-845. DOI: 10.1530/eje.0.1460839

[56] Mueller WM, Gregoire FM, Stanhope KL, Mobbs CV, Mizuno TM, Warden CH, et al. Evidence that glucose metabolism regulates leptin secretion from cultured rat adipocytes. Endocrinology. 1998;**139**:551-558. DOI: 10.1210/endo.139.2.5716

[57] Wang J, Liu R, Hawkins M, Barzilial N, Rossetti L. A nutrient-sensing pathway regulates leptin gene expression in muscle and fat. Nature. 1998;**393**:684-688. DOI: 10.1038/31474

[58] Moreno-Aliaga MJ, Stanhope KL, Havel PJ. Transcriptional regulation of the leptin promoter by insulin-stimulated glucose metabolism in 3T3-L1 adipocytes.

Biochemical and Biophysical Research Communications. 2001;**283**:544-548. DOI: 10.1006/bbrc.2001.4822

[59] Zhang HH, Kumar S, Barnett AH, Eggo MC. Tumour necrosis factor-α exerts dual effects on human adipose leptin synthesis and release. Molecular and Cellular Endocrinology. 2000;**159**: 502-508. DOI: 10.1016/S0303-7207(99)00194-X

[60] Kirchgessner TG, Uysal KT, Wiesbrock SM, Marino MW, Hotamisligil GS. Tumor necrosis factor-α contributes to obesity-related hyperleptinemia by regulating leptin release from adipocytes. The Journal of Clinical Investigation. 1997;**100**:2777-2782. DOI: 10.1172/JCI119824

[61] Considine RV, Sinha MK, Heiman ML, Kriauciunas A, Stephens TW, Nyce MR, et al. Serum immunoreactive-leptin concentrations in normal-weight and obese humans. The New England Journal of Medicine. 1996;**334**:292-295. DOI: 10.1056/nejm199602013340503

[62] Halaas JL, Boozer C, Blair-West J, Fidahusein N, Denton DA, Friedman JM. Physiological response to long-term peripheral and central leptin infusion in lean and obese mice. Proceedings of the National Academy of Sciences of the United States of America. 1997;**94**:8878-8883. DOI: 10.1073/pnas.94.16.8878

[63] Blüher M. Adipokines - removing road blocks to obesity and diabetes therapy. Molecular Metabolism. 2014;**3**:230-240. DOI: 10.1016/j.molmet.2014.01.005

[64] Myers MG, Cowley MA, Münzberg H. Mechanisms of leptin action and leptin resistance. Annual Review of Physiology. 2008;**70**:537-556. DOI: 10.1146/annurev.physiol.70.113006.100707

[65] Scarpace PJ, Matheny M, Tümer N, Cheng KY, Zhang Y. Leptin resistance exacerbates diet-induced obesity and is associated with diminished maximal leptin signalling capacity in rats. Diabetologia. 2005;**48**:1075-1083. DOI: 10.1007/s00125-005-1763-x

[66] Crujeiras AB, Carreira MC, Cabia B, Andrade S, Amil M, Casanueva FF. Leptin resistance in obesity: An epigenetic landscape. Life Sciences. 2015;**140**:57-63. DOI: 10.1016/j.lfs.2015.05.003

[67] Da Silva BA, Bjørbæk C, Uotani S, Flier JS. Functional properties of leptin receptor isoforms containing the gln→pro extracellular domain mutation of the fatty rat. Endocrinology. 1998;**139**:3681-3690. DOI: 10.1210/endo.139.9.6168

[68] Mix H, Manns MP, Wagner S, Widjaja A, Jandl O, Cornberg M, et al. Expression of leptin and leptin receptor isoforms in the human stomach. Gut. 2000;**47**:e7624. DOI: 10.1136/gut.47.4.481

[69] Triantafyllou GA, Paschou SA, Mantzoros CS. Leptin and hormones: Energy homeostasis. Endocrinology and Metabolism Clinics of North America. 2016;**45**:633-645. DOI: 10.1016/j.ecl.2016.04.012

[70] Mullen M, Gonzalez-Perez RR. Leptin-induced JAK/STAT signaling and cancer growth. Vaccine. 2016;**4**:26. DOI: 10.3390/vaccines4030026

[71] Park HK, Ahima RS. Leptin signaling. F1000Prime Reports. 2014;**6**:73. DOI: 10.12703/P6-73

[72] Banks AS, Davis SM, Bates SH, Myers MG. Activation of downstream signals by the long form of the leptin receptor. The Journal of Biological Chemistry. 2000;**275**:14563-14572. DOI: 10.1074/jbc.275.19.14563

[73] Zhou Y, Rui L. Leptin signaling and leptin resistance. Frontiers in Medicine.

2013;7:207-222. DOI: 10.1007/s11684-013-0263-5

[74] Bjørbæk C, Lavery HJ, Bates SH, Olson RK, Davis SM, Flier JS, et al. SOCS3 mediates feedback inhibition of the leptin receptor via Tyr985. The Journal of Biological Chemistry. 2000;**275**:40649-40657. DOI: 10.1074/jbc.M007577200

[75] Gong Y, Ishida-Takahashi R, Villanueva EC, Fingar DC, Münzberg H, Myers MG. The long form of the leptin receptor regulates STAT5 and ribosomal protein S6 via alternate mechanisms. The Journal of Biological Chemistry. 2007;**282**:31019-31027. DOI: 10.1074/jbc.M702838200

[76] Xu AW, Kaelin CB, Takeda K, Akira S, Schwartz MW, Barsh GS. PI3K integrates the action of insulin and leptin on hypothalamic neurons. The Journal of Clinical Investigation. 2005;**115**:951-958. DOI: 10.1172/JCI200524301

[77] Morris DL, Rui L. Recent advances in understanding leptin signaling and leptin resistance. American Journal of Physiology-Endocrinology and Metabolism. 2009;**297**:E1247-E1259. DOI: 10.1152/ajpendo.00274.2009

[78] Duan C, Li M, Rui L. SH2-B Promotes Insulin Receptor Substrate 1 (IRS1)- and IRS2-mediated Activation of the Phosphatidylinositol 3-Kinase Pathway in Response to Leptin. The Journal of Biological Chemistry. 2004;**279**:43684-43691. DOI: 10.1074/jbc.M408495200

[79] Gelen V, Kükürt A, Şengül E, Başer ÖF, Karapehlivan M. Can polyphenols be used as anti-inflammatory agents against Covid-19 (SARS-CoV-2)-induced inflammation? In: Badria FA, editor. Phenolic Compd. [Working Title]. Rijeka: IntechOpen; 2021. pp. 1-21. DOI: 10.5772/intechopen.98684

[80] Kükürt A, Kuru M, Karapehlivan M. Nitrik oksit, nitrik oksit sentaz ve dişi üreme sistemindeki rolleri. In: Evereklioğlu C, editor. Sağlık Bilim. Alanında Akad. Çalışmalar - II, Gece Kitaplığı. Ankara: Gece Publishing; 2020. pp. 113-123

[81] Gelen V, Kükürt A, Şengül E. Role of the renin-angiotensin-aldosterone system in various disease processes: An overview. In: Renin-Angiotensin Aldosterone Syst. [Working Title]. Rijeka: IntechOpen; 2021. DOI: 10.5772/intechopen.97354

[82] Kükürt A. Doğal bir antioksidan olarak propolis tedavisinin koruyucu etkileri. In: Evereklioğlu C, editor. Sağlık Bilim. Teor. ve Araştırmalar II, Gece Kitaplığı. Ankara: Gece Publishing; 2020. pp. 501-515

[83] Kükürt A, Kuru M, Faruk Başer Ö, Karapehlivan M. Kisspeptin: Role in female infertility. In: Marsh C, editor. Reprod. Horm. Rijeka: IntechOpen; 2021. DOI: 10.5772/intechopen.94925

[84] Başer ÖF, Kükürt A, Karapehlivan M. Oksidatif stresin azaltılmasında anjiyotensin dönüştürücü enzimin rolü. In: Evereklioğlu C, editor. Sağlık Bilim. Teor. ve Araştırmalar II, Gece Kitaplığı. Ankara: Gece Publishing; 2020. pp. 243-253

[85] Kükürt A, Gelen V, Faruk Başer Ö, Ahmet Deveci H, Karapehlivan M. Thiols: Role in oxidative stress-related disorders. In: Lipid Peroxidation [Working Title]. Rijeka: IntechOpen; 2021. DOI: 10.5772/intechopen.96682

[86] Kara A, Gedikli S, Sengul E, Gelen V, Ozkanlar S. Oxidative stress and autophagy. In: Free Radicals Disease. Rijeka: InTech; 2016. DOI: 10.5772/64569

[87] Morawietz H, Bornstein SR. Leptin, endothelin, NADPH oxidase, and heart failure. Hypertension. 2006;**47**:20-21. DOI: 10.1161/01.HYP.0000218452.18010.fb

[88] Dong F, Zhang X, Ren J. Leptin regulates cardiomyocyte contractile function through endothelin-1 receptor–NADPH oxidase pathway. Hypertension. 2006;**47**:222-229. DOI: 10.1161/01.HYP.0000198555.51645.f1

[89] Frühbeck G, Catalán V, Rodríguez A, Ramírez B, Becerril S, Portincasa P, et al. Normalization of adiponectin concentrations by leptin replacement in ob/ob mice is accompanied by reductions in systemic oxidative stress and inflammation. Scientific Reports. 2017;7:2752. DOI: 10.1038/s41598-017-02848-0

[90] Niki E, Yoshida Y, Saito Y, Noguchi N. Lipid peroxidation: Mechanisms, inhibition, and biological effects. Biochemical and Biophysical Research Communications. 2005;**338**:668-676. DOI: 10.1016/j.bbrc.2005.08.072

[91] Gelen V, Şengül E. Antioxidant, anti-inflammatory and antiapoptotic effects of naringin on cardiac damage induced by cisplatin. Indian Journal of Traditional Knowledge. 2020; **19**:459-465

[92] Gelen V, Sengul E, Yildirim S, Celebi F, Cinar A. Effects of rutin on bladder contractility and histopathology in cyclophosphamide-induced hemorrhagic cystitis in rats. Atatürk University Journal of Veterinary Sciences. 2018;**13**:337-346

[93] Karamese M, Guvendi B, Karamese SA, Cinar I, Can S, Erol HS, et al. The protective effects of epigallocatechin gallate on lipopolysa ccharide-induced hepatotoxicity: An in vitro study on Hep3B cells. Iranian Journal of Basic Medical Sciences. 2016;**19**:483-489

[94] Sengul E, Gelen V, Yildirim S, Tekin S, Dag Y. The effects of selenium in acrylamide-induced nephrotoxicity in rats: Roles of oxidative stress, inflammation, apoptosis, and DNA damage. Biological Trace Element Research. 2021;**199**:173-184

[95] Gelen V, Şengül E, Yıldırım S, Senturk E, Tekin S, Kükürt A. The protective effects of hesperidin and curcumin on 5-fluorouracil–induced nephrotoxicity in mice. Environmental Science and Pollution Research. 2021;**34**:47046-47055. DOI: 10.1007/s11356-021-13969-5

[96] Sengul E, Gelen V, Gedikli S. Cardioprotective activities of quercetin and rutin in sprague dawley rats treated with 5-fluorouracil. Journal of Animal and Plant Sciences. 2020;**31**:423-431

[97] Şengül E, Gelen V, Gedikli S, Özkanlar S, Gür C, Çelebi F, et al. The protective effect of quercetin on cyclophosphamide-Induced lung toxicity in rats. Biomedicine & Pharmacotherapy. 2017;**92**:303-307. DOI: 10.1016/j. biopha.2017.05.047

[98] Ozata M, Uckaya G, Aydin A, Isimer A, Ozdemir IC. Defective antioxidant defense system in patients with a human leptin gene mutation. Hormone and Metabolic Research. 2000;**32**:269-272. DOI: 10.1055/s-2007-978634

[99] Amos DL, Robinson T, Massie MB, Cook C, Hoffsted A, Crain C, et al. Catalase overexpression modulates metabolic parameters in a new 'stress-less' leptin-deficient mouse model. Biochimica et Biophysica Acta, Molecular Basis of Disease. 2017;**1863**:2293-2306. DOI: 10.1016/j.bbadis.2017.06.016

[100] Erkasap S, Erkasap N, Koken T, Kahraman A, Uzuner K, Yazihan N, et al. Effect of leptin on renal ischemia-reperfusion damage in rats. Journal of Physiology and Biochemistry. 2004; **60**:79-84. DOI: 10.1007/BF03168443

[101] Zwirska-Korczala K, Adamczyk-Sowa M, Sowa P, Pilc K,

Suchanek R, Pierzchala K, et al. Role of leptin, ghrelin, angiotensin II and orexins in 3T3 L1 preadipocyte cells proliferation and oxidative metabolism. Journal of Physiology and Pharmacology. 2007;**58**:53-64

[102] Madhkhoor SR, Ibrahim IR. Evaluation of some stress indicators and their relation with leptin injection in experimentally induced diabetic rats. International Journal of Advanced Research. 2016;**4**:9-13. DOI: 10.21474/IJAR01/102

[103] Gülen Ş, Dinçer S. Effects of leptin on oxidative stress in healthy and Streptozotocin-induced diabetic rats. Molecular and Cellular Biochemistry. 2007;**302**:59-65. DOI: 10.1007/s11010-007-9426-5

[104] Watson AM, Poloyac SM, Howard G, Blouin RA. Effect of leptin on cytochrome P-450, conjugation, and antioxidant enzymes in the ob/ob mouse. Drug Metabolism and Disposition. 1999;**27**:695-700

[105] Sailaja JBK, Balasubramaniyan V, Nalini N. Effect of exogenous leptin administration on high fat diet induced oxidative stress. Pharmazie. 2004;**59**:475-479

[106] Essa Ahmed S, Maher FT, Ahmed NN. Effect of leptin and oxidative stress in the blood of obese individuals. Biochemistry and Analytical Biochemistry. 2016;**5**:3. DOI: 10.4172/2161-1009.1000288

[107] Malti N, Merzouk H, Bouhmama L, Saker M, Elhabiri M, Cherrak S. Time course of changes in leptin levels and their relationships with oxidant status biomarkers in pregnant women with obesity. Journal of Clinical and Diagnostic Research. 2020;**14**:1-5. DOI: 10.7860/JCDR/2020/43475.13640

[108] Ali IMM, Yenzeel JH, Al-ansari HMS. Evaluation of oxidative stress and leptinlevel in samples of Iraqi obese women. Iraqi Journal of Science. 2020;**61**:1565-1570. DOI: 10.24996/ijs.2020.61.7.3

[109] Beltowski J, Wójcicka G, Jamroz A. Leptin decreases plasma paraoxonase 1 (PON1) activity and induces oxidative stress: the possible novel mechanism for proatherogenic effect of chronic hyperleptinemia. Atherosclerosis. 2003;**170**:21-29. DOI: 10.1016/S0021-9150(03)00236-3

[110] Beltowski J, Wójcicka G, Marciniak A, Jamroz A. Oxidative stress, nitric oxide production, and renal sodium handling in leptin-induced hypertension. Life Sciences. 2004;**74**:2987-3000. DOI: 10.1016/j.lfs.2003.10.029

[111] Maingrette F, Renier G. Leptin increases lipoprotein lipase secretion by macrophages: Involvement of oxidative stress and protein kinase C. Diabetes. 2003;**52**:2121-2128. DOI: 10.2337/diabetes.52.8.2121

[112] Bouloumié A, Marumo T, Lafontan M, Busse R. Leptin induces oxidative stress in human endothelial cells. The FASEB Journal. 1999;**13**:1231-1238. DOI: 10.1096/fasebj.13.10.1231

[113] Savini I, Catani MV, Rossi A, Duranti G, Ranalli M, Melino G, et al. Vitamin C recycling is enhanced in the adaptive response to leptin-induced oxidative stress in keratinocytes. The Journal of Investigative Dermatology. 2003;**121**:786-793. DOI: 10.1046/j.1523-1747.2003.12538.x

[114] Alshaheen TA, Awaad MHH, Mehaisen GMK. Leptin improves the in vitro development of preimplantation rabbit embryos under oxidative stress of cryopreservation. PLoS One. 2021;**16**:e0246307. DOI: 10.1371/journal.pone.0246307

[115] Kaeidi A, Hajializadeh Z, Jahandari F, Fatemi I. Leptin attenuates

oxidative stress and neuronal apoptosis in hyperglycemic condition. Fundamental & Clinical Pharmacology. 2019;**33**:75-83. DOI: 10.1111/fcp.12411

[116] Yagishita Y, Uruno A, Fukutomi T, Saito R, Saigusa D, Pi J, et al. Nrf2 improves leptin and insulin resistance provoked by hypothalamic oxidative stress. Cell Reports. 2017;**18**:2030-2044. DOI: 10.1016/j.celrep.2017.01.064

[117] Surmacz E. Leptin and adiponectin: Emerging therapeutic targets in breast cancer. Journal of Mammary Gland Biology and Neoplasia. 2013;**18**:321-332. DOI: 10.1007/s10911-013-9302-8

[118] Jardé T, Caldefie-Chézet F, Goncalves-Mendes N, Mishellany F, Buechler C, Penault-Llorca F, et al. Involvement of adiponectin and leptin in breast cancer: Clinical and in vitro studies. Endocrine-Related Cancer. 2009;**16**:1197-1210. DOI: 10.1677/ERC-09-0043

[119] Khan S, Shukla S, Sinha S, Meeran SM. Role of adipokines and cytokines in obesity-associated breast cancer: Therapeutic targets. Cytokine & Growth Factor Reviews. 2013;**24**:503-513. DOI: 10.1016/j.cytogfr.2013.10.001

[120] Gonzalez-Perez R, Lanier V, Newman G. Leptin's Pro-Angiogenic Signature in Breast Cancer. Cancers (Basel). 2013;**5**:1140-1162. DOI: 10.3390/cancers5031140

[121] Ray A. Adipokine leptin in obesity-related pathology of breast cancer. Journal of Biosciences. 2012;**37**:289-294. DOI: 10.1007/s12038-012-9191-9

[122] Laud K, Gourdou I, Pessemesse L, Peyrat JP, Djiane J. Identification of leptin receptors in human breast cancer: functional activity in the T47-D breast cancer cell line. Molecular and Cellular Endocrinology. 2002;**188**:219-226. DOI: 10.1016/S0303-7207(01)00678-5

[123] Catalano S, Mauro L, Marsico S, Giordano C, Rizza P, Rago V, et al. Leptin Induces, via ERK1/ERK2 Signal, Functional Activation of Estrogen Receptor α in MCF-7 Cells. The Journal of Biological Chemistry. 2004; **279**:19908-19915. DOI: 10.1074/jbc.M313191200

[124] Bruno A, Siena L, Gerbino S, Ferraro M, Chanez P, Giammanco M, et al. Apigenin affects leptin/leptin receptor pathway and induces cell apoptosis in lung adenocarcinoma cell line. European Journal of Cancer. 2011;**47**:2042-2051. DOI: 10.1016/j.ejca.2011.03.034

[125] Song C-H, Liao J, Deng Z-H, Zhang J-Y, Xue H, Li Y-M, et al. Is leptin a predictive factor in patients with lung cancer? Clinical Biochemistry. 2014;**47**:230-232. DOI: 10.1016/j.clinbiochem.2013.12.003

[126] Shen Y, Wang Q, Zhao Q, Zhou J. Leptin promotes the immune escape of lung cancer by inducing proinflammatory cytokines and resistance to apoptosis. Molecular Medicine Reports. 2009;**2**:295-299. DOI: 10.3892/mmr_00000099

[127] Andò S, Catalano S. The multifactorial role of leptin in driving the breast cancer microenvironment. Nature Reviews. Endocrinology. 2012;**8**: 263-275. DOI: 10.1038/nrendo.2011.184

[128] Zheng X-J, Yang Z-X, Dong Y-J, Zhang G-Y, Sun M-F, An X-K, et al. Downregulation of leptin inhibits growth and induces apoptosis of lung cancer cells via the Notch and JAK/STAT3 signaling pathways. Biology Open. 2016;**5**:794-800. DOI: 10.1242/bio.017798

[129] Uddin S, Bavi P, Siraj AK, Ahmed M, Al-Rasheed M, Hussain AR, et al. Leptin-R and its association with PI3K/AKT signaling pathway in

papillary thyroid carcinoma. Endocrine-Related Cancer. 2010;**17**:191-202. DOI: 10.1677/ERC-09-0153

[130] Uddin S, Hussain AR, Siraj AK, Khan OS, Bavi PP, Al-Kuraya KS. Role of leptin and its receptors in the pathogenesis of thyroid cancer. International Journal of Clinical and Experimental Pathology. 2011;**4**:637-643

[131] Ribatti D, Belloni AS, Nico B, Di Comite M, Crivellato E, Vacca A. Leptin–leptin receptor are involved in angiogenesis in human hepatocellular carcinoma. Peptides. 2008;**29**:1596-1602. DOI: 10.1016/j.peptides.2008.05.011

[132] Miyahara K, Nouso K, Tomoda T, Kobayashi S, Hagihara H, Kuwaki K, et al. Predicting the treatment effect of sorafenib using serum angiogenesis markers in patients with hepatocellular carcinoma. Journal of Gastroenterology and Hepatology. 2011;**26**:1604-1611. DOI: 10.1111/j.1440-1746.2011.06887.x

[133] Duan X-F, Tang P, Li Q, Yu Z-T. Obesity, adipokines and hepatocellular carcinoma. International Journal of Cancer. 2013;**133**:1776-1783. DOI: 10.1002/ijc.28105

[134] Cheung OK-W, Cheng AS-L. Gender differences in adipocyte metabolism and liver cancer progression. Frontiers in Genetics. 2016;**7**:5-6. DOI: 10.3389/fgene.2016.00168

[135] Stattin P, Lukanova A, Biessy C, Söderberg S, Palmqvist R, Kaaks R, et al. Obesity and colon cancer: Does leptin provide a link? International Journal of Cancer. 2004;**109**:149-152. DOI: 10.1002/ijc.11668

[136] Pietrzyk L, Torres A, Maciejewski R, Torres K. Obesity and obese-related chronic low-grade inflammation in promotion of colorectal cancer development. Asian Pacific Journal of Cancer Prevention. 2015;**16**:4161-4168. DOI: 10.7314/APJCP.2015.16.10.4161

[137] Riondino S. Obesity and colorectal cancer: Role of adipokines in tumor initiation and progression. World Journal of Gastroenterology. 2014;**20**:5177. DOI: 10.3748/wjg.v20.i18.5177

[138] Tutino V, Notarnicola M, Guerra V, Lorusso D, Caruso MG. Increased soluble leptin receptor levels are associated with advanced tumor stage in colorectal cancer patients. Anticancer Research. 2011;**31**:3381-3383

[139] Yoon K-W, Park S-Y, Kim J-Y, Lee S-M, Park C-H, Cho S-B, et al. Leptin-induced adhesion and invasion in colorectal cancer cell lines. Oncology Reports. 2014;**31**:2493-2498. DOI: 10.3892/or.2014.3128

[140] Ray A, Fornsaglio J, Dogan S, Hedau S, Naik D, De A. Gynaecological cancers and leptin: A focus on the endometrium and ovary. Facts, Views & Vision in ObGyn. 2018;**10**:5-18

[141] Wang D, Chen J, Chen H, Duan Z, Xu Q, Wei M, et al. Leptin regulates proliferation and apoptosis of colorectal carcinoma through PI3K/Akt/mTOR signalling pathway. Journal of Biosciences. 2012;**37**:91-101. DOI: 10.1007/s12038-011-9172-4

[142] Uddin S, Bu R, Ahmed M, Abubaker J, Al-Dayel F, Bavi P, et al. Overexpression of leptin receptor predicts an unfavorable outcome in Middle Eastern ovarian cancer. Molecular Cancer. 2009;**8**:74. DOI: 10.1186/1476-4598-8-74

[143] Ptak A, Kolaczkowska E, Gregoraszczuk EL. Leptin stimulation of cell cycle and inhibition of apoptosis

gene and protein expression in OVCAR-3 ovarian cancer cells. Endocrine. 2013;**43**:394-403. DOI: 10.1007/s12020-012-9788-7

[144] Alshaker H, Sacco K, Alfraidi A, Muhammad A, Winkler M, Pchejetski D. Leptin signalling, obesity and prostate cancer: Molecular and clinical perspective on the old dilemma. Oncotarget. 2015;**6**:35556-35563. DOI: 10.18632/oncotarget.5574

[145] Osório CF, Souza DB de, Gallo CBM, Costa WS, Sampaio FJB. Leptin and leptin receptor expressions in prostate tumors may predict disease aggressiveness? Acta Cirúrgica Brasileira 2014;29:44-48. 10.1590/S0102-86502014001700009.

[146] Calgani A, Delle Monache S, Cesare P, Vicentini C, Bologna M, Angelucci A. Leptin contributes to long-term stabilization of HIF-1α in cancer cells subjected to oxygen limiting conditions. Cancer Letters. 2016;**376**:1-9. DOI: 10.1016/j.canlet.2016.03.027

Chapter 10

Drosophila Central Taste Circuits in Health and Obesity

Shivam Kaushik, Shivangi Rawat and Pinky Kain

Abstract

When there is a perturbation in the balance between hunger and satiety, food intake gets mis-regulated leading to excessive or insufficient eating. In humans, abnormal nutrient consumption causes metabolic conditions like obesity, diabetes, and eating disorders affecting overall health. Despite this burden on society, we currently lack enough knowledge about the neuronal circuits that regulate appetite and taste perception. How specific taste neuronal circuits influence feeding behaviours is still an under explored area in neurobiology. The taste information present at the periphery must be processed by the central circuits for the final behavioural output. Identification and understanding of central neural circuitry regulating taste behaviour and its modulation by physiological changes with regard to internal state is required to understand the neural basis of taste preference. Simple invertebrate model organisms like *Drosophila melanogaster* can sense the same taste stimuli as mammals. Availability of powerful molecular and genetic tool kit and well characterized peripheral gustatory system with a vast array of behavioural, calcium imaging, molecular and electrophysiological approaches make *Drosophila* an attractive system to investigate and understand taste wiring and processing in the brain. By exploiting the gustatory system of the flies, this chapter will shed light on the current understanding of central neural taste structures that influence feeding choices. The compiled information would help us better understand how central taste neurons convey taste information to higher brain centers and guide feeding behaviours like acceptance or rejection of food to better combat disease state caused by abnormal consumption of food.

Keywords: Taste, neural circuits, pharynx, gustatory receptors, feeding behaviour

1. Introduction

The sense of taste is a fundamental sensory modality for all animals. It controls many behavioural decisions by processing and integrating information from the periphery. In all animals, gustatory system plays a critical role in evaluating the nutritional value of food. The sense of taste warms animals against consumption of spoiled/fermented or toxic compounds and orchestrate appetitive responses to energy, protein and calorie-rich food sources.

In humans, taste buds on the tongue can differentiate between the five basic tastes: sweet, sour, salty, bitter, and umami (a savoury taste) by processing the taste information in the brain. These are important building blocks for our understanding of flavour. Animals show attraction towards low salt, sweet and umami taste and aversive behaviour towards high salt, bitter and sour foods. Such responses are innate and largely invariant throughout animal's life suggesting physiological hard-wiring of taste quality to hedonic value.

For decades, flies have been used as a genetically accessible system to study molecular mechanisms that coordinate feeding behaviour with sensory signals. They show an array of feeding characteristics that can be easily exploited for various behavioural and physiological analysis. Identification of gustatory chemosensory receptors has provided a major impetus in understanding taste signal transduction [1–5]. Gustatory sensory neurons located in external mouth region as well as internally in the pharynx project to sub esophageal zone (SEZ-a region implicated in feeding and taste) [5–8]. Much less is known about the organization of the SEZ. Very few neurons that connect SEZ to higher brain centers have been identified. These circuits represent critical higher-order features of gustatory system including various set of interneurons, projection neurons, modulatory neurons and motor neurons that help flies to process and integrate peripheral taste signals. Although recently, many studies have focused on understanding how gustatory neural circuits are spatially organized to represent information about taste quality. Yet, the role of various regions in the central nervous system (CNS) in integrating feeding behaviour with sensory signals on the availability and quality of nutrients is currently insufficiently understood. How central taste circuits play an important role in health and disease is still undetermined. In this chapter, we have assimilated the information together to present a map of various taste circuits identified in the past few years beyond the level of primary taste neurons specifically in *Drosophila melanogaster.* Hopefully the information provided in the chapter would be useful to gain insight into brain structures and the neural networks that control taste and feeding behavior in simple model organisms and may provide information that would be useful in combating obesity or other metabolic disorders in humans.

2. Central taste circuits in humans

Tongue is the peripheral taste organ of the human taste system essential for tasting, chewing, swallowing and speech [9–11]. Tiny bumps present on the tongue called papillae give the tongue its texture. Many thousand taste buds cover the surfaces of the papillae that respond to taste and transmit that information from periphery to the CNS [9]. Different types of papillae are present on the tongue classified as circumvallate, fungiform, filiform and foliate. All except the filiform papillae are associated with taste buds. The most common mushroom-shaped fungiform papillae cover two third of the tongue and are involved in detecting taste. They also contain sensory cells for detecting touch and temperature. The human taste system, along with the olfactory and trigeminal systems, helps in identifying and controlling the nutrient versus toxic compounds that finally leads to acceptance and rejection behaviour [9, 12]. Inside the mouth, the chemical components of food interact with taste receptors cells located inside the taste buds on the tongue and evaluate the quality and intensity of the taste. The other areas where taste cells are present includes the back of the throat, and at the junction of the hard and soft palates, epiglottis, the nasal cavity, and even in the upper part of the esophagus [13, 14]. The current findings also suggest nutrient sensing and presence of taste receptors in the gut [15–18].

Taste buds are generally present as clusters of 50-100 polarized neuro-epithelial cells which can detect nutrients and other chemical compounds. They have numerous sensory cells that are in turn connected to many different nerve fibres [12, 19]. The first stage of gustatory signal processing starts with the taste buds. They communicate using electrical coupling via gap junctions and by cell to cell chemical communication via neurotransmitters including glutamate, serotonin, and ATP among other possible transmitters [20, 21]. Taste receptor cells get consistently replaced in taste buds to compensate the injury of the gustatory epithelia [22]. Several afferent nerves carry specific sensory information from a specific peripheral region. The chorda tympani (CT), a branch of the facial nerve (cranial nerve VII), transmits gustatory information from fungiform papillae, while the lingual branch of the trigeminal nerve (cranial nerve V) carries information from fungiform about pain, tactile, and temperature and filiform papillae in the same area [23, 24]. Multimodal information including taste, tactile, pain, and thermal cues get conveyed from circumvallate papillae by the glossopharyngeal nerve (cranial nerve IX), from palatal taste buds by the greater superficial petrosal nerve (GSP, another branch of VII), and from the throat by the superior laryngeal branch of the vagus (cranial nerve X) [25–28]. Foliate papillae are innervated by the CT (taste) and V (tactile) in anterior regions and by IX (multimodal) in posterior regions [29, 30]. All together taste and oral somatosensory cues combine centrally with retro nasal olfaction to generate the composite experience of taste [31].

The entire human taste system includes both peripheral receptors and central pathways. As afferent taste signals ascend the brain from caudal to rostral, the information flow split between the ventral forebrain and more dorsal thalamo-cortical regions where primary and secondary gustatory cortices (opercular, insular, orbitofrontal) give rise to conscious taste sensation [32–34]. Taste qualities, attention, reward, higher cognitive functions and multiple-modal sensory integration are managed by multiple secondary and tertiary cortices that are involved in the dorsal pathways [20, 35, 36]. While sensory processing at the extent of the taste bud is complex, the information transfer to the CNS via marked line [37]. A gustotopic map has been produced when taste signals extend to the insula of the gustatory cortex [38]. Each individual taste has a representation in the insular cortex by fine-tuned cells organized in a precise and spatially ordered taste map with each taste quality encoded in its own stereotypical cortical field [38].

The final step in perceiving taste is relaying the taste information collected by taste cells to the central nervous system via cranial nerves VII (Facial), IX (Glossopharyngeal), and X (Vagus), where there is a topographical representation of the oral cavity within the first nuclear relay, the solitary tract nucleus, in which brainstem reflexes of acceptance and rejection are controlled (**Figure 1**) [39]. The taste cells within the taste buds transduce the stimuli from the ingested food and provide additional information about the identity, concentration and pleasant or unpleasant quality of the substance [20]. Taste nerve fibers on stimulation by the binding of chemicals to their receptors, depolarize, resulting in an action potential that gets ultimately transmitted to the brain [19]. This information also prepares the gastrointestinal system to receive food by causing salivation and swallowing (or gagging and regurgitation if the substance is noxious). The principal receptors involved to transduce human sweet stimuli are T1R2/T1R3, T1R1/T1R3 for umami stimuli (although mGluR1, mGluR4 and NMDA have been implicated), and T2R family for bitter taste stimuli. Growing evidences have suggested the role of epithelial sodium channel (ENaC) in part, in transducing salty taste, and acid sensing ion channels (ASICs) for sour taste stimuli [20, 40–42].

The ventral pathways are involved in autonomic and visceral functions, affective and emotional processing, memory and learning [43, 44] and ultimately, the

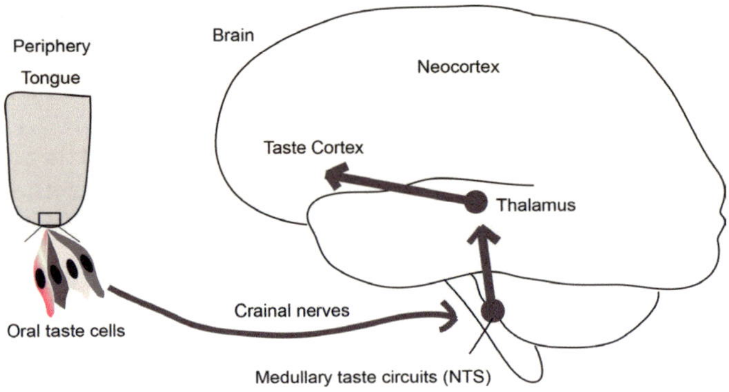

Figure 1.
A portion of the taste pathway in the human brain. Taste information from taste receptor cells on the tongue (peripheral organ) is relayed to the nucleus of the solitary tract (NTS) in the medulla. Gustatory neurons in the NTS send projections to the thalamus, which in turn directs gustatory information to taste cortex in the brain.

informational content and values of the ventral and the dorsal pathways integrate [45]. The circuitry is such that the cells make synaptic connection with primary sensory axons that run in the chorda tympani and greater superior petrosal branches of the facial nerve. The taste cells in fungiform papillae on the anterior tongue are innervated exclusively by the chorda tympani branch of the facial nerve. In circumvallate papillae, the taste cells are innervated entirely by the lingual branch of the glossopharyngeal nerve and in the palate they are innervated by the greater superior petrosal branch of the facial nerve [46]. The lingual branch of the glossopharyngeal nerve and the superior laryngeal branch of the vagus nerve project into the rostral portion of the nucleus of the NST. The central axons of these primary sensory neurons in the respective cranial nerve ganglia project to rostral and lateral regions of the medulla [47, 48]. Secondary cortical taste area in the orbitofrontal cortex, present in the frontal lobe of the brain is responsible for decision making [49]. Here, single neurons respond to combinations of chemosensory, somatic sensory, olfactory, and gustatory stimuli and even visual information [34]. Information about the temperature and texture of food transmit from the mouth via the cranial nerves to the thalamus and somatic sensory cortices [50].

In the orbital cortex, feeding to satiety with one food reduces the responses of those neurons to that particular food only suggesting computation of sensory-specific satiety in the orbitofrontal neurons [51]. Hypothalamic nuclei project to and receive input from other extra hypothalamic brain regions such as the nucleus of the solitary tract (NTS) to regulate food intake and energy expenditure [52–58]. Hunger, satiety and food consumption neural regulations are directly control by the genetic influence on human obesity [34]. High sweet tastes are attractive while high bitter tastes are aversive, even in decerebrate animals and anencephalic humans [59, 60]. The brain ascent from caudal to rostral by the afferent taste signals where the information start breaking between the ventral forebrain and more dorsal thalamo-cortical regions then later opercular, insular, orbitofrontal (primary and secondary gustatory cortices) bring the awareness to taste sensation [32].

Taste pathways in the CNS are intimately connected with general viscero sensory sensory nerves from the cardiovascular, respiratory and, importantly, gastrointestinal systems [61]. Circulating metabolic signals modulate neural responses in relays of the taste system, such as the NTS, and in areas that receive direct or indirect gustatory afferents like the hypothalamic homeostatic centers and reward-related areas in the midbrain [62]. Vagus in particular contain afferent neurons that transfer mechanical and chemical sensory information from the gastrointestinal tract (GIT) to the brain. The neural transmission of chemical information could result from recognizing signalling peptides, such as CCK, produced by enteroendocrine epithelial cells with chemo-sensing properties [63].

Although a great deal of information has been generated but elucidation of how taste intensity is encoded in the insular cortex is necessary to address. It is still unknown whether taste qualities with similar valence project to common targets in the brain. Tracing the connectivity of each basic taste qualities to higher brain areas is still incomplete and will help decipher how these integrate with other modalities and combine with internal and external state for the final behavioural output. Hopefully understanding taste circuits in simple invertebrate model systems like *Drosophila* can help addressing these mysteries of the central taste system in higher animals.

3. *Drosophila* gustatory system and circuits

In the olfactory system of the adult fruit fly, the structure and function of the neural circuits involved in detecting and processing olfactory information are well known. Approximately 50 different classes of olfactory receptors neurons express a particular type of olfactory receptor. The olfactory sensory neurons expressing the same receptor projects its axon to a single glomerulus in the antennal lobe of the fly where synaptic association with projection neurons and local interneurons occurs. The projection neurons transfer processed sensory information from the glomeruli to higher order brain centers including mushroom bodies (MB) and lateral horn (LH) which further process olfactory information for behavioural functions such as learning and memory or appetitive and inhibitory response control [64–66].

On the other hand, the identified central taste circuits of the gustatory system of *Drosophila* involved in sensory processing i.e. from detection to behavior are very few. The gustatory system of *Drosophila* is a commendable system for learning taste perception, taste modulation and behavior due to its simple brain architecture of the fly, gustatory receptor neurons (GRNs), vigorous behavioural responses that are flexible to probe molecular genetics and electrophysiological dissection [67]. Different aspects of feeding behavior include finding a food source, evaluating food for nutritional suitability, choosing between different food sources, and deciding to initiate or terminate feeding. Like mammals, taste helps *Drosophila* to detect the potential edible food sources and to decide whether to accept it or not. The fruit fly can detect and sense all the distinct taste modalities that mammals can i.e., sweet, bitter, salts, water, sour and umami. Flies attract to sweet substances and show aversive behavior towards bitter making final feeding decisions [68]. The taste neurons house inside the hair like structures known as sensilla (**Figure 2B**) present on different peripheral organs of the fly body i.e., labellum, legs, wing margins, ovipositor and pharyngeal organs lining the esophagus (**Figure 2A**). The small sensory structures known as taste pegs are also present in the labellum [69]. Taste neurons of tarsal segments are the first that come in contact with food source and then on the labellum (**Figure 2A**) [70]. The GRN axons from various peripheral taste organs transmit the taste information to the higher brain area, the primary taste processing center called SEZ (**Figure 2A**) [71]. SEZ is the first relay for taste information in the fly brain just below the antennal lobe where axons of gustatory receptor neurons (GRNs) of peripheral organs terminate [67, 72, 73].

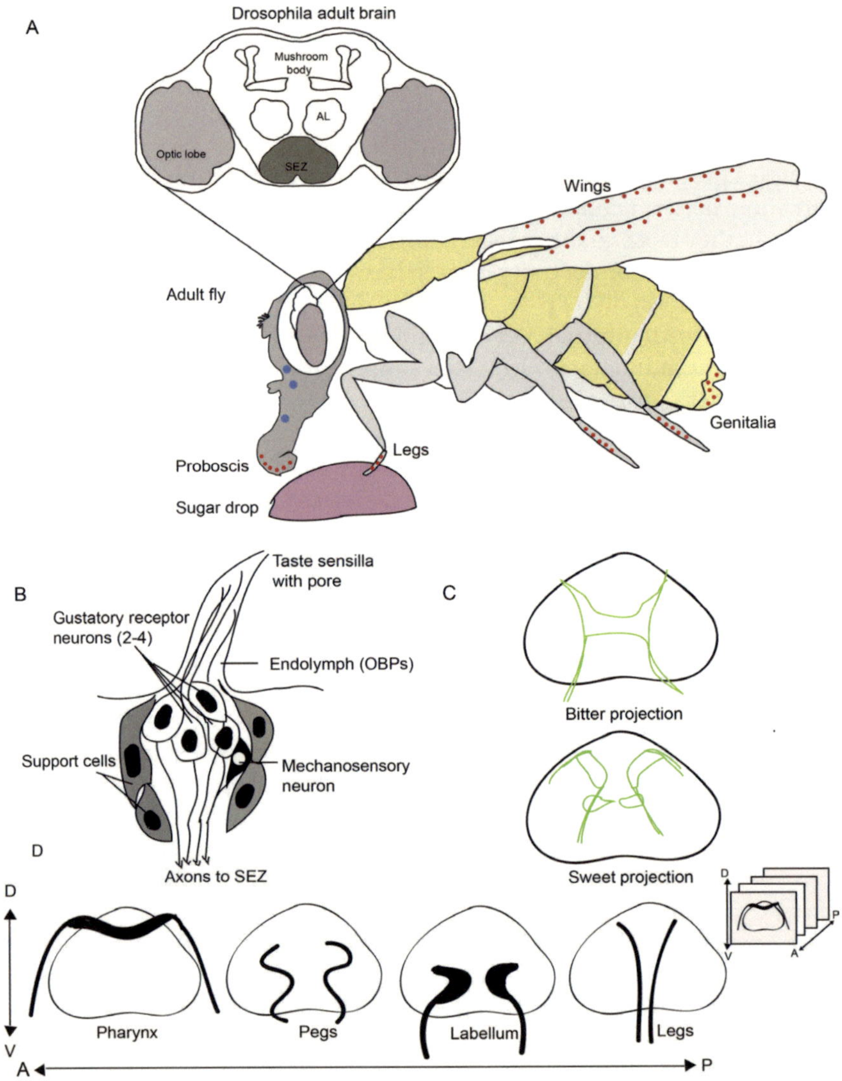

Figure 2.
Drosophila *taste system. (A) Adult fly accessing sugar drop with the tarsi. Proboscis, legs, wing margins, and genitalia are peripheral taste organs where taste receptor cells house in taste sensillae. The taste information from various taste organs goes to the brain. SEZ is a first relay of taste processing (shown in the magnified version of brain). Antennal lobe (AL) receive information about volatile chemicals from the periphery and mushroom bodies are learning and memory centers. (B) Taste sensillum containing gustatory receptor neurons, mechanosensory neurons and support cells. (C and D) Taste representation in the SEZ. Projection map in the SEZ in accordance with the taste modalities (C) and taste organs (D).*

4. *Drosophila* SEZ is the first relay of taste information

The adult *Drosophila* bears approximately 135,000 neurons in the central nervous system and thousands of neurons in ventral nerve cord (alike mammalian spinal cord). Taste neurons transmit their input (**Figure 2B**) to SEZ in the CNS, where the inputs received from different organs and taste modalities are refined and united [74] (**Figure 2C** and **D**). The gustatory neuropil of the SEZ includes the sub esophageal zone, gnathal ganglia (GNG), and parts of the periesophageal neuropil [75], and is relatively disorganized compared to the olfactory and visual neuropils. Immunohistochemistry and microscopy visualization of axonal termini of distinct categories of GRNs has exposed a spatial representation of taste quality within SEZ for example sweet taste neurons from proboscis terminate in discrete regions of the SEZ that do not overlap with axonal projections of bitter taste neurons (**Figure 2C**) [67, 72]. There is a distinct projection map in the SEZ in accordance with the taste modalities (**Figure 2C** and **D**) [67, 72] and taste organs i.e. gustatory axons of the mouth part ends in the dorsal anterior SEZ, axons from labellum ends in the medial SEZ, and axons from legs ends in dorsal posterior SEZ (**Figure 2C** and **D**) [67, 71]. Motor neurons and modulatory neurons that guide proboscis extension are also found in the SEZ [71, 76] indicating that the SEZ carry local circuits that connect sensory, motor, modulatory and command neurons that have processes in this region [71, 76–78] suggesting its role as a sensorimotor center for feeding. Taste information is also integrated with other internal and external sensory cues, but where this occurs is not known. Later the taste information get conveyed to higher brain centers, including the mushroom body, which contains neurons activated upon sucrose ingestion [79, 80]. Recently found various central neurons that may or may not synapse with taste sensory neurons and/or play modulatory roles have been identified which are discussed in further sections.

5. *Drosophila* sweet taste feeding circuits in the brain

SEZ has been shown to play a key role in gustatory signal transduction and feeding responses in different insects. *Drosophila* larval neurons expressing neuropeptide gene (referred as *hugin* neuron) are identified as probable interneurons that modulates taste mediated feeding behavior [77]. These are about 20 neurons in the SEZ. The connectivity pattern of *hug* neurons in larvae and adult flies is similar. Blocking *hug* neurons activity results in alteration of food intake initiation which depends on previous nutrient condition. The *hug* neurons send axons to three distinct targets - to the ring gland (central neuroendocrine organ), pharyngeal muscles, and higher brain center protocerebrum. The extension to the ring gland and the pharyngeal muscles depicts that *hug* neurons correlate sensory information with growth, metabolism, and feeding. The axon tracts to the protocerebrum indicates a role of *hug* neurons in transducing sensory signals for higher brain processing. The connectivity pattern of *hug* neurons suggest a role of incorporating gustatory sensory signals with higher brain functions and feeding behavior [77].

Additionally, to understand the central taste circuits in the fly brain that are involved in feeding decisions and different aspects of feeding behavior few second order neurons have been identified in the past few years. The first set of sweet gustatory projection neurons (sGPNs) marked by *NP1562* have been identified in a genetic screen (**Figure 3A**) [81]. Suppression of sGPNs activity results in decrease food intake and inhibition of PER responses. The sGPNs activation by applying sucrose and other sugars to the labellum suggested a functional link with Gr5a+ sweet taste neurons. These neurons relay sweet information from the SEZ to the antennal and mechanosensory motor center (AMMC) in the deutocerebrum of fly brain. Starvation and dopamine signaling increases the sucrose sensitivity of the sGPNs providing direct confirmation for state dependent alterations in sweet taste circuit activity [81]. The AMMC is known to receive input from sensory axons of the basal antennal segments involved in sensing gravity, sound and [82–85] olfactory inputs from a class of olfactory projection neurons [86]. It remains to determine if AMMC acts as a secondary center for sweet taste and receive inputs from other categories of taste neurons, such as water [87, 88], bitter [67, 72], and salty [89, 90], sour [91] and fat [92] and, if so, whether the representation of different tastes remains distinct in AMMC. Little is understood about the wiring where information from the AMMC is transmitted, but single-cell tracing experiments in

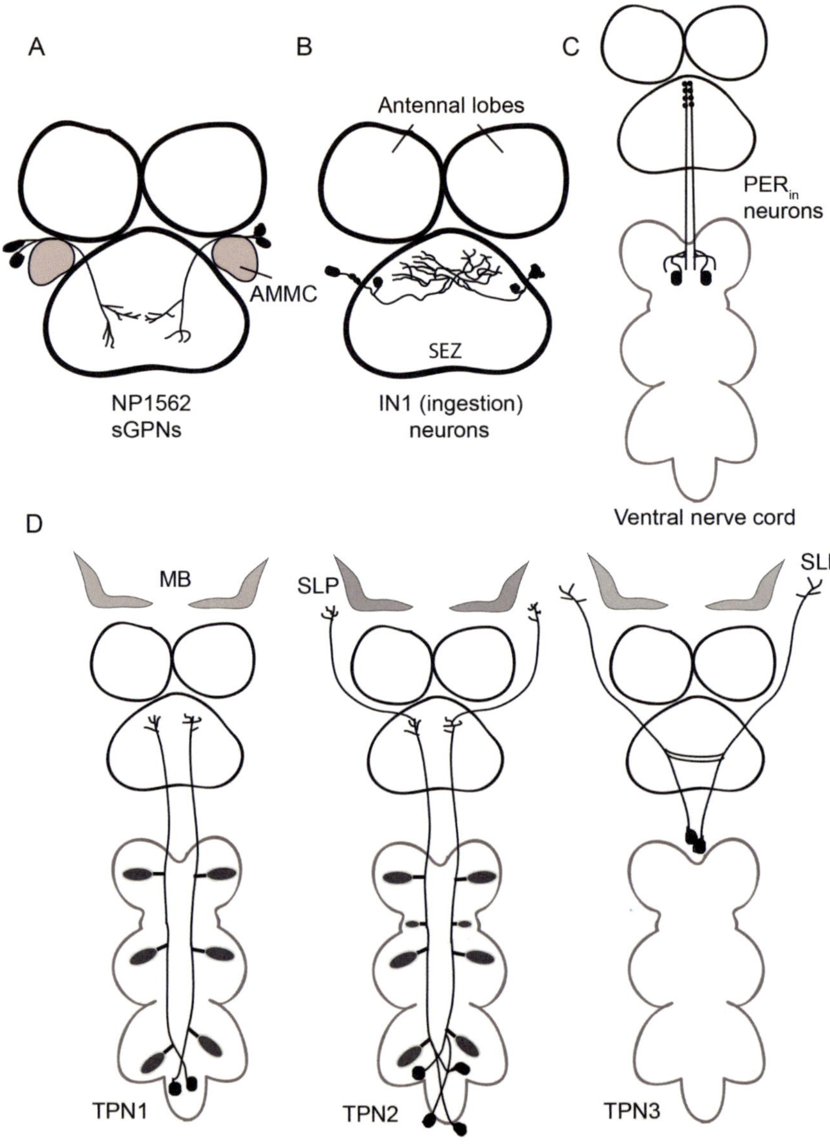

Figure 3.
Examples of few taste circuits in the Drosophila *brain. (A) Sweet gustatory projection neurons (*NP1562+ *sGPNs). (B) IN1 Cholinergic Local Taste Interneurons (ingestion neurons). (C) PER$_{in}$ neurons. (D) TPN1, TPN2, TPN3 neurons. TPN2 and TPN3 neurons terminate in the SLP (superior lateral protocerebrum) and in and around lateral horn area. Both SLP and lateral horn are nearby structure.*

flies reveal the caudal ventrolateral protocerebrum (CVLP) as a possible target [93] as some Gr32a+ GRNs involved in pheromone sensing appear to terminate directly in the VLP [94]. It is still undetermined whether AMMC conveys information from sGPNs to higher brain centers or back to the SEZ, where it can be transferred to motor neurons connecting to proboscis muscles.

Another genetic screen identified pair of 12 cholinergic local interneurons to characterize *Drosophila* ingestion circuit. These neurons namely IN1 (ingestion neurons, **Figure 3B**) controls the dynamics of ingestion in flies regulated by hunger state and sucrose concentration [95]. Upon sucrose ingestion, IN1 interneurons show persistent increase in activity in fasted flies. The activity drops in response to subsequent feeding bouts. Conversely IN1 interneurons in fed flies show smaller responses to sucrose which lacked persistent activity. In a satiated fly, insensitive sucrose IN1 neurons show decrease drive to ingest and results in shorter ingestion episodes. IN1 SEZ second-order interneurons monitor ingestion by receiving presynaptic input from sugar sensitive taste neurons in the pharynx [95]. Hence, the IN1 probably be the second- order neurons for a particular subprogram of feeding behavior i.e. ingestion that provides a fast feedback mechanism to regulate sucrose ingestion by integrating taste and hunger signals. The study proposes IN1 neurons as a key node in the circuit that governs rapid food intake decisions.

6. Bitter taste circuit in the brain

The bitter taste modality is conserved in insects and mammals. It plays a key role in evoking aversive behavior in animals [32, 66, 68, 96]. Bitter sensitive gustatory interneurons (*VGN6341*) in the adult SEZ are identified by performing a functional behavioural screen and shown to be involved in aversive gustatory responses [97]. These neurons receive direct synaptic input from *Gr66a* labelled bitter-sensitive GRNs. The *VGN6341* neurons are single bilaterally symmetric pair of SEZ interneurons responsible for the inhibition of the appetitive PER responses and gets activated by natural or transgenic stimulation of bitter GRNs [97]. Identified bitter gustatory local interneurons (bGLNs) play an important role in the aversive bitter-sensitive gustatory circuitry of the adult fly and represent a significant step towards understanding how bitter taste modalities are processed by the gustatory circuitry in the brain. Identifying their postsynaptic targets in the bitter gustatory circuitry of the SEZ will reveal new players of the bitter higher order taste circuits. And whether they will receive excitatory or inhibitory input from these new player's cells await further investigation [97].

Three classes of taste projection neurons (TPNs) have been identified based on their morphology and taste selectivity [98] named as TPN1, TPN2 and TPN3 (**Figure 3D**). TPN1/TPN2 neurons respond to sweet taste and promotes PER (innate feeding behavior) while TPN3 is bitter responsive and inhibits PER. TPNs are long-range projection neurons that separately carry sweet (TPN1 and TPN2 selectively relay sugar taste detection from the legs) or bitter information to higher brain demonstrating modality-specific relays. TPN3 responds to bitter taste on the legs and the proboscis, suggesting aversion to bitter compounds may not require specific location. Their data suggests that taste detection from different organs serves different functions, consistent with other studies where interneurons sense sweet taste from the mouthparts and drive ingestion [95]. The organ-specific and modality-specific connectivity of TPNs demonstrates a mechanism to encode both taste location and taste quality. As both TPN2 and TPN3 send axons to the superior lateral protocerebrum (SLP) (**Figure 3D**) suggesting that information from the higher brain feeds back onto sensorimotor circuits for PER. Functional link from TPNs to mushroom body (learning and memory centers) has been postulated based on the presence of their arbors in the SLP and lateral horn, which further excite or inhibit MB extrinsic neurons. Reciprocal and bidirectional interactions between SLP and MBs for learned associations have also been shown previously [99]. Conditional silencing of TPNs suggested that TPNs are not essential for proboscis extension and contribution from other neurons must contribute to this behavior but TPN2 and TPN3 are essential for conditioned taste aversion. Inhibition of synaptic transmission in sugar-sensing TPN2 during either training or testing decreased conditioned aversion, whereas inhibiting bitter TPN3 decreased aversion only if inhibition occurred during training. The modulatory role played by TPNs without being essential components of PER circuits require future investigation. These studies demonstrate modality-selective taste pathways to higher brain.

In a separate study, a pair of interneurons (PER_{in} neurons, **Figure 3C**) are identified that activate by stimulation of mechanosensory neurons inhibiting feeding initiation. Conversely, inhibition of activity promotes feeding initiation and inhibits locomotion suggesting such neurons suppress feeding while the fly is walking [100]. The dendrites of these neurons reside in the first leg neuromeres whereas axons are found in both SEZ and first leg neuromeres suggesting that they process information from the legs and convey to SEZ. These neurons do not make synaptic connections with known neurons that regulate proboscis extension. This study highlights that feeding initiation and locomotion are mutually exclusive behaviours and identified pair of interneurons influence this behavioural choice.

A receptor-to-neuron maps of pharyngeal taste organs reveals the presence of multiple classes of taste neurons [101], consistent with the knowledge that the pharynx may independently assess food quality. In this study use of *Pox-neuro* (*Poxn*) mutants (mutants in which all external taste bristles are transformed into mechanosensory bristles but all pharyngeal taste neurons retain) [101–104] suggests how pharyngeal taste input affects feeding behaviours. It is found that high salt inhibits sucrose-evoked activity of pharyngeal *Gr43a*+ sweet GRNs. Furthermore, feeding avoidance of denatonium, tartaric acid, or high salt eliminates only when both inhibition of pharyngeal *Gr43a* sweet GRNs and activation of different combinations of aversive pharyngeal GRNs are absent. Tracing experiments reveals that both appetitive and aversive pharyngeal GRNs convey inputs to two common brain areas (pars intercerebralis and lateral protocerebrum), suggesting that pharyngeal taste is represented across brain regions. This study demonstrates an important role of pharyngeal taste in controlling food choice and intake [105].

7. Central neurons controlling regurgitation

In another genetic screen to understand how sensory information is translated into behavior, a subset of higher order neurons labeled by *VT041723-GAL4* transgenic line are identified that controls regurgitation after food ingestion [105]. The neurons labeled by *VT041723-GAL4* receive sensory input from peripheral *Ir76b*+ taste neurons in the pharynx. Optogenetics activation of these neurons produce "proboscis holding" behavior (extrusion of the mouthpart without withdrawal). Flies pre-fed with either sugar or water before neuronal activation shows regurgitation indicative of an aversive response. However, motor circuits controlling regurgitation and if PER and regurgitation share common motor programs are not known. Identification of *VT041723-GAL4* neurons provide a ground to address such questions [105].

8. Higher order taste circuits involved in taste learning and memory

In *Drosophila*, MBs are the central sites for experiential learning that are composed of approx. 2,000 Kenyon cells (KCs) which have dendrites in a region known as calyx (**Figure 4A**) [106–108]. Pairing of sugar with a deterrent compound creates aversion to sugar in flies although for the short duration [109]. The conditioned taste aversion involves MBs [80, 109]. How the diversity of sensory information that the MB integrates is still undetermined. Anatomical studies have suggested that visual, tactile and gustatory cues are processed in different compartments of MB as conditional stimulus (CS) [110]. The MBs also receives multimodal inputs as they are required for courtship, taste conditioning and visual learning [109, 111].

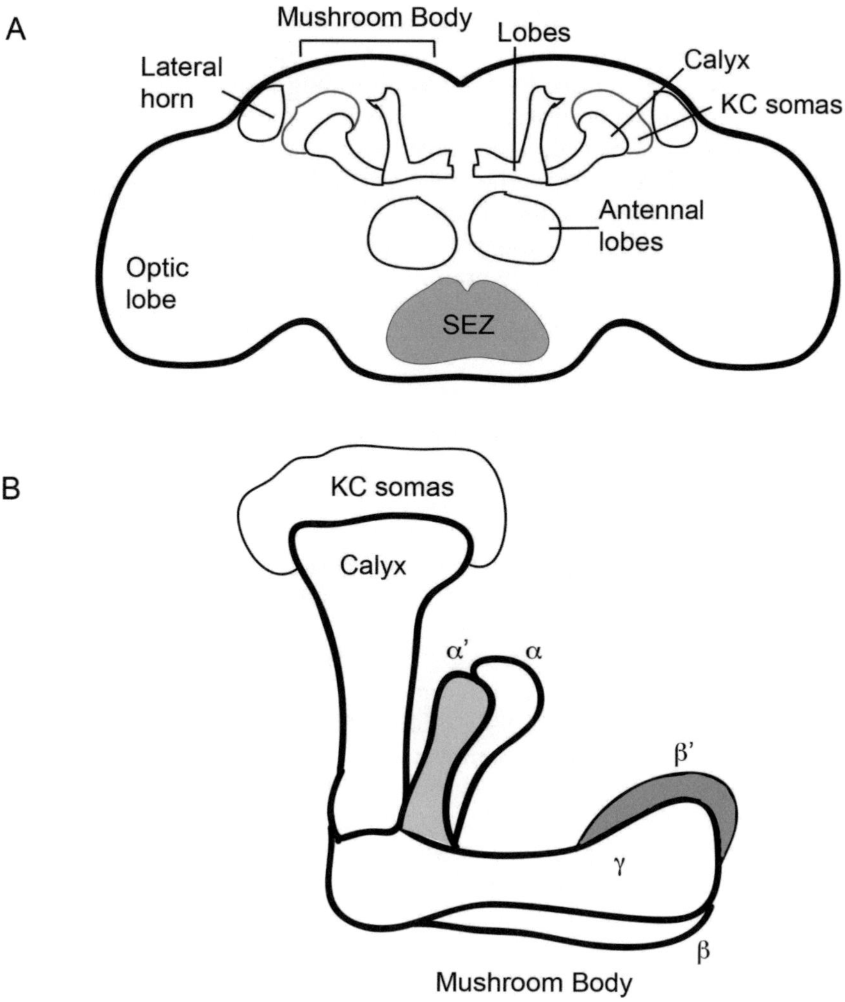

Figure 4.
Adult Drosophila *brain showing higher brain areas. (A) Learning and memory centers in adult fly brain includes mushroom body, calyx, Kenyon cells (KC) and lateral horn. (B) Structure of MB lobes. There are three different classes of neurons that make up the MB lobes (α/β, α'/β' and γ).*

Based on their axonal arborizations in the α/β, α'/β', and γ lobes, the KCs of the MB are divided into three main classes (**Figure 4B**). Evidences have identified that functional specializations among and within the classes, with different subsets playing different roles in the phase, type, and length of associative memory [112]. Evidence that the MB processes tastes as CS and US (unconditional stimulus) comes from behavioural taste conditioning experiments [109, 113]. A simple taste behavior is the proboscis extension response (PER): when leg gustatory neurons detect sucrose, the fly extends its proboscis to eat. Pairing sucrose stimulation to the leg (CS) with an aversive stimulus (US) causes short-term inhibition of proboscis extension. This learned behavior requires the MB, but the neural processing in the MB that underlies taste conditioning is unknown. To gain insight into sensory processing, taste representation and role of these structures in aversive taste conditioning in the MB, behavioural and high end imaging studies reveal that the gustatory information in the main calyx are segregated and have unique representation by different taste modalities and different taste organs [80]. Such inputs get differentially and independently modified by learning. Selectively blocking the γ lobe neurons leads to complete elimination of conditioned aversion suggesting role γ lobe as the site for aversive taste memory formation in the MB. The study also demonstrates the requirement of MB neurons for taste conditioning and taste information relayed to the MB is via multiple pathways. Only taste stimulation (bitter compounds and sucrose) activates the dorsal accessory calyx which has been implicated in gustatory processing in other insects earlier [114] providing evidences that gustatory MB representation is distinct from olfactory cues. These studies have extended the understanding of the neural coding underlying conditioned learning in the MB as a sensory integration center in the fly brain.

9. Motor neuron circuit

Interneurons are the local circuit neuron of CNS that relays impulses between sensory neuron and motor neuron while a neuron that passes from CNS or a ganglion towards a muscle and conducts a nerve impulse resulting in movement is known as motor neuron. The process by which brain process the sensory information into motor actions is not well acknowledged. A major step in most of the sensory-motor transformations is to convert the coordinates of sensory system into a map of spatially directed motor actions.

Proboscis is the primary feeding organ of flies and also plays an important role for taste cue detection and food ingestion and show reliable PER by applying positive gustatory stimulus to GRNs [67, 109, 115, 116]. PER represents an innate, sequential behavior involving many movement steps [78]. PER sequence may require activation of different muscle groups at distinct time points, implying a defined temporal organization of upstream motor neuron (MN) activity. It has been proposed that the relay of gustatory sensory information from GRNs to MNs occurs mainly within the SEZ [67, 72, 117–119]. The motor neurons innervating proboscis musculature have been portrayed in fruit fly and blow fly [120, 121]. There are 15 paired proboscis muscles found in blowfly and 17 in *Drosophila*, illustrating 13 prime muscle groups. These muscles control action of 3 segments of the proboscis i.e. rostrum, haustellum and labellum with distinct muscles intricate in extension or retraction. The central and dorsal dilator muscle, forms the cibarial pump, which dilates the pharynx to coordinate fluid intake [122]. Twenty pairs of motor neurons innervate proboscis muscles [120, 121] and each proboscis muscle is innervated by 1 to 3 motor neurons. On the basis of the nerve through which their axons depart the CNS, the proboscis motor neurons are categorized as labial, pharyngeal, or accessory pharyngeal. The Cibarial muscles, forming the oral pump, are innervated by pharyngeal motor neurons, while the proboscis muscles required for the placement of proboscis during feeding are innervated by labial motor neurons.

A pair of neurons that generate feeding motor program and induces the entire feeding sequence when activated are identified in *Drosophila* [78]. The interneurons called feeding neurons (*fdg*) located in the SEZ are required for feeding as their suppression eliminates the sugar-induced feeding behaviour (**Figure 5B**). Activation of a single *Fdg*-neuron leads to asymmetric feeding behavior. *Fdg*-neurons respond to food only in starved condition suggesting this response is dependent on the metabolic state of the animal. The asymmetric regulation of proboscis extension by the *Fdg*-neuron suggests that each *Fdg*-neuron may selectively regulate the strength of proboscis muscle contraction on the same side of the body. These results are consistent with the observation that presentation of food to gustatory receptors on one side of the body leads to proboscis extension on that side demonstrate that *Fdg*-neurons operate firmly within the sensori-motor watershed, downstream of sensory and metabolic cues and at the top of the feeding motor hierarchy to execute

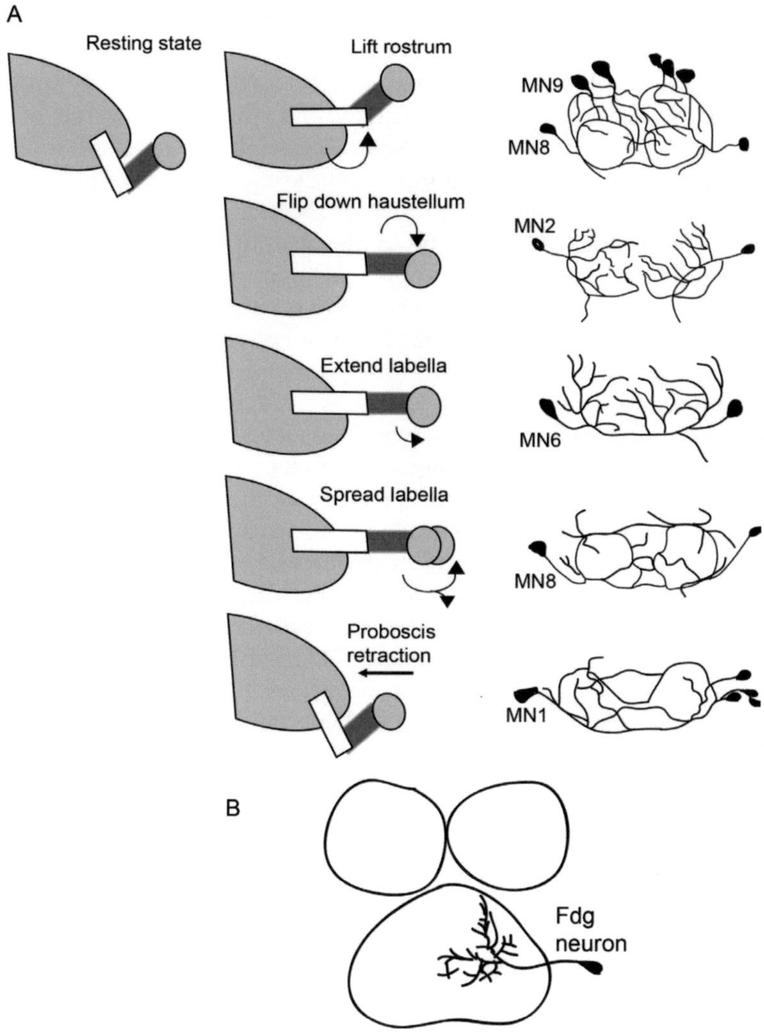

Figure 5.
Examples of motor neurons in adult fly that are involved in proboscis extension. (A) Five motor neuron types that control the key steps of proboscis extension were identified, lifting of the rostrum (MN9), extension of the haustellum (MN2), extension of the labella (MN6), spreading of the labella (MN8) and proboscis retraction (MN1). (B) Fdg *neurons.*

the decision to feed. How the *Fd*g-neurons coordinate the various motor patterns involved in feeding remains to be determined.

One of a study revealed that the mouth mechano-reception can ease and end feeding by two distinct central motor circuits and these two mechanosensory circuits merge with bitter taste in opposing manners to shape feeding behavior. Mechanosensory neurons (MSNs) were identified in taste pegs and taste bristles of the labella which rely on the same mechanoreceptor, NOMPC (No mechanoreceptor potential C) to transduce mechanical drift. The optogenetic arousal of bristle MSNs induce labellar spread, while activation of peg MSNs induces proboscis retraction [123].

Another pair of motor neurons involved in taste behavior has been identified to identify the components of the PER circuits. These neurons activate by sugar stimulation and inhibit by bitter stimuli [76]. The bilateral pair of E49 motor neurons are both necessary and adequate to initiate proboscis extension reflex. Although these neurons synapse on proboscics musculature and show wide dendritic field in SEZ but otherwise are shown to make no direct connections with GRNs [76].

In *Drosophila*, feeding is achieved by a pump that draws fluid into the esophagus. It has been shown that the cibarial motor neurons play a key role in such a pumping behavior [124]. The inhibition of these motor neurons decrease the feeding and pump frequency, while activation induce arrhythmic pumping. The rate of pumping is shown not to be affected by sucrose concentration or hunger but is changed by fluid viscosity. These neurons respond to taste stimuli and show prolonged prolonged to palatable substances. The open question is how cibarial pump motor neurons talk to rest of the feeding circuit in flies. How rhythmic motor activity is generated together with other feeding motor program such as proboscis extension and retraction and the neural circuits involved in such a behavior will provide insight in their role in the feeding circuit. There is a possibility that different chemosensory inputs may trigger PER and pumping as stimulation of tarsal taste neurons elicit PER but not pumping [115, 125]. Further studies revealed four GABAergic interneurons in the fly brain that impose feeding restraint in *Drosophila*. Inactivation of these neurons results in excessive ingestion of all compounds regardless of taste quality or nutritional state while severe activation of these neurons decreases ingestion of water and nutrients. These neurons act upstream of motor neurons for multiple feeding subprograms such as meal initiation and ingestion. Hence, this study unfolds how central inhibitory control regulates feeding behaviors and is required to inhibit a latent state of uncontrolled and nonselective consumption [125].

In a separate study, analysis of sequential features of the motion pattern of PER provided morphological description of proboscis motor neurons and muscles [121]. By implying genetic manipulations along with artificial activation and silencing process, five motor neuron types that control the key steps of proboscis extension are identified, lifting of the rostrum (MN9), extension of the haustellum (MN2), extension of the labella (MN6), spreading of the labella (MN8) and proboscis retraction (MN1) (**Figure 5A**). The above-mentioned steps are independently controlled in a one-to-one manner with the majority of MNs both sufficient and required for the execution of one individual step of the forward reaching behavior.

Remarkable specificity has been observed for candidate higher-order neurons in terms of the sensory neurons that activate them (proboscis versus mouthparts) and the behavioural subprograms they generate i.e. proboscis extension versus ingestion. The identification of these neurons suggest taste information is processed by parallel labelled lines via several different neural streams that coordinate different aspects of feeding behavior. Another behavioural study of the function of different taste neurons on the legs found that some cause inhibition of locomotion whereas others promote proboscis extension [72]. This study highlights that sweet taste receptor neurons of legs are essential for sugar choice and highlighted a functional dissociation between and within taste organs of *Drosophila*.

10. Modulation of feeding behaviors via taste circuits

Taste preference and sensitivity are two most essential elements of food evaluation. Such criteria are not always constant and often change depending on internal states such as hunger and satiety. Recent evidences reveal that starvation induces increased sweet taste preference and sensitivity at the periphery and in the CNS in various species from fruit flies to humans [81, 126, 127]. Electrical recordings of various neurons in central brain areas in mice and monkeys including amygdala, orbital frontal cortex, and hypothalamus have indicated the existence of neurons that can respond to taste stimuli in a state (hunger/satiety)-dependent manner [128–130]. However, the key neuronal pathway(s) responsible for hunger-induced taste modification are still unknown.

Neuromodulators such as neurotransmitters, neuropeptides, and endocrine hormones, play an important role in changing the morphological and functional characteristics of neural circuits to achieve behavioural flexibility. The changes in taste preference could occur through variation in the peripheral taste receptor cells, or in higher order neural circuits controlling food intake in the brain. To understand how changes in the internal state influence behavioural decisions in flies, various neurons in the SEZ whose activity depends on starvation state have been identified. It has been suggested that Dopamine is a potent modulator of a variety of behaviors in mammals and flies. Tyrosine hydroxylase ventral unpaired medial (TH-VUM) dopaminergic neurons modulate feeding in response to nutritional needs (**Figure 6A**) [131] and feeding (*Fdg)* interneurons (**Figure 5B**) integrate gustatory input with the internal state to command a feeding behaviour routine [78]. Even in mice mutant for Tyrosine hydroxylase show failure in initiating feeding in spite of intact motor ability to consume [132]. It has been shown that TH-VUM neurons can drive proboscis extension and neuronal activity of TH-VUM corresponds with the starvation duration. Silencing TH-VUM neurons decrease PER in starved flies to sucrose whereas increasing the activity of TH-VUM elevates PER in both fed and starved flies [131].

Role of various neuromodulators in regulating feeding responses in starved adult *Drosophila* [125, 133–135] has shown that dNPF and sNPF, neuropeptides related to mammalian NPY, modulate multiple feeding related behaviours, including the formation and expression of food-associated memory, enhancement of food-related olfactory sensitivity, and control of food intake during starvation [136–140]. During energy deficit conditions, animals become less selective in their food choices by enhancing their sensitivity to nutritious resources, such as sugar [115, 141–145]. Hunger enhances behavioural sensitivity to sweet taste, at least in part, via increased dopamine (DA) release onto Gr5a-expressing sugar-sensing GRNs, which increases calcium responses to GR activation in flies [131, 144]. Starvation also reduces sensitivity to unpalatable and potentially toxic compounds, such as bitter tastants. In PER assay, sensitivity to bitter tastants reduce in fasting flies', in part, independently of the increase in sugar sensitivity [126]. Both dopamine and $dNPF^+$ modulates sugar and show enhanced sugar sensitivity during starvation. dNPF act upstream of dopamine to control sugar. This study also suggests that subsets of sNPF expressing neurons regulate bitter sensitivity under starvation and sNPF as well as dNPF-dopamine pathways independently regulate bitter- and sugar sensitivity at the neuronal circuit level suggesting neuromodulatory cascades serve as key mediators of state-dependent control [134, 146–148]. Separately it has been shown that starvation reduces Octopaminergic/tyraminergic OA-VL activity and results in depotentiation of bitter taste in flies (**Figure 6B**) [149].

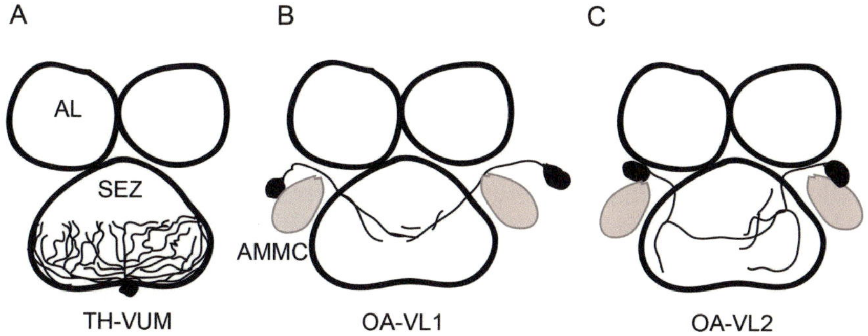

Figure 6.
Examples of few modulatory neurons in the adult fly brain. (A) TH-VUM neurons. (B) OA-VL1 and OA-LV2 (B) neurons that send projections to SEZ.

Recent identification of second-order sweet taste neurons [81] has enabled investigations into the interplay between sweet taste circuits and other sweet- and starvation responsive neurons to understand the neural basis of feeding behavior. Both starvation state and an increase in dopamine signaling brings about an enhancement of sGPN sensitivity to sucrose. In both cases, increases in sucrose-induced calcium activity occurs in the absence of corresponding changes in peripheral sweet Gr5a+ neural activity. Other studies have detected that starvation leads to increases in sucrose-evoked electrophysiological [150, 151] or calcium activity in Gr5a+ taste neurons [144]. In most cases, the observed increases in GRN sensitivity was comparatively small in magnitude compared with the alterations in *NP1562+* sGPN activity of starved flies.

There are several other neurons that have been identified as modulating sugar feeding. A pair of *Fdg* (feeding) neurons (**Figure 5B**) act as command neurons in the fly, is also required for normal feeding behavior as the ablation of the neurons distort the sugar prompt feeding behavior. These neurons activate by sugar taste but only in starved flies [78]. Moreover, twelve cholinergic interneurons, IN1 in the SEZ form synapse with sugar sensing neurons. The activity of these neurons is also regulated by hunger state/starvation but unlike feeding neurons that respond to sweet taste, ingestion neuron is triggered by sucrose ingestion. Also, the activation of IN1 neurons increases the chance of sugar ingestion upon presenting a drop of sucrose solution in close proximity instead of directly triggering the feeding behavior [95].

In another study, it has been shown that only sweet neurons express $GABA_B$ receptor ($GABA_BR$) [152]. $GABA_BR$ mediates presynaptic inhibition of calcium responses in sweet GRNs, and both sweet and bitter stimuli evoke GABAergic neuron activity in the vicinity of GRN axon terminals. Blockage of $GABA_BR$ both lead to increased sugar responses and decreased suppression of the sweet response by bitter compounds. This study propose a model in which GABA acts via $GABA_BR$ to expand the dynamic range of sweet GRNs through presynaptic gain control and suppress the output of sweet GRNs in the presence of opposing bitter stimuli [152].

Further evidences [77] show that *hug* neurons function within a neural circuit that modulates taste mediated feeding behavior. Suppression of *hug* neurons activity, cause a change in particular feeding behavior response. As a result of this alteration the control flies when shifted to a new food medium, they hold back for a period of time before feeding, on contrary the experimental flies initiate feeding promptly. The size of the crop after a long feeding period does not change in both cases, implying that there is no difference in the termination phase of feeding. There is a possibility that the *Drosophila* link feeding with a familiar source of food and when they experience different food source, they first re-examine it before feeding. Hence, the *hug* neurons seem to regulate feeding initiation based on earlier food encounter.

It has also been shown that starvation of amino acid stimulates yeast feeding by regulating central brain circuits. Two dopaminergic neurons (DA-WED) in each hemisphere of the adult brain innervating the "Wedge" neuropil are suggested to encode protein hunger. The suppression of these neurons results in decrement of yeast intake but elevates the sucrose consumption, whereas if these neurons are triggered they enhances the yeast intake but minimizes the sucrose consumption. Thus, like overall hunger and thirst, nutrient specific hunger motive may also compete for behavioral expression [153].

Mating has also been shown to be responsible for modifying the feeding behavior in female *Drosophila*, and the sex peptide is a key molecule involved in this modulation [154]. Mating improves female's interest in valuable nutrient source (polyamines such as spermine and putrescine). The mated females attract more to the taste and smell of polyamines than virgin females. This modulation in behavior is regulated through sex peptide receptor (SPR) and its conserved ligands MIPs (myoinhibitory peptides) that directly act on chemosensory neurons [155]. Another modulation in feeding was shown by Walker and colleagues that mating induces a salt appetite in *Drosophila*. Mating promote chances of salt appetite by increasing gustatory response to sodium. It is induced by male-derived Sex Peptide acting on the SPR (Sex peptide receptor) in female reproductive tract neuron [156]. In has been suggested that mating is a pivotal modulator of the decision-making process in female flies and depends on the action of the SPR in internal *ppk+* sensory neurons along with a neuronal TOR /S6K act as an essential input to this decision. The SPR signaling in *ppk+* neurons trigger a robust inclination for yeast in mated females while neuronal TOR/S6K signaling modulates food choices [157].

It has been studied and shown that mushroom body controls the responses of adult flies to learned odours as well as regulates their innate food seeking behavior elicit by food odours. A study depicted that 5 of the 21 types of MBONs (Mushroom body output neurons) are required for starved flies to seek food odours. Four other MBONs (MBON-a3, MBON-b2b02a, MBON-a02 and MBON-g2a01) and their corresponding dopaminergic neurons (DANs) also regulate innate food seeking behavior. Obstructing MBONs and DANs reduce innate food seeking behavior in starved flies, and activation of dopaminergic neurons is sufficient to evoke food seeking behavior in fed flies. The results from RNAi knock-down of different receptors for various hunger and satiety cues illustrates that the MB innervating dopaminergic neurons are modulated by many of these signals, making the MB an integrative center for hunger and satiety signals in the fly brain [158].

11. Influence of taste on food intake and obesity in humans

High calories (especially overconsumption of energy from high fat and sugar foods) and low nutrition density (poor nutrition) are associated with many chronic metabolic diseases including cardiovascular diseases, obesity, diabetes mellitus type 2 and eating disorders in humans. It's a great burden on healthcare system in any country and effective intervention strategies are yet to be found to control them. Past research has suggested that taste impacts the selection of food and its intake in animals as well as other factors like satiation and palatability. Obese and overweight individuals show a tendency of selecting energy-dense-food [159]. In humans, pleasure achieved by food can stimulate "non- homoeostatic" eating making it a prospective player contributing obesity [160]. Nonetheless, factors like previous food experiences, liking, wanting, taste sensitivities and depressed sense of taste cannot be ignored. Many pathways, neural circuits and neurohormones involved as discussed in *Drosophila* section, regulate food intake and decision to stop eating. Internal and external cues also trigger immediate desire to eat specific foods and can impact the final outcome of how much to eat. Similarly, in humans as well several conserved pathways and genes have been observed to play a significant role in controlling feeding behavior.

Although it has been seen that smell also plays a key role in modulating taste perception and influence food intake in individuals [161], but alteration in reward, dopamine signaling, homeostatic signals and affective circuits lead to hedonic eating causing obesity [162, 163]. Various neuroimaging methods have provided insights into central mechanisms underlying taste and hedonic eating highlighting the role of taste circuits in obesity. It has been found food stimuli causes different neural brain responses in obese individuals compared to normal weight people showing striking structural and functional brain circuitry alterations [164–170]. A recent review by [171] and others [172, 173] have beautifully described neural correlates of sweet, fat, umami, bitter, salty, and sour tastes across brain areas implicated in obesity. Although more conclusive neuroimaging outcomes are required to confirm the role of various taste neural circuits but experimental data indicates different hedonic responses to taste information in obesity. Dysregulations in brain reward circuitry in response to fat and sugar has been associated with obesity [165, 168, 174–177] suggesting fat and sugar affect brain reward circuitry differently. Similarly, high salt consumption has been linked to obesity engaging different brain areas which modulate taste processing and reward [178, 179]. These brain circuits also encode salt taste intensity [178, 180]. Data showing convincing differences in higher salt sensitivities between obese and normal individuals is still insignificant [181, 182]. Studies on neural responses to salt taste in case of obesity are still limited.

Another taste studied in the context of obesity is Umami which contributes to a sense of satiety [183, 184]. Obese individuals show reduced sensitivity but higher preference for umami taste [185, 186] than healthy controls. Since, umami and salt taste both activate primary gustatory cortex circuits in case of umami high tasters compared to low tasters suggest that both tastes share common processing system and may contribute to feeding behaviors implicated in obesity in a similar manner [179]. Bitter taste influence dietary fat consumption suggesting its relevance in obesity [187]. Bitter taste linked with appetite reduction affect many brain areas [188–190]. Conditioning to bitter taste modulates Hedonic evaluation [191]. Alterations in brain activation patters associated with bitter taste in individuals with obesity [190] compared to people without obesity have been observed but more consistent and reliable findings are needed to understand the interaction between brain responses and hedonic ratings of bitter taste [192, 193]. Sour taste is least explored in context of obesity but it plays major role in food selection and consumption and recruit brain regions in sex, age and internal state, condition dependent manner [194, 195]. Neural correlates of sour taste in obesity are limited and require further investigations. dysregulation of gut to brain neural connections and chemosensory pathways along this axis may also contribute to increased risk of obesity [196] suggesting gut could offer potential therapeutic targets in obesity [197]. Nutritional interventions to target neural pathways involved in taste behaviors and perception could offer solutions for prevention and treating obesity in humans.

Further detailed neuroimaging studies to understand taste response, taste physiology and dietary intake in humans and higher animal model systems are required to illustrate the neurobiological underpinnings of taste modalities and their relevance in obesity. Further research to characterize the influence of gut taste receptors and neural circuits on brain responses following food consumption and its modulation by smell in obese individuals that influence food intake are also needed. Collectively, research on invertebrate model system like *Drosophila* shows potential in understanding neurobiological basis of metabolic diseases like obesity at level of neural circuits that regulate feeding behaviors.

12. Conclusion

For the animal fitness, feeding is regulated by peripheral and central feeding circuits to help in acquiring a necessary and balanced dietary input for energy and nutrient homeostasis. It is subjected to intense regulation by multiple neuromodulator systems. In this chapter, we have illustrated recent progress in understanding neural circuits and its modulation in the feeding behavior including local circuits and motor neurons of adult flies which links various internal energy and nutrient needs to adaptive behaviors. This chapter has integrated information about the structure, function, and molecular regulation of fly taste and feeding circuits. The fruit fly *Drosophila melanogaster*, with many fewer neurons, is ideally suited to understand the complex interactions between neural circuits and genetics that ultimately control behavior. Countless studies have demonstrated the conservation of critical genes between flies and humans, and striking similarities in the organization of the brain, particularly the circuits that process sensory information. A number of functionally distinct populations of neurons in the fly taste circuits have been identified recently in flies that regulate various aspects of feeding behavior. We emphasize on the set or individual neurons that directly or indirectly affects steps in feeding behavior which can be independently adjusted by neuromodulatory cues. How newly identified interneurons that regulate feeding motor program, suppress non- selective ingestion and regulate fluid ingestion connect taste sensory input to the motor output of ingestion as well as interpret top-down information about hunger state is not known. The fruit fly shares the basic metabolic regulation that is conserved throughout evolution. Therefore, simple genetic models like *Drosophila* can provide reliable insights to advance studies in more complex vertebrates, and enhance understanding of specific feeding-related neurological and metabolic disorders in humans. Tracing taste neural circuits in the fly brain, understanding the contribution of taste-independent calorie sensing to feeding, and uncovering novel regulators of neuronal remodeling in the taste system can help elucidate similar principals in higher animals including humans. Together, such studies may provide important clues to how feeding circuits may function in mammals, and lay the groundwork for understanding genetic factors that affect feeding control and body weight.

Humans live in a society very different from the ones that shaped the evolution of our brains. Easy access to cheap, calorie-rich foods has resulted in widespread obesity and an explosion of obesity-related diseases such as type 2 diabetes, hypertension, and heart disease. A detailed understanding of how feeding behaviour is controlled at the level of neural circuits is an important step towards developing new ways to treat and prevent obesity. Humans consume more calories when their diets consist of processed foods [198]. It has been shown that reducing taste sensation at the periphery, a high sugar diet impairs the central Dopamine processing of sensory signals and weakens satiation [199]. Given the importance of sensory changes in initiating this cascade of circuit dysfunction, understanding how diet composition mechanistically affects taste is imperative to understand how the food environment directs feeding behavior and metabolic disease.

Funding

This work is supported by Wellcome trust/DBT India Alliance Fellowship (grant number IA/I/15/2/502074) awarded to PK.

Declaration of conflicting interests

The authors declares no potential conflicts of interest with respect to authorship and publication of this article.

Author details

Shivam Kaushik†, Shivangi Rawat† and Pinky Kain*
Regional Centre for Biotechnology, NCR Biotech Science Cluster,
Faridabad, Haryana, India

*Address all correspondence to: pinkykain@gmail.com; pksharma@rcb.res.in

† These authors have contributed equally.

References

[1] Clyne PJ, Warr CG, Freeman MR, Lessing D, Kim J, Carlson JR. A novel family of divergent seven-transmembrane proteins: candidate odorant receptors in Drosophila. Neuron. 1999;22(2):327-38.

[2] Gao Q, Chess A. Identification of candidate Drosophila olfactory receptors from genomic DNA sequence. Genomics. 1999;60(1):31-9.

[3] Vosshall LB, Amrein H, Morozov PS, Rzhetsky A, Axel R. A spatial map of olfactory receptor expression in the Drosophila antenna. Cell. 1999;96(5):725-36.

[4] Clyne PJ, Warr CG, Carlson JR. Candidate taste receptors in Drosophila. Science. 2000;287(5459):1830-4.

[5] Scott K, Brady R, Jr., Cravchik A, Morozov P, Rzhetsky A, Zuker C, et al. A chemosensory gene family encoding candidate gustatory and olfactory receptors in Drosophila. Cell. 2001;104(5):661-73.

[6] Stocker RF, Schorderet M. Cobalt filling of sensory projections from internal and external mouthparts in Drosophila. Cell Tissue Res. 1981;216(3):513-23.

[7] Singh RN. Neurobiology of the gustatory systems of Drosophila and some terrestrial insects. Microsc Res Tech. 1997;39(6):547-63.

[8] Gendre N, Luer K, Friche S, Grillenzoni N, Ramaekers A, Technau GM, et al. Integration of complex larval chemosensory organs into the adult nervous system of Drosophila. Development. 2004;131(1):83-92.

[9] Gravina SA, Yep GL, Khan M. Human biology of taste. Ann Saudi Med. 2013;33(3):217-22.

[10] Logemann JA, Pauloski BR, Rademaker AW, McConnel FM, Heiser MA, Cardinale S, et al. Speech and swallow function after tonsil/base of tongue resection with primary closure. J Speech Hear Res. 1993;36(5):918-26.

[11] Pauloski BR, Logemann JA, Rademaker AW, McConnel FM, Heiser MA, Cardinale S, et al. Speech and swallowing function after anterior tongue and floor of mouth resection with distal flap reconstruction. J Speech Hear Res. 1993;36(2):267-76.

[12] Chaudhari N, Roper SD. The cell biology of taste. J Cell Biol. 2010;190(3):285-96.

[13] Bradbury J. Taste perception: cracking the code. PLoS Biol. 2004;2(3):E64.

[14] Snyder DJ, Bartoshuk LM. Oral sensory nerve damage: Causes and consequences. Rev Endocr Metab Disord. 2016;17(2):149-58.

[15] Rozengurt E. Taste receptors in the gastrointestinal tract. I. Bitter taste receptors and alpha-gustducin in the mammalian gut. Am J Physiol Gastrointest Liver Physiol. 2006;291(2):G171-7.

[16] Iwatsuki K, Ichikawa R, Uematsu A, Kitamura A, Uneyama H, Torii K. Detecting sweet and umami tastes in the gastrointestinal tract. Acta Physiol (Oxf). 2012;204(2):169-77.

[17] Janssen S, Depoortere I. Nutrient sensing in the gut: new roads to therapeutics? Trends Endocrinol Metab. 2013;24(2):92-100.

[18] Livovsky DM, Pribic T, Azpiroz F. Food, Eating, and the Gastrointestinal Tract. Nutrients. 2020;12(4).

[19] Roper SD, Chaudhari N. Taste buds: cells, signals and synapses. Nat Rev Neurosci. 2017;18(8):485-97.

[20] Breslin PA. An evolutionary perspective on food and human taste. Curr Biol. 2013;23(9):R409-18.

[21] Roper SD. Taste buds as peripheral chemosensory processors. Semin Cell Dev Biol. 2013;24(1):71-9.

[22] Yee KK, Li Y, Redding KM, Iwatsuki K, Margolskee RF, Jiang P. Lgr5-EGFP marks taste bud stem/progenitor cells in posterior tongue. Stem Cells. 2013;31(5):992-1000.

[23] Lewis D DW. The Course of the Nerve Fibers Transmitting Sensation of Taste. Archives of Surgery. 1930;21:249-88.

[24] Zahm DS, Munger BL. The innervation of the primate fungiform papilla--development, distribution and changes following selective ablation. Brain Res. 1985;356(2):147-86.

[25] Fay T. Observations and Results from Intracranial Section of the Glossopharyngeus and Vagus Nerves in Man. J Neurol Psychopathol. 1927;8(30):110-23.

[26] R. N. Central Neural Mechanisms of Taste. American Physiological Society; Washington, DC. 1927; 8:110-23.

[27] Reichert F. Neuralgias of the Glossopharyngeal Nerve: With Particular Reference to the Sensory, Gustatory, and Secretory Functions of the Nerve. Archives of Neurology and Psychiatry. 1934;32:1030-7.

[28] Kanagasuntheram R, Wong WC, Chan HL. Some observations on the innervation of the human nasopharynx. J Anat. 1969;104(Pt 2):361-76.

[29] Oakley B. Reformation of taste buds by crossed sensory nerves in the rat's tongue. Acta Physiol Scand. 1970;79(1):88-94.

[30] Pritchard T. The Primate Gustatory System. In: Getchell Tv, Doty Rl, Bartoshuk Lm, Snow Jb, Editors. Smell and Taste in Health and Disease. Raven Press; New York. 1991 109-25.

[31] DH. M. Taste, smell, and flavor terminology: Taking the confusion out of fusion. . In: Meiselman HL, Rivlin RS, editors Clinical Measurement of Taste and Smell Macmillan; New York. 1986:pp. 117-25.

[32] Breslin PA, Spector AC. Mammalian taste perception. Curr Biol. 2008;18(4):R148-55.

[33] de Araujo IE, Simon SA. The gustatory cortex and multisensory integration. Int J Obes (Lond). 2009;33 Suppl 2:S34-43.

[34] Oliveira-Maia AJ, Roberts CD, Simon SA, Nicolelis MA. Gustatory and reward brain circuits in the control of food intake. Adv Tech Stand Neurosurg. 2011;36:31-59.

[35] Zald DH. Orbitofrontal cortex contributions to food selection and decision making. Ann Behav Med. 2009;38 Suppl 1:S18-24.

[36] Veldhuizen MG, Albrecht J, Zelano C, Boesveldt S, Breslin P, Lundstrom JN. Identification of human gustatory cortex by activation likelihood estimation. Hum Brain Mapp. 2011;32(12):2256-66.

[37] Hellekant G, Ninomiya Y, Danilova V. Taste in chimpanzees. III: Labeled-line coding in sweet taste. Physiol Behav. 1998;65(2):191-200.

[38] Chen X, Gabitto M, Peng Y, Ryba NJ, Zuker CS. A gustotopic map of taste qualities in the mammalian brain. Science. 2011;333(6047):1262-6.

[39] Sofia M. The Physiology of Taste in Fish: Potential Implications for Feeding Stimulation and Gut Chemical Sensing. Reviews in Fisheries Science & Aquaculture. 2017;25:133-49.

[40] Shigemura N, Shirosaki S, Sanematsu K, Yoshida R, Ninomiya Y. Genetic and molecular basis of individual differences in human umami taste perception. PLoS One. 2009;4(8):e6717.

[41] Torii K, Uneyama H, Nakamura E. Physiological roles of dietary glutamate signaling via gut-brain axis due to efficient digestion and absorption. J Gastroenterol. 2013;48(4):442-51.

[42] Kurihara K. Umami the Fifth Basic Taste: History of Studies on Receptor Mechanisms and Role as a Food Flavor. Biomed Res Int. 2015;2015:189402.

[43] Piette CE, Baez-Santiago MA, Reid EE, Katz DB, Moran A. Inactivation of basolateral amygdala specifically eliminates palatability-related information in cortical sensory responses. J Neurosci. 2012;32(29):9981-91.

[44] Tandon S, Simon SA, Nicolelis MA. Appetitive changes during salt deprivation are paralleled by widespread neuronal adaptations in nucleus accumbens, lateral hypothalamus, and central amygdala. J Neurophysiol. 2012;108(4):1089-105.

[45] Small DM. Flavor is in the brain. Physiol Behav. 2012;107(4):540-52.

[46] Purves D AG, Fitzpatrick D, et al., editors. . Neuroscience. 2nd edition. . Sunderland (MA): Sinauer Associates. 2001.

[47] Frank ME, Hettinger TP, Mott AE. The sense of taste: neurobiology, aging, and medication effects. Crit Rev Oral Biol Med. 1992;3(4):371-93.

[48] Spector AC, Glendinning JI. Linking peripheral taste processes to behavior. Curr Opin Neurobiol. 2009;19(4):370-7.

[49] Kennerley SW, Walton ME. Decision making and reward in frontal cortex: complementary evidence from neurophysiological and neuropsychological studies. Behav Neurosci. 2011;125(3):297-317.

[50] Haggard P, de Boer L. Oral somatosensory awareness. Neurosci Biobehav Rev. 2014;47:469-84.

[51] Rolls ET. Brain mechanisms underlying flavour and appetite. Philos Trans R Soc Lond B Biol Sci. 2006;361(1471):1123-36.

[52] Sohn JW, Elmquist JK, Williams KW. Neuronal circuits that regulate feeding behavior and metabolism. Trends Neurosci. 2013;36(9):504-12.

[53] Morton GJ, Meek TH, Schwartz MW. Neurobiology of food intake in health and disease. Nat Rev Neurosci. 2014;15(6):367-78.

[54] Schneeberger M, Gomis R, Claret M. Hypothalamic and brainstem neuronal circuits controlling homeostatic energy balance. J Endocrinol. 2014;220(2):T25-46.

[55] Waterson MJ, Horvath TL. Neuronal Regulation of Energy Homeostasis: Beyond the Hypothalamus and Feeding. Cell Metab. 2015;22(6):962-70.

[56] Roh E, Kim MS. Brain Regulation of Energy Metabolism. Endocrinol Metab (Seoul). 2016;31(4):519-24.

[57] Roh E, Song DK, Kim MS. Emerging role of the brain in the homeostatic regulation of energy and glucose metabolism. Exp Mol Med. 2016;48:e216.

[58] Timper K, Bruning JC. Hypothalamic circuits regulating appetite and energy homeostasis: pathways to obesity. Dis Model Mech. 2017;10(6):679-89.

[59] Steiner JE. The gustofacial response: observation on normal and anencephalic newborn infants. Symp Oral Sens Percept. 1973(4):254-78.

[60] Grill HJ, Norgren R. Neurological tests and behavioral deficits in chronic thalamic and chronic decerebrate rats. Brain Res. 1978;143(2):299-312.

[61] Lundy RF, Jr., Norgren R. Activity in the hypothalamus, amygdala, and cortex generates bilateral and convergent modulation of pontine gustatory neurons. J Neurophysiol. 2004;91(3):1143-57.

[62] Zheng H, Berthoud HR. Neural systems controlling the drive to eat: mind versus metabolism. Physiology (Bethesda). 2008;23:75-83.

[63] Cummings DE, Overduin J. Gastrointestinal regulation of food intake. J Clin Invest. 2007;117(1):13-23.

[64] Masse NY, Turner GC, Jefferis GS. Olfactory information processing in Drosophila. Curr Biol. 2009;19(16):R700-13.

[65] Hong W, Luo L. Genetic control of wiring specificity in the fly olfactory system. Genetics. 2014;196(1):17-29.

[66] Joseph RM, Carlson JR. Drosophila Chemoreceptors: A Molecular Interface Between the Chemical World and the Brain. Trends Genet. 2015;31(12):683-95.

[67] Wang Z, Singhvi A, Kong P, Scott K. Taste representations in the Drosophila brain. Cell. 2004;117(7):981-91.

[68] Yarmolinsky DA, Zuker CS, Ryba NJ. Common sense about taste: from mammals to insects. Cell. 2009;139(2):234-44.

[69] Falk R, Bleiser-Avivi N, Atidia J. Labellar taste organs of Drosophila melanogaster. J Morphol. 1976;150(2):327-41.

[70] Ling F, Dahanukar A, Weiss LA, Kwon JY, Carlson JR. The molecular and cellular basis of taste coding in the legs of Drosophila. J Neurosci. 2014;34(21):7148-64.

[71] Rajashekhar KP, Singh RN. Neuroarchitecture of the tritocerebrum of Drosophila melanogaster. J Comp Neurol. 1994;349(4):633-45.

[72] Thorne N, Chromey C, Bray S, Amrein H. Taste perception and coding in Drosophila. Curr Biol. 2004;14(12):1065-79.

[73] Vosshall LB, Stocker RF. Molecular architecture of smell and taste in Drosophila. Annu Rev Neurosci. 2007;30:505-33.

[74] Freeman EG, Dahanukar A. Molecular neurobiology of Drosophila taste. Curr Opin Neurobiol. 2015;34:140-8.

[75] Ito K, Shinomiya K, Ito M, Armstrong JD, Boyan G, Hartenstein V, et al. A systematic nomenclature for the insect brain. Neuron. 2014;81(4):755-65.

[76] Gordon MD, Scott K. Motor control in a Drosophila taste circuit. Neuron. 2009;61(3):373-84.

[77] Melcher C, Pankratz MJ. Candidate gustatory interneurons modulating feeding behavior in the Drosophila brain. PLoS Biol. 2005;3(9):e305.

[78] Flood TF, Iguchi S, Gorczyca M, White B, Ito K, Yoshihara M. A single pair of interneurons commands the Drosophila feeding motor program. Nature. 2013;499(7456):83-7.

[79] Liu Q, Liu S, Kodama L, Driscoll MR, Wu MN. Two dopaminergic neurons signal to the dorsal fan-shaped body to promote wakefulness in Drosophila. Curr Biol. 2012;22(22):2114-23.

[80] Kirkhart C, Scott K. Gustatory learning and processing in the Drosophila mushroom bodies. J Neurosci. 2015;35(15):5950-8.

[81] Kain P, Dahanukar A. Secondary taste neurons that convey sweet taste and starvation in the Drosophila brain. Neuron. 2015;85(4):819-32.

[82] Homberg U, Christensen TA, Hildebrand JG. Structure and function of the deutocerebrum in insects. Annu Rev Entomol. 1989;34:477-501.

[83] Kamikouchi A, Shimada T, Ito K. Comprehensive classification of the auditory sensory projections in the brain of the fruit fly Drosophila melanogaster. J Comp Neurol. 2006;499(3):317-56.

[84] Kamikouchi A, Inagaki HK, Effertz T, Hendrich O, Fiala A, Gopfert MC, et al. The neural basis of Drosophila gravity-sensing and hearing. Nature. 2009;458(7235):165-71.

[85] Yorozu S, Wong A, Fischer BJ, Dankert H, Kernan MJ, Kamikouchi A, et al. Distinct sensory representations of wind and near-field sound in the Drosophila brain. Nature. 2009;458(7235):201-5.

[86] Awasaki T, Kao CF, Lee YJ, Yang CP, Huang Y, Pfeiffer BD, et al. Making Drosophila lineage-restricted drivers via patterned recombination in neuroblasts. Nat Neurosci. 2014;17(4):631-7.

[87] Inoshita T, Tanimura T. Cellular identification of water gustatory receptor neurons and their central projection pattern in Drosophila. Proc Natl Acad Sci U S A. 2006;103(4):1094-9.

[88] Cameron P, Hiroi M, Ngai J, Scott K. The molecular basis for water taste in Drosophila. Nature. 2010;465(7294): 91-5.

[89] Zhang YV, Raghuwanshi RP, Shen WL, Montell C. Food experience-induced taste desensitization modulated by the Drosophila TRPL channel. Nat Neurosci. 2013;16(10):1468-76.

[90] Jaeger AH, Stanley M, Weiss ZF, Musso PY, Chan RC, Zhang H, et al. A complex peripheral code for salt taste in Drosophila. Elife. 2018;7.

[91] Chen Y, Amrein H. Ionotropic Receptors Mediate Drosophila Oviposition Preference through Sour Gustatory Receptor Neurons. Curr Biol. 2017;27(18):2741-50 e4.

[92] Masek P, Keene AC. Drosophila fatty acid taste signals through the PLC pathway in sugar-sensing neurons. PLoS Genet. 2013;9(9):e1003710.

[93] Chiang AS, Lin CY, Chuang CC, Chang HM, Hsieh CH, Yeh CW, et al. Three-dimensional reconstruction of brain-wide wiring networks in Drosophila at single-cell resolution. Curr Biol. 2011;21(1):1-11.

[94] Miyamoto T, Amrein H. Suppression of male courtship by a Drosophila pheromone receptor. Nat Neurosci. 2008;11(8):874-6.

[95] Yapici N, Cohn R, Schusterreiter C, Ruta V, Vosshall LB. A Taste Circuit that Regulates Ingestion by Integrating Food and Hunger Signals. Cell. 2016;165(3): 715-29.

[96] Liman ER, Zhang YV, Montell C. Peripheral coding of taste. Neuron. 2014;81(5):984-1000.

[97] Bohra AA, Kallman BR, Reichert H, VijayRaghavan K. Identification of a Single Pair of Interneurons for Bitter Taste Processing in the Drosophila Brain. Curr Biol. 2018;28(6):847-58 e3.

[98] Kim H, Kirkhart C, Scott K. Long-range projection neurons in the taste circuit of Drosophila. Elife. 2017;6.

[99] Aso Y, Hattori D, Yu Y, Johnston RM, Iyer NA, Ngo TT, et al. The neuronal architecture of the mushroom body provides a logic for associative learning. Elife. 2014;3:e04577.

[100] Mann K, Gordon MD, Scott K. A pair of interneurons influences the choice between feeding and locomotion in Drosophila. Neuron. 2013;79(4):754-65.

[101] Chen YD, Dahanukar A. Molecular and Cellular Organization of Taste Neurons in Adult Drosophila Pharynx. Cell Rep. 2017;21(10):2978-91.

[102] Nottebohm E, Dambly-Chaudiere C, Ghysen A. Connectivity of chemosensory neurons is controlled by the gene poxn in Drosophila. Nature. 1992;359(6398):829-32.

[103] Awasaki T, Kimura K. pox-neuro is required for development of chemosensory bristles in Drosophila. J Neurobiol. 1997;32(7):707-21.

[104] Chen YD, Park SJ, Ja WW, Dahanukar A. Using Pox-Neuro (Poxn) Mutants in Drosophila Gustation Research: A Double-Edged Sword. Front Cell Neurosci. 2018;12:382.

[105] Chen YD, Ahmad S, Amin K, Dahanukar A. A subset of brain neurons controls regurgitation in adult Drosophila melanogaster. J Exp Biol. 2019;222(Pt 19).

[106] Heisenberg M. Mushroom body memoir: from maps to models. Nat Rev Neurosci. 2003;4(4):266-75.

[107] Davis RL. Olfactory memory formation in Drosophila: from molecular to systems neuroscience. Annu Rev Neurosci. 2005;28:275-302.

[108] Keene AC, Waddell S. Drosophila olfactory memory: single genes to complex neural circuits. Nat Rev Neurosci. 2007;8(5):341-54.

[109] Masek P, Scott K. Limited taste discrimination in Drosophila. Proc Natl Acad Sci U S A. 2010;107(33):14833-8.

[110] Menzel R. The insect mushroom body, an experience-dependent recoding device. J Physiol Paris. 2014;108(2-3):84-95.

[111] Zars T. Behavioral functions of the insect mushroom bodies. Curr Opin Neurobiol. 2000;10(6):790-5.

[112] van Swinderen B. Fly memory: a mushroom body story in parts. Curr Biol. 2009;19(18):R855-7.

[113] Keene AC, Masek P. Optogenetic induction of aversive taste memory. Neuroscience. 2012;222:173-80.

[114] Farris SM. Tritocerebral tract input to the insect mushroom bodies. Arthropod Struct Dev. 2008;37(6): 492-503.

[115] Dethier VG. The Hungry Fly: A Physiological Study of the Behavior Associated with Feeding. Harvard U Press 1976.

[116] Shiraiwa T, Carlson JR. Proboscis extension response (PER) assay in Drosophila. J Vis Exp. 2007(3):193.

[117] Altman J.S. KJ. A Model for Decision Making in the Insect Nervous System. . In: Ali MA (eds) Nervous Systems in Invertebrates Springer, Boston, MA. 1987.

[118] Stocker RF. The organization of the chemosensory system in Drosophila melanogaster: a review. Cell Tissue Res. 1994;275(1):3-26.

[119] Dunipace L, Meister S, McNealy C, Amrein H. Spatially restricted expression of candidate taste receptors in the Drosophila gustatory system. Curr Biol. 2001;11(11):822-35.

[120] Rajashekhar KP SR. Organization of Motor Neurons Innervating the Proboscis Musculature in Drosophila Melanogaster Meigen (Diptera : Drosophilidae). Int J Insect Morphol & Embryol 1994b;23:225-42.

[121] Schwarz O, Bohra AA, Liu X, Reichert H, VijayRaghavan K, Pielage J. Motor control of Drosophila feeding behavior. Elife. 2017;6.

[122] Rice MJ. Cibarial stretch receptors in the tsetse fly (Glossina austeni) and the blowfly (Calliphora erythrocephala). J Insect Physiol. 1970;16(2):277-89.

[123] Zhou Y, Cao LH, Sui XW, Guo XQ, Luo DG. Mechanosensory circuits coordinate two opposing motor actions in Drosophila feeding. Sci Adv. 2019;5(5):eaaw5141.

[124] Manzo A, Silies M, Gohl DM, Scott K. Motor neurons controlling fluid ingestion in Drosophila. Proc Natl Acad Sci U S A. 2012;109(16):6307-12.

[125] Pool AH, Kvello P, Mann K, Cheung SK, Gordon MD, Wang L, et al. Four GABAergic interneurons impose feeding restraint in Drosophila. Neuron. 2014;83(1):164-77.

[126] Inagaki HK, Panse KM, Anderson DJ. Independent, reciprocal neuromodulatory control of sweet and bitter taste sensitivity during starvation in Drosophila. Neuron. 2014;84(4):806-20.

[127] Hanci D, Altun H. Hunger state affects both olfactory abilities and gustatory sensitivity. Eur Arch Otorhinolaryngol. 2016;273(7):1637-41.

[128] Burton MJ, Rolls ET, Mora F. Effects of hunger on the responses of neurons in the lateral hypothalamus to the sight and taste of food. Exp Neurol. 1976;51(3):668-77.

[129] Rolls ET, Sienkiewicz ZJ, Yaxley S. Hunger Modulates the Responses to Gustatory Stimuli of Single Neurons in the Caudolateral Orbitofrontal Cortex of the Macaque Monkey. Eur J Neurosci. 1989;1(1):53-60.

[130] de Araujo IE, Gutierrez R, Oliveira-Maia AJ, Pereira A, Jr., Nicolelis MA, Simon SA. Neural ensemble coding of satiety states. Neuron. 2006;51(4):483-94.

[131] Marella S, Mann K, Scott K. Dopaminergic modulation of sucrose acceptance behavior in Drosophila. Neuron. 2012;73(5):941-50.

[132] Szczypka MS, Rainey MA, Kim DS, Alaynick WA, Marck BT, Matsumoto AM, et al. Feeding behavior in dopamine-deficient mice. Proc Natl Acad Sci U S A. 1999;96(21):12138-43.

[133] Nassel DR, Wegener C. A comparative review of short and long neuropeptide F signaling in invertebrates: Any similarities to vertebrate neuropeptide Y signaling? Peptides. 2011;32(6):1335-55.

[134] Taghert PH, Nitabach MN. Peptide neuromodulation in invertebrate model systems. Neuron. 2012;76(1):82-97.

[135] Itskov PM, Ribeiro C. The dilemmas of the gourmet fly: the molecular and neuronal mechanisms of feeding and nutrient decision making in Drosophila. Front Neurosci. 2013;7:12.

[136] Lee KS, You KH, Choo JK, Han YM, Yu K. Drosophila short neuropeptide F regulates food intake and body size. J Biol Chem. 2004;279(49):50781-9.

[137] Krashes MJ, DasGupta S, Vreede A, White B, Armstrong JD, Waddell S. A neural circuit mechanism integrating motivational state with memory expression in Drosophila. Cell. 2009;139(2):416-27.

[138] Root CM, Ko KI, Jafari A, Wang JW. Presynaptic facilitation by neuropeptide signaling mediates odor-driven food search. Cell. 2011;145(1):133-44.

[139] Hergarden AC, Tayler TD, Anderson DJ. Allatostatin-A neurons inhibit feeding behavior in adult Drosophila. Proc Natl Acad Sci U S A. 2012;109(10):3967-72.

[140] Beshel J, Zhong Y. Graded encoding of food odor value in the Drosophila brain. J Neurosci. 2013;33(40):15693-704.

[141] Page RE, Jr., Erber J, Fondrk MK. The effect of genotype on response thresholds to sucrose and foraging behavior of honey bees (Apis mellifera L.). J Comp Physiol A. 1998;182(4):489-500.

[142] Gillette R, Huang RC, Hatcher N, Moroz LL. Cost-benefit analysis potential in feeding behavior of a predatory snail by integration of hunger, taste, and pain. Proc Natl Acad Sci U S A. 2000;97(7):3585-90.

[143] Kawai K, Sugimoto K, Nakashima K, Miura H, Ninomiya Y. Leptin as a modulator of sweet taste sensitivities in mice. Proc Natl Acad Sci U S A. 2000;97(20):11044-9.

[144] Inagaki HK, Ben-Tabou de-Leon S, Wong AM, Jagadish S, Ishimoto H, Barnea G, et al. Visualizing neuromodulation in vivo: TANGO-mapping of dopamine signaling reveals appetite control of sugar sensing. Cell. 2012;148(3):583-95.

[145] Sengupta P. The belly rules the nose: feeding state-dependent modulation of peripheral chemosensory responses. Curr Opin Neurobiol. 2013;23(1):68-75.

[146] Bargmann CI. Beyond the connectome: how neuromodulators shape neural circuits. Bioessays. 2012;34(6):458-65.

[147] Flavell SW, Pokala N, Macosko EZ, Albrecht DR, Larsch J, Bargmann CI. Serotonin and the neuropeptide PDF initiate and extend opposing behavioral states in C. elegans. Cell. 2013;154(5):1023-35.

[148] Komuniecki R, Hapiak V, Harris G, Bamber B. Context-dependent modulation reconfigures interactive sensory-mediated microcircuits in Caenorhabditis elegans. Curr Opin Neurobiol. 2014;29:17-24.

[149] LeDue EE, Mann K, Koch E, Chu B, Dakin R, Gordon MD. Starvation-Induced Depotentiation of Bitter Taste in Drosophila. Curr Biol. 2016;26(21):2854-61.

[150] Meunier N, Belgacem YH, Martin JR. Regulation of feeding behaviour and locomotor activity by takeout in Drosophila. J Exp Biol. 2007;210(Pt 8):1424-34.

[151] Nishimura A, Ishida Y, Takahashi A, Okamoto H, Sakabe M, Itoh M, et al. Starvation-induced elevation of taste responsiveness and expression of a sugar taste receptor gene in Drosophila melanogaster. J Neurogenet. 2012;26(2):206-15.

[152] Chu B, Chui V, Mann K, Gordon MD. Presynaptic gain control drives sweet and bitter taste integration in Drosophila. Curr Biol. 2014;24(17):1978-84.

[153] Liu Q, Tabuchi M, Liu S, Kodama L, Horiuchi W, Daniels J, et al. Branch-specific plasticity of a bifunctional dopamine circuit encodes protein hunger. Science. 2017;356(6337):534-9.

[154] Yapici N, Kim YJ, Ribeiro C, Dickson BJ. A receptor that mediates the post-mating switch in Drosophila reproductive behaviour. Nature. 2008;451(7174):33-7.

[155] Hussain A, Ucpunar HK, Zhang M, Loschek LF, Grunwald Kadow IC. Neuropeptides Modulate Female Chemosensory Processing upon Mating in Drosophila. PLoS Biol. 2016;14(5):e1002455.

[156] Walker SJ, Corrales-Carvajal VM, Ribeiro C. Postmating Circuitry Modulates Salt Taste Processing to Increase Reproductive Output in Drosophila. Curr Biol. 2015;25(20): 2621-30.

[157] Ribeiro C, Dickson BJ. Sex peptide receptor and neuronal TOR/S6K signaling modulate nutrient balancing in Drosophila. Curr Biol. 2010;20(11):1000-5.

[158] Tsao CH, Chen CC, Lin CH, Yang HY, Lin S. Drosophila mushroom bodies integrate hunger and satiety signals to control innate food-seeking behavior. Elife. 2018;7.

[159] Mela DJ. Determinants of food choice: relationships with obesity and weight control. Obes Res. 2001;9 Suppl 4:249S-55S.

[160] Mela DJ. Eating for pleasure or just wanting to eat? Reconsidering sensory hedonic responses as a driver of obesity. Appetite. 2006;47(1):10-7.

[161] Riera CE, Tsaousidou E, Halloran J, Follett P, Hahn O, Pereira MMA, et al. The Sense of Smell Impacts Metabolic Health and Obesity. Cell Metab. 2017;26(1):198-211 e5.

[162] Lindgren E, Gray K, Miller G, Tyler R, Wiers CE, Volkow ND, et al. Food addiction: A common neurobiological mechanism with drug abuse. Front Biosci (Landmark Ed). 2018;23:811-36.

[163] Volkow ND, Wise RA, Baler R. The dopamine motive system: implications for drug and food addiction. Nat Rev Neurosci. 2017;18(12):741-52.

[164] Wang GJ, Volkow ND, Felder C, Fowler JS, Levy AV, Pappas NR, et al. Enhanced resting activity of the oral somatosensory cortex in obese subjects. Neuroreport. 2002;13(9):1151-5.

[165] Wang GJ, Volkow ND, Thanos PK, Fowler JS. Similarity between obesity and drug addiction as assessed by neurofunctional imaging: a concept review. J Addict Dis. 2004;23(3):39-53.

[166] Volkow ND, Wang GJ, Telang F, Fowler JS, Thanos PK, Logan J, et al. Low dopamine striatal D2 receptors are associated with prefrontal metabolism in obese subjects: possible contributing factors. Neuroimage. 2008;42(4): 1537-43.

[167] Patriarca L, Magerowski G, Alonso-Alonso M. Functional neuroimaging in obesity. Curr Opin Endocrinol Diabetes Obes. 2017;24(3):260-5.

[168] Barry RL, Byun NE, Williams JM, Siuta MA, Tantawy MN, Speed NK, et al. Brief exposure to obesogenic diet disrupts brain dopamine networks. PLoS One. 2018;13(4):e0191299.

[169] Schlogl H, Horstmann A, Villringer A, Stumvoll M. Functional neuroimaging in obesity and the potential for development of novel treatments. Lancet Diabetes Endocrinol. 2016;4(8):695-705.

[170] Zhang B, Tian D, Yu C, Zhang J, Tian X, von Deneen KM, et al. Altered baseline brain activities before food intake in obese men: a resting state fMRI study. Neurosci Lett. 2015;584:156-61.

[171] Kure Liu C, Joseph PV, Feldman DE, Kroll DS, Burns JA, Manza P, et al. Brain Imaging of Taste

Perception in Obesity: a Review. Curr Nutr Rep. 2019;8(2):108-19.

[172] Iwata S, Yoshida R, Ninomiya Y. Taste transductions in taste receptor cells: basic tastes and moreover. Curr Pharm Des. 2014;20(16):2684-92.

[173] Freeman CR, Zehra A, Ramirez V, Wiers CE, Volkow ND, Wang GJ. Impact of sugar on the body, brain, and behavior. Front Biosci (Landmark Ed). 2018;23:2255-66.

[174] Bohon C. Brain response to taste in overweight children: A pilot feasibility study. PLoS One. 2017;12(2):e0172604.

[175] Tzieropoulos H, Rytz A, Hudry J, le Coutre J. Dietary fat induces sustained reward response in the human brain without primary taste cortex discrimination. Front Hum Neurosci. 2013;7:36.

[176] Stice E, Burger KS, Yokum S. Relative ability of fat and sugar tastes to activate reward, gustatory, and somatosensory regions. Am J Clin Nutr. 2013;98(6):1377-84.

[177] Alsio J, Olszewski PK, Norback AH, Gunnarsson ZE, Levine AS, Pickering C, et al. Dopamine D1 receptor gene expression decreases in the nucleus accumbens upon long-term exposure to palatable food and differs depending on diet-induced obesity phenotype in rats. Neuroscience. 2010;171(3):779-87.

[178] Mun C KS, Choi K, Lee H, Shin W, Eun C. . Salty-taste Activation of Human Brain Disclosed by Gustatory fMRI Study. J Korean Soc Magn Reson Med. 2005;9(1):30-5.

[179] Han JE, Frasnelli J, Zeighami Y, Larcher K, Boyle J, McConnell T, et al. Ghrelin Enhances Food Odor Conditioning in Healthy Humans: An fMRI Study. Cell Rep. 2018;25(10):2643-52 e4.

[180] Zald DH, Lee JT, Fluegel KW, Pardo JV. Aversive gustatory stimulation activates limbic circuits in humans. Brain. 1998;121 (Pt 6):1143-54.

[181] Bertoli S, Laureati M, Battezzati A, Bergamaschi V, Cereda E, Spadafranca A, et al. Taste sensitivity, nutritional status and metabolic syndrome: Implication in weight loss dietary interventions. World J Diabetes. 2014;5(5):717-23.

[182] Simchen U, Koebnick C, Hoyer S, Issanchou S, Zunft HJ. Odour and taste sensitivity is associated with body weight and extent of misreporting of body weight. Eur J Clin Nutr. 2006;60(6):698-705.

[183] Masic U, Yeomans MR. Umami flavor enhances appetite but also increases satiety. Am J Clin Nutr. 2014;100(2):532-8.

[184] Magerowski G, Giacona, G., Patriarca, L. et al. Neurocognitive effects of umami: association with eating behavior and food choice. Neuropsychopharmacol. 2009-2016 (2018);43.

[185] Overberg J, Hummel T, Krude H, Wiegand S. Differences in taste sensitivity between obese and non-obese children and adolescents. Arch Dis Child. 2012;97(12):1048-52.

[186] Pepino MY, Finkbeiner S, Beauchamp GK, Mennella JA. Obese women have lower monosodium glutamate taste sensitivity and prefer higher concentrations than do normal-weight women. Obesity (Silver Spring). 2010;18(5):959-65.

[187] Keller KL, Adise S. Variation in the Ability to Taste Bitter Thiourea Compounds: Implications for Food Acceptance, Dietary Intake, and Obesity Risk in Children. Annu Rev Nutr. 2016;36:157-82.

[188] Wabnegger A, Schwab D, Schienle A. Aversive aftertaste changes visual food cue reactivity: An fMRI study on cross-modal perception. Neurosci Lett. 2018;673:56-60.

[189] Bembich S, Lanzara C, Clarici A, Demarini S, Tepper BJ, Gasparini P, et al. Individual differences in prefrontal cortex activity during perception of bitter taste using fNIRS methodology. Chem Senses. 2010;35(9):801-12.

[190] Zald DH, Hagen MC, Pardo JV. Neural correlates of tasting concentrated quinine and sugar solutions. J Neurophysiol. 2002;87(2):1068-75.

[191] Kishi M, Sadachi H, Nakamura J, Tonoike M. Functional magnetic resonance imaging investigation of brain regions associated with astringency. Neurosci Res. 2017;122:9-16.

[192] Wichchukit S, O'Mahony M. The 9-point hedonic scale and hedonic ranking in food science: some reappraisals and alternatives. J Sci Food Agric. 2015;95(11):2167-78.

[193] Kalva JJ, Sims CA, Puentes LA, Snyder DJ, Bartoshuk LM. Comparison of the hedonic general Labeled Magnitude Scale with the hedonic 9-point scale. J Food Sci. 2014;79(2):S238-45.

[194] Haase L, Green E, Murphy C. Males and females show differential brain activation to taste when hungry and sated in gustatory and reward areas. Appetite. 2011;57(2):421-34.

[195] Hoogeveen HR, Dalenberg JR, Renken RJ, ter Horst GJ, Lorist MM. Neural processing of basic tastes in healthy young and older adults - an fMRI study. Neuroimage. 2015;119:1-12.

[196] Depoortere I. Taste receptors of the gut: emerging roles in health and disease. Gut. 2014;63(1):179-90.

[197] Steensels S, Depoortere I. Chemoreceptors in the Gut. Annu Rev Physiol. 2018;80:117-41.

[198] Hall KD, Ayuketah A, Brychta R, Cai H, Cassimatis T, Chen KY, et al. Ultra-Processed Diets Cause Excess Calorie Intake and Weight Gain: An Inpatient Randomized Controlled Trial of Ad Libitum Food Intake. Cell Metab. 2019;30(1):67-77 e3.

[199] May CE, Rosander J, Gottfried J, Dennis E, Dus M. Dietary sugar inhibits satiation by decreasing the central processing of sweet taste. Elife. 2020;9.